A HISTORY OF UNCERTAINTY

A HISTORY OF UNCERTAINTY
Bovine Tuberculosis in Britain
1850 to the Present

The Winchester University Press
New Perspectives on
Veterinary History

The early twenty-first century has seen a dramatic growth in both scholarly and public interest in all aspects of the health and illness of domesticated animals. The aim of this series is to provide an international forum of academic publications that explore veterinary history from a range of multi-disciplinary perspectives. By doing so, the series sheds new light on various aspects of veterinary history and makes a contribution to the growing scholarship in this area.

How shall we know the dancer from the dance?

W. B. Yeats, 1928

A HISTORY OF UNCERTAINTY

Bovine Tuberculosis In Britain
1850 To The Present

Peter J. Atkins

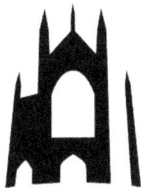

WINCHESTER UNIVERSITY PRESS

Published by the Winchester University Press 2016

First Published in Great Britain in 2016 by
The Winchester University Press
University of Winchester
Winchester SO22 4NR

British Library Cataloguing-in-Publication Data
A CIP catalogue record for this book is available from the British Library.

ISBN: 978-1-906113-17-9

Printed and Bound in Great Britain

CONTENTS

LIST OF FIGURES

LIST OF TABLES

LIST OF ABBREVIATIONS

AHVLA	Animal Health and Veterinary Laboratories Agency (2011-14)
APHA	Animal and Plant Health Agency (2014-)
AHWBE	Animal Health and Welfare Board for England
BCG	Bacillus Calmette-Guérin
BoA	Board of Agriculture (1889-1903)
BoAF	Board of Agriculture and Fisheries (1903-1919)
BPP	British Parliamentary Papers
BSE	Bovine spongiform encepalopathy
bTB	Bovine tuberculosis
BMA	British Medical Association
BVA	British Veterinary Association (1952-)
CCA	Central and Affiliated Chambers of Agriculture
CLA	Country Landowners' Association
CMO	Chief Medical Officer
CVL	Central Veterinary Laboratory (1894-1995)
CVO	Chief Veterinary Officer
DC	Departmental Committee
Defra	Department of Environment, Food and Rural Affairs
DIT	Double Intradermal Test
GRO	General Register Office
HC Deb	UK Parliament, House of Commons Debates
HL Deb	UK Parliament, House of Lords Debates
HRA	High Risk Area
HTST	High temperature short time
IDC	Inter-Departmental Committee
LCC	London County Council
LGB	Local Government Board

LRA	Low Risk Area
LTLT	Low temperature long time
MAF	Ministry of Agriculture and Fisheries (1919-55)
MAFF	Ministry of Agriculture, Fisheries and Food (1955-2001)
MAC	Milk Advisory Committee
MF	Ministry of Food (1916-21, 1939-55)
MH	Ministry of Health
MISS	Milk in Schools Scheme
MMB	Milk Marketing Board
MMS	Milk Marketing Scheme
MOH	Medical Officer of Health
MP	Member of Parliament
MRC	Medical Research Committee (1913-20), Medical Research Council (1920 to present)
M. bovis	*Mycobacterium bovis*
M. tuberculosis	*Mycobacterium tuberculosis*
NCMS	National Clean Milk Society
NFU	National Farmers' Union
NFDA	National Federation of Dairymen's Associations
NIRD	National Institute for Research in Dairying
NMPC	National Milk Publicity Campaign
NVMA	National Veterinary Medical Association (1919-1952)
NVA	National Veterinary Association (1882-1919)
OTF	Officially Tuberculosis Free
OTF-S	Officially Tuberculosis Free Status Suspended
OTF-W	Officially Tuberculosis Free Status Withdrawn
PJMC	Permanent Joint Milk Committee
PLH	People's League of Health
PPD	Purified Protein Derivative
RBCT	Randomised Badger Culling Trial
RC	Royal Commission

RC1	Royal Commission to inquire into Effect of Food from Tuberculous Animals on Human Health (1890-95)
RC2	Royal Commission to Inquire into Administrative Procedures for Controlling Danger to Man Through Use as Food of Meat and Milk of Tuberculous Animals (1896-98)
RC3	Royal Commission on the Relation between Human and Animal Tuberculosis (1901-11)
RoI	Republic of Ireland
RVC	Royal Veterinary College
SICT	Single Intradermal Cervical Test
SICCT	Single Intradermal Comparative Cervical Test
SIR	Standard Interpretation Inconclusive Reactor
SIT	Single Intradermal Test
TB	Tuberculosis
TBEAG	Tuberculosis Eradication Advisory Group
TNA	The National Archives, Kew
TT	Tuberculin Test(ed)
UFAW	Universities Federation for Animal Welfare
UHT	Ultra high temperature processing
UK	United Kingdom
VLA	Veterinary Laboratories Agency (1995-2011)

PREFACE

Introduction

What have we shared since the middle of the nineteenth century? It certainly isn't wealth or happiness. It is exposure to one of the most widespread and successful organisms on earth, tuberculosis. In its various forms this mycobacterium has left its DNA in one third of humans alive and also in the bodies of a wide spectrum of other species.[1] Tuberculosis has been one of the most important killer diseases in history. In 2013 it was responsible for an estimated 1.5 million deaths globally, probably the most ever in a single year, and it infected another nine million people.[2]

In addition to active disease, tuberculosis has the ability to lie dormant in the human body for years, sometimes reactivating under conditions of stress or compromised immunity. The mycobacteria have therefore become part of the human condition, constant companions, blurring the boundary with the non-human world. Rather than 'out there' this part of nature is now 'in here', creating a strange hybrid form of life, the 'more-than-human'. In general terms Timothy LeCain suggests that the idea of bodies bounded and distinct from the material world is anyway an illusion of modernism resulting from our dreams of mastery over nature.[3] *Mycobacterium bovis (M. bovis)* has punctured this fantasy in a brutal fashion in the United Kingdom (UK) in the last 150 years, leading to large-scale mortality.

Several members of the *Mycobacterium tuberculosis* family cause tuberculosis in the human body: *M. tuberculosis hominis*, *M. bovis*, *M. caprae*, *M. africanum*, *M. cannettii*; and also rarely *M. microti*, *M. pinnepedii* and *M. mungi*.[4] Of these, *M. cannettii* is probably the original organism, from which the others have split over the millennia by small deletions in their DNA; but there was certainly a full range of the present-day species of the *M. tuberculosis* complex active 40,000 years ago.[5]

---

[1] WHO 2014a.
[2] Westergaard 2007; WHO 2014b.
[3] LeCain 2014.
[4] Grange 2014; Rodriguez-Campos et al. 2014; Thoen, LoBue and Enarson 2014.
[5] Drewe and Smith 2014; Grange 2014; Gordon and Behr 2015.

Recent genetic investigation has shown that there remains a 99.95 per cent identity between *M. tuberculosis* and *M. bovis* - the two strains that will receive most attention in this book - yet they have many significant differences in host specificity and pathogenicity.[6] What we don't know is the relative proportions of human infections that they cause because attempts to make the distinction are not routinely performed in the laboratory.[7] Informed guesswork has tuberculosis of bovine origin at ten to twenty per cent of TB cases in those countries where milk is not systematically pasteurized and 0.5-1.0 per cent where it is.[8]

Paul Virilio spoke of the 'original accident' where the 'invention' of the train wreck followed the invention of the train.[9] Similarly zoonotic disease was arguably inevitable once livestock became a vital component of agrarian economies. In fact the zoonotic hazard has increased with the greater intensity of modern livestock husbandry and in recent decades has accelerated and taken on a qualitatively different guise with the speed of connections worldwide.[10] Of the 1,407 species of human pathogen, fifty-eight per cent are known to be zoonotic, while seventy-three per cent of emerging or re-emerging pathogens are zoonotic.[11] As a result of the obvious connexions between human and animal disease, a One World One Health movement has emerged in recent years to provide a context for interdisciplinary knowledge at the animal-human disease interface and also a platform for coordinated action by way of mitigation, mainly in the Global South.

The hazard of bovine tuberculosis (bTB) to cattle in Europe seems to have been taken seriously first in the late eighteenth century. Before that its symptoms were not perceived to be separate from those of other diseases. Because *M. bovis* seems to prosper in intensive group situations, the rise of commercial dairy farming for butter and cheese and in urban cowsheds for liquid drinking milk was its threshold of opportunity. There were larger herds and greater interconnections in the cattle economy gave possibilities for infection when animals were

---

[6] Thoen and Barletta 2014.

[7] Humblet et al. 2009.

[8] Cosivi et al. 1998; Ashford et al. 2006.

[9] Virilio 2007.

[10] Greger 2007; Coker et al. 2011; Kaneene et al. 2014.

[11] Woolhouse and Gowtage-Sequeria 2005; Jones et al. 2008.

gathered at markets or moved over long distances. BTB is particularly insidious because infected animals may remain asymptomatic, making it difficult to judge the risks.

At one point, in the interwar years of the twentieth century, the rate of bTB infection in the UK milking herd was running at about forty per cent. A concerted effort in the 1950s, using compulsory slaughter in an area eradication drive, brought this proportion down to manageable levels, and the whole country was declared free of bTB in 1960. Since then most other European states have dealt with the issue, including some that have eliminated it altogether (Table 0.1).

Table 0.1 The proportion of tested European cattle herds infected with *M. bovis*, 2012

Country	% herds infected	Country	% herds infected
Austria	OTF	Lithuania	0
Belgium	OTF	Luxembourg	OTF
Bulgaria	0	Malta	OTF
Cyprus	0	Netherlands	OTF
Czech Republic	OTF	Norway	OTF
Denmark	OTF	Poland	OTF
Estonia	OTF	Portugal	0.36
Finland	OTF	Romania	0.01
France	OTF	Slovakia	OTF
Germany	OTF	Slovenia	OTF
Greece	0.41	Spain	1.31
Hungary	OTF	Sweden	OTF
Ireland	4.37	Switzerland	OTF
Italy	0.76	United Kingdom	16.16
Latvia	OTF	EU	4.72

Source: EFSA 2014.
Note: OTF, Officially Tuberculosis Free.

A recrudescence of bTB in British cattle began in the 1980s and accelerated in the first decade of the twenty-first century, so that now the country has by far the worst bovine infection rate in Europe, especially concentrated in the South West and West Midlands of England, and in South Wales. According to the European Food Safety Authority, 16.2 per cent (Table 1.1) of herds tested in the UK have bTB, a serious enough figure but even more shocking in comparative terms when one considers that together the UK and the Republic of Ireland (RoI) between them have eighty-nine per cent of the infected herds in Europe (UK 60.8 per cent and RoI 28.2 per cent) that have been tested. This is not just a matter of national embarrassment; it has economic consequences for international trade. Officially Tuberculosis Free

(OTF) status is granted only when the percentage of OTF-withdrawn herds has not exceeded 0.1 per cent nationally for six consecutive years.[12] Within the UK only Scotland has this status.

Globally fifty million cattle are infected with bTB leading to annual losses of around $3 billion.[13] This widespread distribution is probably the result of cattle being sent around the world originally at the encouragement of the colonial powers, in the nineteenth and early twentieth centuries as they sought to establish agricultural economies in their empires that resembled those at home.[14]

Nowadays bTB in cattle in developed countries rarely advances to the point of disease generalised in the animal's body. Most reactors to the tuberculin test are asymptomatic and there no evidence of suffering or pain. Milk yields fall by about ten per cent and there is a six to twelve per cent reduction in meat production among infected cattle but in the UK those animals that do not earn their keep are anyway speedily despatched to the abattoir irrespective of whether they are diseased.[15] The risk to the consumers of meat, milk and other dairy products is small since most milk is pasteurized and any lesions are cut out of carcases.

Why then is there such concern about bTB? If the purchase of raw milk were further restricted, the risk to consumers would be negligible and the economic consequences would be entirely for the farming community to deal with. But the real answer is the obligation of European countries under EU law to have active regimes of containment and eradication. In the UK bTB is estimated to have cost the taxpayer £500 million over the last ten years and is likely to cost a further £1 billion over the next decade.[16] In annual terms this is about £150 million in Britain, £23 million in Northern Ireland, and £50 million in the RoI, a substantial burden for the authorities in these countries.[17] By comparison there is no other cattle disease for which the annual cost of surveillance exceeds £1m.

In bTB then we have a disease that is an economic challenge and a

---

[12] Reviriego Gordejo and Vermeersch 2006.
[13] Schiller et al. 2010.
[14] Salmon 1906; Michel et al. 2010.
[15] Zinsstag, Schelling et al. 2006.
[16] EFRA Select Committee 2013.
[17] Abernethy et al. 2013.

political minefield for governments in European governments into the latter half of the twentieth century. Of these it is the UK that continues to suffer, for reasons that are debatable but some claim is due to a wildlife reservoir of infection. *M. bovis* has resisted efforts in the UK to eradicate it and this makes it interesting, along with the shocking toll of human life in the era before effective vaccination and drug therapies.

A plan of the book

In *Liquid Materialities* I referred to my plans for a quartet of volumes on the history of milk.[18] The first volume was on the materiality of the commodity: an archaeology of its qualities and a biography of its emergence as a valued and trusted element of the diet. That complex series of stories is taken forward in this, the second volume, by reversing the story's direction. Here we will be looking at the dark side of the food system, the disease and ill-health that sometimes follow the act of consumption. A principal conceit of the present volume, for instance, is that bTB was a significant cause of human mortality in the British Isles in the period 1850 to 1960: above 600,000 deaths in total. That makes it one of the most deadly of native zoonotic diseases, spread mainly through raw cow's milk. As a result, one might have thought that at some point in that century the government would have reacted quickly and decisively to control it but interventions on the whole were slow and ineffective.

While I have published on this disease before, the way it is presented in this book is new. Here in the 165 years since 1850 we will treat bTB as an episystem.[19] This approach is inclusive, extending the usual epidemiological factors of host, agent and environment to include social, economic and political factors. Beyond that we will also argue that the indeterminate materiality of *M. bovis* is a crucial consideration. Chapter 1 discusses the uncertainty surrounding *M. bovis* through the lens of the New Materialism and other schools of thought that take materials seriously. The review includes Actor Network Theory (ANT), assemblages and the ontological complexity of the more-than-human,

---

[18] Atkins 2010a.
[19] O'Connor et al. 2012.

concluding that a new kind of onto-political ecology is desirable for a more intensive engagement with the mycobacterium.

Chapter 2 addresses the knowability of *M. bovis*. This was not just a matter of laboratory expertise in its isolation and its differentiation from the human mycobacterium, *M. tuberculosis*; there was also the problem of whose knowledge of bTB counted as a basis for action. The power of the medical establishment overwhelmed veterinary science and practice through most of the nineteenth century and into the twentieth. A hinge point was Koch's controversial statement in 1901 that there was only a minor risk of catching the disease from infected bovine milk or meat. The resulting controversy highlighted the fragile power of veterinary medical expertise and stimulated years of intensive research seeking to regain the pre-1901 consensus.

The impact of bTB upon the human body is the focus of Chapter 3. This stretches from the surveys of scrofula by Phillips in the 1840s, through the mortality data collected by the Registrars General, and the body site information from hospitals in the late nineteenth century, to the bacteriological research of Stanley Griffith and others in the twentieth century. The point of the various calculations we will make is to demonstrate that bTB was principally a disease of milk drinkers, for instance those aged under four years, and that it presented especially as an abdominal and cervical disease. An estimate of overall mortality for the period 1850 to 1960 is attempted and some comments are also made about regional concentrations of infection.

In Chapter 4 there is a discussion of the evolving veterinary science of bovine tuberculosis. This begins with the pathogenesis of the disease in cattle and then moves on to the many uncertainties that accompanied early versions of the skin test that was used in the field as a diagnostic tool. This story of indeterminacy is later taken up for the modern era in Chapter 14.

Chapters 5 and 6 seek to build upon the recent, heightened interest in our food environment by demonstrating that a continuing controversy about food standards – whether milk should or should not be compulsorily pasteurized – had a prehistory before the Second World War. There was a public debate from about 1900 to 1945, sometimes fierce in terms of the passionate arguments deployed, about whether it was appropriate for there to be any intervention at all, even though the risks to health were well-known. We will examine this through an account of the views of the two camps, the pro- and the anti-pasteurization lobbies. It will be argued that essentially this was a clash between discourses which were opposed in their views in the broader sense about the desirability of modernism and its impact on food systems.

Chapter 7 then looks at diseased meat. Contemporary estimates indicate that a substantial proportion of the indigenous beef consumed in Britain in the late nineteenth and early twentieth centuries came from tuberculous animals. If properly cooked, this meat presented less of a risk to human health than infected raw milk but concerns were nevertheless expressed by many public health professionals, especially in the 1880s and 1890s. The chapter looks at the interests of the various parties in the debate about diseased meat that evolved between 1889 and 1924. It investigates the solutions proposed and comments on the nature of central government policy-making. Much depended on a notorious case in 1889 in Glasgow. The local authority there prosecuted a butcher and a meat wholesaler for displaying diseased meat illegally, thereby creating a precedent and placing the responsibility for quality at the feet of particular actors in the food system. This unleashed a heated debate between the local state and the meat trade but it also created friction between farmers and butchers. The National Federation of Meat Traders wished to shift blame for unfit meat to the producers and discussed the possibility of requiring a warranty from their suppliers. Finding a negotiated compromise between the various parties proved to be difficult and finally, in 1924, the government felt the need to impose its own solution in the form of the Public Health (Meat) Regulations.

The story of tuberculous milk before the age of pasteurization is the subject of Chapter 8. The proposition is that this can be understood by reflection on the science and milk politics of one city, Manchester. It was here that the bacteriological laboratory of Sheridan Delépine was established and rose to prominence in the 1890s. He was a pioneer of a number of techniques that later became industry standards and it was his checking of samples for many local authorities that popularised the idea of laboratory support for the aims of the public health movement. Manchester as a progressive local authority also pioneered administrative intervention and control of bTB in milk and in cattle.

Chapter 9 covers bTB politics in the fifteen years after the start of the First World War. In 1914 Herbert Samuel replaced John Burns at the Local Government Board (LGB) and in a short period legislation was enacted. The implementation of this was postponed after the war, however, for complex reasons that were mainly to do with cost saving. The 1920s were then a decade of boisterous trade politics that made any producer-led initiatives to reduce bTB unlikely. It is intriguing to note the rise of the National Farmers' Union (NFU) in that decade as a power in the politics of vested interest. Chapter 10 charts this and demonstrates the internecine strife in Whitehall over milk-borne disease between the Ministry of Agriculture and Fisheries (MAF) and the Ministry of Health (MH). The former was pro-farmer and the latter had great difficulty in promoting the interests of the consumer. Chapter 11 completes the trio of chapters on these early politics with an analysis of the area eradication programme of the 1950s. This was an extraordinary accomplishment that was notionally completed in the 1960s but which unfortunately left a substantial pocket of disease in South West England.

The epidemiology of bTB is examined in Chapter 12. Although there is now a large literature, much of which uses sophisticated numerical and statistical modes of analysis, the identification of well calibrated and truly independent variables has proved to be difficult. The nature of farming systems and of their ecological and environmental contexts are obvious starting points. Then herd size and management, along with cattle movement, and the role of enclosed cattle sheds are all discussed.

The unspoken factor before 1971 was the role of badgers. Chapter 13 investigates the story behind this, including the emotional, polarised and entrenched positions taken up by those (mainly farmers and vets) who would cull badgers and those who oppose such interventions (ninety per cent of the general public). A number of attempts by scientists have been made to test the impact of the wildlife reservoir, most famously the Randomised Badger Culling Trial (1998-2007), but some politicians and farmers have chosen to ignore the published advice that culling can make no contribution to the reduction (in the UK) of bTB in cattle.

To the surprise and disappointment of all concerned, *M. bovis* made a come-back from the 1980s onwards. This was the great recrudescence of bTB that is anchored in a swathe of territory from the West Midlands to the South West of England, and also in South Wales. Chapter 14 deals with this and the messy associated politics. It highlights the uncertainty surrounding the skin test for cattle and also looks at one of the mooted solutions, the vaccination of cattle and badgers, but it gives little hope of a speedy resolution. Some improved government-inspired interventions have been introduced since 2005 but the whole country will not achieve OFT status for at least another two decades.

Chapter 15 suggests that uncertainty is the future of bTB, which has material characteristics that make it much more challenging for would-be control than most other livestock diseases. Embracing this uncertainty and being open and transparent with all stakeholders seems to be the only sensible way forward. In addition, *M. bovis* is a good example of a microbe with ample 'possibility spaces' at the more-than-human margin between society and environment. Its resilience and withdrawn stance make it a formidable opponent.

Overall the book is candidly about one of the messiest and least heartening stories in the anthology of UK agricultural and veterinary history. The politics are murky and there has so far been no resolution proposed that can guarantee a long-term improvement. We will argue though that a retreat to explanations emphasising vested interests or political incompetence simply will not do. The argument presented here will be that a focus upon the particular characteristics of the mycobacterium is the best starting point for an inclusive politics that recognises the possibility spaces of all of the agents that play a part in the emergence of zoonotic disease.

Acknowledgements and apologies

It seemed like a good idea at the time. I would write a biography of a neglected but re-emergent zoonotic disease and provide an estimate of the number of people who died from it over a 150 year period. I particularly wanted to know about the 'fissiparous liveliness' of bTB that is withheld from human perception and is somehow beyond human control to the extent it has still not been eliminated from the British Isles, 130 years after its zoonotic potential was first identified.[20]

---

[20] Henry and Roche 2013, 204.

To achieve this I would have to burgle bTB's house, crack the safe and there hidden away I expected to find all of the documentation I needed to write my biography. How long would it take? Maybe a couple of years? There were other projects, other responsibilities of course, so maybe five at the outside.

It was Tony Benn who said that he had to retire to go into politics. When I finally reached the point of superannuation in 2014 I had still not finished the book, now fifteen years late. Freed at last from teaching and administration, I was also divested of any lingering excuses. Being on permanent research leave certainly lightens the spirits and I newly gained the perspective to judge when the research and the writing had to stop. I can only apologise to those who may have felt that my enthusiasm for the archives was stronger than my willpower to finish the job. This includes the legions who have listened to and commented on seminar and conference papers, and also the kindly funders at the Wellcome Trust who provided small grants and a Research Leave Fellowship. Thank you all for your patience.

Thanks are also due to my colleagues in the Department of Geography, Durham University for providing a superb research environment. Their dedication to excellence and the intellectual stimulation over a thirty-five year period have been greatly appreciated. Part of this environment has been the privilege of supervising doctoral students of the highest quality. Although Philip Robinson was the only one to show an interest in bTB, his enthusiasm, his range of skills and his dedication have all been an inspiration. As a qualified vet he taught me a great deal about the disease and as an ethnographer he renewed my conviction that talking to farmers on the ground is essential if we are to understand *M. bovis* and then eliminate it.

As ever I am grateful to Dr Nick Cox for his willingness to discuss statistical matters, and to Dr Christine Dunn and Professors Richard Hall and Derek Oddy for their humorous scepticism. They are living proof that banter is an essential element of the scientific method. Paul Laxton was supportive when the going was tough, especially through his extensive knowledge of the history of public health. Chris Orton drew the art work with his usual professionalism and skill.

Because of the space limitations in this volume, further information will be published online. The reader is referred to my pages on the websites ResearchGate and Academia.edu.

Dedication

This book is dedicated to Ned, Jasper, Henry, Romy and Xander, the next but one generation. And also to Liz, with love – I can't say that often enough.

CHAPTER 1.

TELLING THE STORIES OF BOVINE TUBERCULOSIS

The history of bTB is complex in two senses. First it is multi-perspectival because science, politics, economics, geography and the social history of medicine all have legitimate claims on explaining important elements of its unfolding, and yet these different voices are at times cacophonous and contradictory. Second, the complexity also arises from the uncertainty and the indeterminacy surrounding *M. bovis* itself. The activities and the impacts of the mycobacterium are difficult to tie down and as an 'epistemic thing' it leaves knowledge open-ended.[1] The best we can do overall is to write a complicated simplification - a history that selects but at no time promises or delivers closure.

How then shall we tell our story? We could attempt a political history of the decisions (and indecisions) surrounding the governance of the disease. This approach would focus principally upon the human agency of regulation and control, and might spend time considering the institutional and administrative contexts within which policy emerged. It would need to show a sensitivity to the individuals involved and no doubt also to their underlying and potentially contested interests. The problem is that the politicians, administrators, farmers, veterinarians and public health officials all had difficulties in building a knowledge consensus about the science of bTB, and the generally successful frameworks of intervention used for other livestock diseases in the nineteenth and early twentieth centuries simply did not work for bTB. We are not talking about one set of interests blocking progress or about inadequate processes of governance. No, this was a disease that was fundamentally incompatible with all of the weapons brought to bear upon it. It was 'in excess' of the institutions and tools of veterinary public health, and to some extent still is.

If a history of politics and governance is insufficient on its own, how about shifting the emphasis to a social history of medicine, perhaps with the addition of a constitutive role for animals and zoonotic microbes?

---

[1] Rheinberger 1997.

Here at least we would be on the familiar territory of the 'centred' social science in which the duality of culture and nature is maintained and the core of the explanatory agenda is in the social realm.[2] There would be scope for a social constructivist interpretation of veterinary knowledge acquisition and its associated expertise, perhaps in the Science and Technology Studies style that has been so influential in the last two decades. In that vein there is certainly an attraction in the 'dance of agency' between humans and objects outlined by Pickering in the action-oriented approach he calls 'the mangle of practice'.[3] Pickering maintains the ontological duality in his associative thought experiment but, as we will see, it is difficult to see how this could be applied productively to our history with its great complexity.

Third, we could try a conscious step towards taking materiality seriously. The reason for this move is a general dissatisfaction with the assumption that the human domination of nature is sufficient to enable us to read off a list of greater and lesser triumphs without recourse to the material. The posthuman turn, familiar by now to all in social science and many in the humanities, has set a new agenda in which social factors are no longer the sole priority. At the extreme, gone are bare class and sectional interests, replaced by an understanding of agency as pooled between the social and the material. As stated in *Liquid Materialities*, my taste is for a light version of these metaphysics.[4] I will argue here that, while recognising the emergent potencies and capacities of matter, a fully flattened ontology for bTB would actually be counterproductive because I wish to discuss the 'possibility spaces' of infection and, as I hope will become clear, these are not symmetrically distributed.

The affordances of materials depend upon their capacity to yield an effect when acted upon. They are not independent properties but are shared relationally. Thus we could say that the human or bovine subject infected with bTB is an 'assembled social being' that takes on the properties of both, and is therefore a body-mycobacterium hybrid.[5] The disease affordance of badgers depends, for instance, upon the content and structure of the agro-ecologies created by pastoral farmers.

---

[2] Pickering 2005.

[3] Pickering 1995.

[4] Atkins 2010a.

[5] Dant 2004.

It therefore varies spatially. The implication is one of causality but affordances are contingent and they play an important part in uncertainty because they are inherently indeterminate. Thus the affordances of the bovine body for *M. bovis* are many and varied. The mycobacterium seeks to multiply and spread and in some cases this happens quickly; but in others the infection progresses slowly or lies quiescent until the internal bovine body chemistry stimulates a renewal. This unpredictability is frustrating for the authorities who then blame their failure to find infection upon the testing regime, the testing equipment or even the testers themselves. But the point is that the affordances of the various environments in which *M. bovis* can survive – bodies, water, manure, saliva – are sometimes favourable and provide it with a possibility space. These spaces can be nodal (a cattle shed with poor ventilation), or extensive (a pasture spread with infective slurry); they can be hidden (badger setts), or transparent (the moment that callipers are used to measure a tuberculin test swelling); they can be static (a farm where reactors are discovered at successive testings), or mobile (cattle with sub-clinical symptoms moved from one farm to another). The microbe is exceptionally adaptable to the circumstances it is presented with and appears to make the most of these opportunities.

In addition to the materials, some awareness is required of a materialized theory of practice. Schatzki helpfully talks of material 'arrangements' and he sees social phenomena as slices through the practice-arrangement nexuses that constitute human coexistence with materiality.[6] His arrangements are not unlike the networks of Actor Network Theory (ANT) but, in addition, he goes on to talk about practices, a poorly developed aspect of some versions of ANT.

The New Materialism: real or virtual objects?

The position adopted in this book is that there is a *real* world beyond thought. This is not meant in the naive voice of descriptive empiricism but rather with a view to taking objects seriously. Thinking through objects is also an objective of the New Materialism, a recent turn in the social sciences and humanities, so in this section we will explore the extent to which inspiration can be drawn from this rapidly expanding

---

[6] Schatzki 2010, 2015.

field. In *Liquid Materialities* I argued that the material qualities of milk are emergent and best explained by a genealogical method. In this way the biographies of commodities can be understood as human artefacts but within the limits of material affordances.[7] The present volume is different because here we are dealing with a bad (bTB) rather than a good (milk). While in the constructivist sense we could claim that the spread of zoonoses is an unintended consequence of human actions, emphasis will rather be given to attempts by society to rid itself of this particular deadly disease. *M. bovis* has resisted a suite of eradication efforts; our focus is therefore flipped to the mycobacterium and the material qualities that have placed it beyond control.

The 'things' of interest in this book are not just technical objects; they also include warm bodies and the bacteria in them. How does this compare with the priorities of the New Materialists? First in their conceptual queue was ANT, which for twenty years was a major influence on thinking about objects. More a field with divergent views than a coherent theory, ANT in sum adopts a flattened ontology in which agency is shared symmetrically and the nature/culture duality is dissolved. Its vision is one of networks in which the world is organized via the linkages between, say, bacteria, bovine bodies, raw milk and human tuberculosis, and their effects upon each other.

Having been subjected to a fierce scrutiny, the tide eventually turned against ANT. It was accused of a 'leaden view of stuff' and of being 'bereft of energy and materials'.[8] Maybe commentators have been a little hard on Bruno Latour, the most famous actor networker. Contrary to the excesses of the early ANT, the pronouncements of the later Latour have been positively emollient. In *Reassembling the Social*, for instance, material agency is little more than authorizing, allowing, encouraging, permitting, suggesting, influencing, blocking, or rendering possible.[9] For the reconstructed Latour, 'the project of ANT is simply to extend the list and modify the shapes and figures of those assembled as participants and to design a way to make them act as a durable whole'.

---

[7] Atkins 2010a.

[8] Shove et al. 2012, 10; Ingold 2012, 436.

[9] Latour 2005.

And it is not 'the establishment of some absurd symmetry between humans and non-humans.'[10]

Theorists interested in relational, material-oriented explanations have moved on, in different directions. Some who found actor networks antiseptic and limiting have switched to Deleuze's assemblages as reformulated by Manuel DeLanda.[11] The dispersed, multiple and heterogeneous nature of agencies from ANT is still there, as is the conviction that objects exist in a relational and emergent world.[12] But assemblages have a more holistic understanding of agency and the assemblage literature employs a different vocabulary. There are connexion words such as infection, influence, sympathy, citation, association, synthesis, linkage, network; force words like alloying, catalysis, symbiosis; and process words such as blending, collating, gathering and joining. Assemblages also encompass 'ontic indeterminacy' and the 'messiness and complexity of phenomena' that imply 'a resistance to closure'.[13]

John Allen and others convincingly show influenza to be an example of the power of assemblages. As it spreads the virus mutates into different strains, including versions that are zoonotic and can be devastating. Bird flu and swine flu are examples of this genetic drift and they have the potential to exceed beyond control into global pandemics.[14] Allen's assemblages, though, are 'post-relational' because they take entities seriously in spatially patterned entanglements. His position overall is that assemblages need a version of realism to give them an explanatory cutting edge, and this would be at least one counter to the common criticism of assemblages that they avoid 'both individuals and actuals as the basis for ontology, replacing them with the virtuality of the genus'.[15] Further to this, Harman complains that DeLanda 'grants too little dignity to specific things, and shifts the problem of causal relations away from its true scene: the duel between specific objects'.[16]

Maintaining the heritage of ANT, now rebranded as material semiotics, John Law and his various collaborators have continued with

---

10 Ibid, 72, 76.
11 DeLanda 2006.
12 Anderson and McFarlane 2011.
13 Anderson et al. 2012a.
14 Allen 2012.
15 Harman 2008, 379.
16 Ibid, 380.

the notion of relational hybridity.[17] Law has shown that such analyses are relevant at different scales, from the farming of salmon in Norway to the global links embedded in the Foot and Mouth Disease (FMD) outbreak in Britain in 2001. In *The Body Multiple*, Annemarie Mol in particular has shown how such an ontology opens a space for difference, something not satisfactorily addressed by assemblages.[18] She shows how a diagnosis of atherosclerosis arises, not just from a doctor in a white coat, but from the relations between equipment, physical examinations and expertise. It is a networked achievement that depends upon its components and may fall out differently according to the various dispositions of those objects and performances at any one moment.

Although impressed by the work of Law, Mol and the assemblagers, many of us would baulk at the claim that the constitution of the social is entirely relational. As Hinchliffe points out: 'Things persist despite their relations, they can detach, withdraw, they have histories and geographies in that they are made in and make time-spaces'.[19] But there is certainly attraction in the observation that 'an assemblage approach demands an empirical focus on how these spatial forms and processes are themselves assembled, are held in place, and work in different ways to open up or close down possibilities'. These plain words are close to what many historians do anyway without ever considering the 'A' word, and the slow development of explicitly relational work by historians themselves suggests that the conceptual language may be seen as limiting rather than extending.

Another fork in the road away from ANT has been Jane Bennett's material vitalism, which includes bacteria in the human microbiome as illustrative of the alien quality of our flesh. The vital materiality of her bodies is not fully or exclusively human; it is also a battleground because of the fractious relationship between the human and the non-human.[20] The vibrancy of Bennett's materials also extends to inanimate objects. Although a philosophically sophisticated manoeuvre, for some commentators this extension of materiality is problematic and lacking

---

[17] Law and Lien 2013.
[18] Mol 2002.
[19] Hinchliffe 2011, 398.
[20] Bennett 2010.

in the necessary political leverage that is required when thinking with objects.[21]

À la Bennett, we might see bTB as an animate-inanimate assemblage of bacteria whose epidemiology and pathogenesis are not fully known, breeds of cattle that genetically are susceptible to TB, tuberculin testing that lacks sensitivity, contested parliamentary debate, abattoir slaughter, frequently infected milk, scrofula as a principal symptom in the human body, dairy company profit, lack of trust in veterinary expertise, civil servant rivalries, the use of laboratory guinea pigs, and inefficient pasteurization machinery. In such an assemblage matter is permanently engaged in a network of relationals and it is through series of linkages, and sometimes the lack of them, that the mycobacterium has been able to prosper through a series of (for it) positive links.

Jane Bennett's famous example of the 2003 electricity blackout in the north east of North America is about the (temporary) non-alignment of material objects. More relevant for us, their agential forms as vital assemblages are examples involving the living components of an epidemic: the bacteria and their unwitting hosts. There is nothing more provisional and rapidly emergent than a widespread infection that is out of control. Here the notion of relational hybridity is easy to grasp. According to Ben Anderson, such assemblages form, mutate and disperse with the power that is exerted through them and they are accommodating or resistant to that force field according to the contingent circumstances in which they are participants.[22] The direction and reach depends upon the capacities of the elements.

Myra Hird has a clear bacterial/viral vision, which she terms 'microontology'. This draws upon biosemiotics and other disciplines to formulate a new ethics and (she hopes) a new future for social science. The new ethics is about 'how we could all live together', which of course is not to say that we should accept tuberculosis or draw back from our attempts to eliminate bTB in humans, cattle and badgers.[23] Rather the suggestion is that it is time to accept microontological indeterminacy. In other words, the knowing of microbes is never going to be complete and the acceptance of this is not a defeat for positive science but

---

[21] Gregson 2011.

[22] Anderson et al. 2012b.

[23] Hird 2009; Greenhough 2014, 105.

instead is an important onto-political gesture. The next step after that is to note that the acceptance of bacterial indeterminacy helps us to appreciate difference, a key aspect of the outcomes of encounters in microontology.

In a different register but with similar objectives, Rosalyn Diprose talks of 'corporeal generosity' by which she means the mixing of humans and non-humans.[24] This expansion of the notion of 'self' can encompass bacteria, although often with negative consequences for the host. As early as 1872 Samuel Butler recognised this when he made the prescient comment that '[man] is such a hive and swarm of parasites that it is doubtful whether his body is not more theirs than his'.[25]

Throughout our study of *M. bovis* we will find it difficult to translate Hird's microontology into anything meaningful in terms of epidemiology and pathogenesis. Fortunately, however, some thought has been given in what are called more-than-human studies to materialising the apparently invisible. Hinchliffe, for instance, in his work on urban wildlife discussed the need for the activities of black redstarts or otters to be 'made present' through the triangulation of multiple methods, including the use of surrogate traces.[26] Very often there is little that can be done in such circumstances in the way of direct observation, so it is the shadow that has to stand in as a fugitive yet emergent impression. In our case this is through the collection of tuberculous badger corpses, geo-statistical modelling, the analysis of archival documentation, or even guesswork about infections in live bovine bodies. All of these are legitimate tools it seems to me, along with qualitative fieldwork methods and even art. As a result, 'in practice, researchers can only theorise bacteria as the cause of disease retroductively and abductively by examining their consequences in the world'.[27]

According to Coole and Frost 'there are a number of indications that critical social theory is reorienting toward more realist approaches to political analysis'. And yet at the same time the 'new materialists stubbornly insist on the generativity and resilience of the material forms with which social actors interact, forms which circumscribe, encourage,

---

[24] Diprose 2002.

[25] Butler 1872, 199.

[26] Hinchliffe 2008.

[27] Speake 2011, 534.

and test their discourses'. They argue that 'it is entirely possible ... to accept social constructionist arguments while also insisting that the material realm is irreducible to culture or discourse and that cultural artefacts are not arbitrary vis-à-vis nature'.[28]

Where are we now then with the New Materialists? Without adopting their full theoretical vocabulary or a strong version of their metaphysics, this book is influenced by those new materialisms in social science that acknowledge a need to consider materials and objects as co-sponsors of performance. As a result, we will meet some agents of technoscience, such as pasteurizing machinery and tuberculin testing equipment, and we will doff our cap to their powers of resistance and catalysis during entanglements with human intentionality. But our main focus will remain biocentric, with a principal concern for human and bovine health, while also remaining alert to the relentless agency and astonishing resilience of the pathogenic microbe known as *M. bovis*.

Indeterminacy and difference

Although BSE (Bovine Spongiform Encephalopathy) is a prion disease and therefore very different in its aetiology and epidemiology from bacterial, viral and other livestock diseases, nevertheless there are parallels to bTB in our difficulty in grasping its risk to humans. At first it was thought to be a cattle-only disease; then similarities were noticed with the centuries-old sheep affliction, scrapie, and a human transmissible spongiform encephalopathy from New Guinea known as kuru. Finally, a decision threshold of major significance was crossed in 1996, in a combination of frankly uncertain science and pragmatic public health politics, when it was announced that BSE in cattle was the likely cause of new variant Creutzfeld-Jakob Disease in humans. Steve Hinchliffe reviewed the government BSE Inquiry that reported in the year 2000 on the background to what proved to be a very costly (in human and animal life, treasure and political fall-out) zoonotic disease. His conclusion is that 'knowing prions is ... a knowing of indeterminacy.'[29] Hinchliffe points out that uncertainty is not just a knowledge deficit that will eventually be overcome by the scientific method, the issue being one of a temporary

---

[28] Coole and Frost 2010, 26-7.
[29] Ibid 192.

problem of making accurate representations. There are indeterminacies that continually resist knowing and are apparently in excess of scientific realism. His approach has been dubbed a genealogical assemblage: 'a technique where contemporary conditions and knowledges are shown to be the product of associations that together stabilize or destabilize reliable ways of knowing'.[30]

Knowing is a two-way street and in a sense microbes also seek knowledge. Thus the various mycobacteria of the tuberculosis family have been active over the millennia adapting to their hosts. As a result, *M. bovis* has found that cattle are the optimum species for it to infect. This is the result of an evolutionary learning experience that is on-going, not just in its various modes of pathogenicity but also at the microbiological level. As we will see, mutations are common, resulting in mycobacterial 'fingerprints' being left in the living bodies of its victims. These are the individuated traces of changes in DNA.

Our objects of study, here *M. bovis* and later the badger, are largely withdrawn from our daily world, microscopic or underground. Both depend for their being largely upon the opportunities presented to them by humans, but being out of sight generates issues of knowability and measurability that impinge upon the confidence we place in our knowledge of them. Can we be sure that we understand the mechanisms of infection? The NFU's members say that they 'know' that badgers spread the disease but how can they be sure, and anyway is that a pathway that we need to worry about? This is just the beginning of what turns out to be a story shot through with indeterminacies. Pity the poor policy maker who needs to be seen to act decisively when so many of the so-called facts turn out to be hazy, slippery or even imaginary.

Bacteria: epistemic things?

Historical epistemologists are interested in the past contexts in which knowledge was produced and for bTB they would probably claim that bacteria as objects are not found ready-made as natural phenomena but are constituted in the specific settings of, say, laboratories.[31] As we will see, the 'tubercle bacillus' may have Robert Koch's name firmly

---

[30] Robbins and Marks 2010, 190.

[31] Rheinberger 2010.

attached to it but a hagiography of even such a great scientist would be profoundly inadequate as an expression of the joint effort required by the experimenters, their equipment, their conceptual frameworks, and of course the objects of research, as to whether there will be cooperation or resistance in the process of knowing.

As Rheinberger observes, there are 'epistemic things' with unknown and maybe unknowable characteristics that produce excess.[32] One such, we will assert, is *M. bovis*, which has not yet been fully captured and tamed. Hinchliffe, writing about BSE, argues that 'epistemic things embody what one does not know. They are vague and they are absent in their experimental presence. They present themselves in a characteristic, irreducible vagueness'.[33] Knowing them has to begin with an acknowledgement of their indeterminacy. Knorr Cetina adds that they 'are always in the process of being materially defined, they continually acquire new properties and change the ones they have. But this also means that objects of knowledge can never be fully attained, that they are, if you wish, never quite themselves'.[34] Such epistemic objects are to an extent 'unfolding structures of absences'.[35]

According to Gilbert Simondon, acknowledging absence and uncertainty is best achieved through the concept of emergence. Although usually associated in the anglophone literature with technical objects, Simondon's philosophy was in fact broadly based. He argued, for instance, that the living object is a 'theatre of individuation ... Within the living itself, there is a more complete regime of internal resonance, one that requires permanent communication and that maintains a metastability that is a condition of life ... The living individual is a system of individuation, an individuating system and a system individuating itself'.[36]

Simondon's ontogenetic vision of matter is lubricated by his suggestion that all forms are emergent through this process of individuation. Similarly Ingold argues that the properties of materials

---

[32] Rheinberger 1997.
[33] Hinchliffe 2001, 189.
[34] Knorr Cetina 2001, 190.
[35] Ibid 182.
[36] Simondon 2009, 7.

are histories.[37] Following this we can say that bacteria, such as *M. bovis*, are constantly becoming in two senses. In the present-and-now they are spreading and multiplying but not in any pre-determined fashion – predicting the outcome of a TB infection is exceptionally difficult in both bovine and human bodies. Second, in the longer term the DNA of *M. bovis* is dynamic, creating new sub-strains that leave their genetic footprints behind.

Simondon is well-known for his morphogenetic analogy of the coral reef in which the present is built on the skeletons of the past. Another is the seed, which in effect contains a programme of its future growth but which, as Lopez reminds us, as a pre-individual 'needs allies in order to become a plant, namely water and light'.[38] Similarly *M. bovis* starts in a small way in either bovine of human bodies. Even one mycobacterium is enough to initiate an infection that then multiplies and spreads slowly, exploiting weaknesses in each body's defences. A well nourished individual with a strong immune system can often localise and then destroy the invaders but others will succumb and may then become a hazard themselves. We will see in Chapters 12 and 13 that environmental factors are important in the epidemiology of bTB, and the possibility spaces of diseases have for at least one hundred years been partly shaped by political decisions (Chapters 9-11). It will therefore be profitable for us to consider developing an explanatory framework that has a foothold in 'political ecology'.

Onto-political ecology

The study of political ecology began in the 1970s with the degradation of environmental resources in the Global South and the degree to which this was entangled with the neo-liberal forces studied by political economists. Since then it has become a broad field. Paul Robbins identifies five themes and the political ecology introduced in the present volume falls into his fifth category: the 'political objects and actors thesis'. Here the material characteristics of non-human nature and its components (dung, climate, refrigerators, bacteria, lawn grass, road salt,

---

[37] Ingold 2012.
[38] López 2014.

goats, tropical soil) impinge on the world of human struggles and are entwined within them, and so are inevitably political.39

Tim Forsyth has recently argued for a switch in emphasis in political ecology away from 'the *social interests* of science (who benefits), and instead focus on the *explanatory potential* of science (how we explain problems)'.[40] He wants 'a more politicized engagement with how environmental cause-and-effect statements are made'. If this call is heeded it may well mean a fading of the social constructivism that has been standard among political ecologists, with greater attention to the material. In our case this would mean greater attention to *M. bovis* and the politics associated with its particular ecological characteristics.

The onto-politics of bTB are multiple. First, as we will hear many times in this book, there is the epidemiological and pathogenetic complexity of *M. bovis*, the shy but relentless microbe. Once we can agree that its material characteristics make it hard to know and hard to eliminate, at last we can map out a political ecology in which agency is no longer human-centred. The centre of gravity is shifted to a hybrid politics of both bugs and bodies. This then leads us on to the second politics, which is the 'ontological disorder' that is implicit in the sharing of disease between animals and humans.[41] Zoonoses by their very nature undermine, then redefine our understandings of ourselves. Do our bodies have limits or should we drop such naive realism and see them as meeting grounds of the many forces of nature, both friendly and unfriendly to our long-term welfare? There is something deeply unsettling existentially about the notion of being open to animal disease, but in the twenty-first century this is a risk of rising probability.

The third onto-politics is the more familiar one of human action and inaction. Because bTB is a slow-burn disease it has none of the 'focusing events' that force policy change or speed implementation because of the glare of publicity and the need for politicians to be seen to be doing something. It is therefore different from salmonella in eggs, BSE, FMD, classical swine fever, or even the novel livestock diseases that temporarily hit the headlines, such as blue tongue. Very few of the modern-day infected animals ever develop visible symptoms of TB.

[39] Robbins 2012, 23.

[40] Forsyth 2011, 31. Emphasis as in original.

[41] For a fuller treatment of this point, see Nimmo 2010.

Even in the past when it sometimes proceeded to a more advanced stage, veterinarians were only able to pick it up by inspection of a proportion of the cows yielding bacteria in their milk. Today when considering a vaccine against bTB, it is the Bacillus Calmette-Guérin (BCG) that has most of the desirable properties, although it requires further testing and development before it can be released on to the market. There is no therapy for bTB in cattle and so we are thrown back on the use of testing technologies, which are used in conjunction with slaughter. But none of the available tests is wholly satisfactory and there is no immediate prospect of improvements. Administrative solutions tried in the past have included restrictions on the movement of animals, the separation of infected and health animals, the isolation of incomers for a period of quarantine, restrictions at markets and shows, and the culling of infected wildlife. None of these measures has proved to be decisive, in the UK context at least. Even the eradication campaign of the 1950s was ultimately to be only a temporary success.

We will investigate all of these points in depth. While it is possible to argue that there have been some failings of political will and in the speed and technicalities of policy in the past, our principal argument will be that bTB has emerged as a threat from a combination of human practices and animal ecologies. In particular it is the special characteristics of the mycobacteria that have proven to be resistant to interventions and we will investigate these in depth in the chapters on aetiology, epidemiology and pathogenesis. In short, *M. bovis* is extraordinarily flexible in its exploitation of possibility spaces and so far it has proved to be beyond the control of interventions, both public and private.

Conclusion

In the UK bTB today has become a zoonosis without many human victims. In animals there is also a difference from a century ago in that it rarely progresses to the point that there are visible symptoms. Both these changes represent progress but remarkably we cannot say that there have been commensurate technological improvements. Three continuing problems make this point:

- diagnostic procedures cannot guarantee accurate measurement of *M. bovis* in cattle;
- bTB is connected in an unknown way to an invisible wildlife reservoir;
- bTB is untreatable in animals and, as yet, there is no accepted cattle vaccine by way of prophylaxis.

On the basis of the same set of scientific evidence, successive UK governments have implemented very different policies. In fact, the only solid, stable and knowable element of bTB is the public's opposition to badger culling, which at one point approached North Korean levels of consensus.

None of this is meant as a counsel of despair. The history of bTB may be one of indeterminacy and uncertainty but it is possible to argue that a study of this most difficult disease to understand and control can help us to think differently about other zoonoses. Our onto-political ecology of the relations between humans and non-humans is an attempt to analyse a merged hybrid of the two worlds. This is the infected person or bovine, whose newly individuated form may be unknown to herself, her companions or keepers but represents both an achievement and an opportunity for the mycobacterium. The stories we will tell are therefore a new way of simultaneously writing veterinary and medical history. Ultimately we will argue that these histories have relevance for examining the present crisis of tuberculosis in UK cattle and that they question some of the assumptions behind government policy.

CHAPTER 2.

'YOUR ENEMY THE COW': THE CONSTRUCTION OF EARLY MEDICAL AND VETERINARY KNOWLEDGE ABOUT BOVINE TUBERCULOSIS

Introduction: Koch and the 1901 Congress

It was 3 p.m. on Tuesday 23 July 1901 and Robert Koch was called to speak.[1] Because he was revered as the discoverer of the tubercle bacillus and one of the greatest laboratory scientists of the age, he was received with 'great applause'.[2] It was the occasion of the International Congress on Tuberculosis in London, one of the most important conferences held to that date on a disease that had been a major killer in the preceding century. The venue was St James's Hall, Piccadilly, and in the audience were two thousand clinical experts on tuberculosis, including four hundred from overseas and a strong representation of the public health professionals who were involved in the administration of preventative environmental interventions. Some of Koch's audience had printed copies of his talk and, judging by their ability to give an immediate and powerful response, the key figures must have orchestrated their counterblast in order to maximise publicity.

Koch's paper is modest enough on the page but there are certain sentences which carry a heavy weight of meaning. He asserted in short that tuberculosis was unlikely to be transmitted from cattle to humans and that milk and meat infected with tubercle mycobacteria were therefore safe. He confirmed in subsequent writings and conference papers that this interpretation was correct and that he had fully intended to state an opinion that stood outside of the then accepted wisdom on the relationship between tuberculosis and the food supply. The minute textual analysis to which his 1901 statement was subjected in both the popular and academic media demonstrates the importance that all sections of the community put upon it, and Koch was immediately at the centre of a storm of

---

[1] *The Times* 24 July 1901, 8a-c.
[2] *Transactions of the British Congress on Tuberculosis* 1901, vol. 1, 23.

controversy. It is difficult to exaggerate the consternation he caused in the medical community. A volcanic dispute erupted that continued in its primary form for a decade, with after-shocks for a further fifty years beyond that.

There are three foundational points to make. First, Koch was already a figure of controversy who, despite his celebrity and later his Nobel Prize-winning status, found it difficult to build a full consensus for some of his ideas - that tuberculosis was not a zoonosis was one and the therapeutic effect of tuberculin was another. In this he was different from his contemporary Louis Pasteur, who was adopted by the hygienists of his day and who turned into a figurehead of their movement. This translation of interests was gradually built into a powerful assemblage of elements that drew its initial momentum from Pasteur's laboratory and then from his successful strategy of communicating the significance of his results.[3] Second, tuberculosis by its very nature was a disease whose aetiology, epidemiology, pathogenesis and therapeutics were somewhat opaque at this time. The scientific problems flowing from this were matters of factual instability. As a result, no one authority such as Koch could be relied upon to have a satisfactory set of prescriptions for intervention. Third, because bTB was associated with the food system, commercially and politically one of the most highly charged areas of modern life due to its intersection of many chains of interest, claims about its impact generated clashes between the various concerned parties. In the British context it seems to have taken until 1960 for these to have been resolved, even partially.

Since at least the late eighteenth century a link had been suspected between milk and one specific form of tuberculosis commonly known as scrofula (Figure 2.1). In more general terms, an account of 'phthisis' in the dairy cattle in suburban Paris had been given in 1795 by Jean-Baptiste Huzard.[4] Then in 1831 Gurlt in Berlin identified similarities between tubercles (nodules) in the bodies of cattle and those of humans, and Carmichael in 1810 and Klencke in 1843 and 1846 both reported their suspicions about the infectivity of cow's milk.[5] Collectively these observations made little headway in the era before the germ theory of

---

[3] Latour 1988.

[4] Huzard 1795; Huzard 1834; Hubscher 1999; Blancou 2003.

[5] Carmichael 1810; Gurlt 1831.

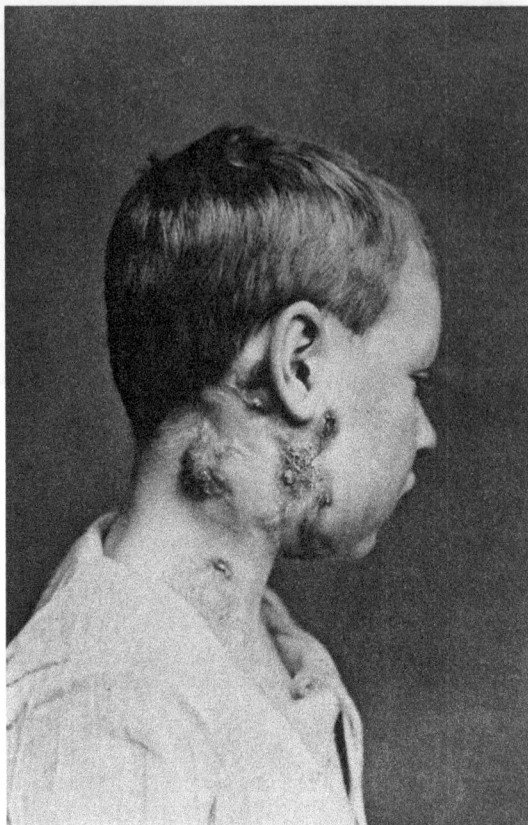

Fig 2.1
Young man with a typical case
of scrofula
(Source: Bramwell 1893, 5,
courtesy of Wellcome Images)

disease, however.[6] It was not until the 1860s that experimental work by Villemin demonstrated that the injection of tuberculous material from humans and cows into rabbits and guinea pigs could induce the disease. He reported this to the Académie Nationale de Médecine in Paris in 1865 and 1868 and his findings were confirmed shortly after by Chauveau and Cohnheim feeding their experimental animals with tubercular tissue, and then by Gerlach and Klebs feeding theirs with infected milk.[7] This proved the possibility of trans-species infection but there were many doubters, for instance those still under the influence of Broussais and the German school of histopathologists who believed most diseases to be based on cellular disorders, with no specific infective agent involved. Under certain anatomical conditions they thought that any accumulation of inflammatory products in the lungs was liable to

[6] Duguid 1890; Moore 1913; Basset 1952; Grange and Yates 1994.
[7] Nocard 1895; Ernst 1914; Dubos 1953; Hardy 2003a; Waddington 2006.

undergo caseous degeneration, leading to phthisis.[8] They also refused to acknowledge any analogy between the bovine and human diseases.[9] As Worboys shows, these beliefs continued into the 1880s and 1890s, the era of microbiological discoveries, because physicians did not necessarily see existing ideas about hereditary predisposition and cellular susceptibility as incompatible with the notion of infection. After all, Laënnec in his unitary theory had pioneered the notion of internal dissemination within the body via tubercles some 60 years before.[10]

In Britain, George Fleming, the army's chief veterinarian, was already warning in the 1870s and early 1880s of the possible dangers of catching tuberculosis from infected meat and milk.[11] He believed the evidence of the zoonotic power of bTB to be 'strong and decisive'. In 1881 Creighton expressed what by then was probably the majority view that 'there already exist grounds, of a certain kind, for suspecting that the tuberculosis of the bovine species may have communicated itself to man', and he was the first to differentiate the bovine from the human disease at post mortem.[12] It therefore came as no surprise when Koch announced the discovery of the tubercle bacillus to the Physiological Society of Berlin in March 1882. The sensation was more in the unleashing of a flood of research into tuberculosis which lasted for several decades. Thus in 1890 Duguid commented that 'during the past eight or ten years tuberculosis ... has received more attention than any other disease of either man or animals'.[13]

If Koch's tubercle bacillus was the cause of disease in both humans and animals, then surely the consumption of diseased meat, milk, and dairy products such as butter and cream, must be dangerous. In 1882 Koch himself certainly seemed to think so:

> Bovine tuberculosis is identical with human tuberculosis, and is thus a disease transmissible to man ... Be the danger which arises from the consumption of the flesh or milk of tuberculosis cattle ever so great or ever so small, it exists, and it must therefore be prevented.[14]

---

[8] Delépine 1920.

[9] Blancou 2003; Seyfarth and Seyfarth 1998.

[10] Worboys 2000.

[11] Fleming 1874, 1875, 1880, 1888; Lydtin et al. 1883.

[12] Creighton 1880, 1881a.

[13] Duguid 1890, 305.

[14] Pattison 1981, 118.

Subsequently many others thought that a large proportion of 'human phthisis comes from the butcher's stall' or the cow byre and this became the well-established view of the medical, veterinary and public health professions.[15] The National Veterinary Medical Association agreed upon the possibility of contagion at its meetings in London in 1883 and Manchester in 1884, as did the International Medical Congress in Copenhagen, also in 1884.[16] In 1886 a survey by the Association of Municipal Corporations found that 85 per cent of English MOsH (Medical Officers of Health) believed that tuberculosis was communicable via raw milk and undercooked meat, a view endorsed subsequently by various parliamentary enquiries in the 1890s.

In the later 1890s there seemed little room left for debate. In 1896 Sheridan Delépine observed that 'for thirty years it has been known that tuberculosis was a disease easily communicable, but it is only of late that belief in the infectiousness of tuberculosis has become universal', and five years earlier Sims Woodhead had reported that the gist of discussions at the recent International Congress of Hygiene and Demography was 'that there is grave danger arising from the use of tuberculous milk must be accepted as proved without any shadow of doubt'. At the same meeting Sir John Burdon-Sanderson observed that 'the identity of bovine and human tuberculosis is a thing to be accepted as a fundamental proposition'.[17] In December 1898 Sir Richard Thorne Thorne presided over a meeting of National Association for Prevention of Consumption at which there was 'absolute unanimity' that the greatest danger of infection in milk came from tuberculous cows.[18]

In hindsight a knowledge stabilization concerning bovine tuberculosis was not quite achieved by 1900. Up to that point there were a number of lingering issues. First, tuberculosis is not a dramatic disease in the sense of quickfire epidemics and so 'proving' a link with milk was not as easy as the assertions quoted above seem to imply. In the 1890s there was even a group of doctors called before the Royal Commissions on Tuberculosis who were willing to give evidence contrary to the microbiological theory. These were senior men who had probably qualified before

---

[15] McFadyean 1898, 344-50.

[16] BPP 1888 (C. 5461-I) xxxii.Q.7528.

[17] Delépine 1896, 81; Delépine 1901; Sims Woodhead 1891.

[18] Thorne Thorne 1899; *The Times* November 11, 1898, 12b; Newsholme 1935, 241.

the contagionist era and who clung to environmental notions of disease or to the idea of heredity. Thomas Barlow, Physician to University College Hospital and the Hospital for Sick Children, Great Ormond Street, for instance, claimed that the possibility infection from milk 'has been a very new suggestion to us, I do not think that our minds have been always sufficiently alive to that point'.[19] Dr James Goodhart was convinced that everyone had tubercle bacilli in their bodies but that these only took 'root' if the host was susceptible to the disease. He took no special precautions against tuberculosis on behalf of his patients at Guy's Hospital since he did not believe the disease to be infectious and saw no advantage in boiling milk.[20] Overall we see here the continuation of the heredity and seed and soil ideas that were dominant through the earlier part of the nineteenth century.[21]

A common belief in the 1880s and 1890s was that the bacteria causing tuberculosis in humans and in animals were the same. Nevertheless there was persistent curiosity about the apparent difference in virulence between the bacteria isolated from human and bovine subjects.[22] In America Theobald Smith researched this between 1896 and 1898 and described slight morphological differences between a human strain of bacillus, nowadays termed *Mycobacterium tuberculosis* and a bovine type, *Mycobacterium bovis*.[23] The latter is shorter and its growth is slow in glycerol. It is less aerobic and produces smaller, flatter colonies by comparison with the luxuriant, heaped colonies of *M. tuberculosis*.[24]

Smith's observations may have furthered medical knowledge about the complexity of the disease but in the process he also shattered the consensus that tuberculosis was the same for all mammals. Further seeds of doubts were sown when Koch showed at this time, correctly as we now know, that the human mycobacterium was weak in producing disease in calves and other animals. His error was in then going on to assume that the reverse would also be true, that *M. bovis* would not migrate successfully to the human body. It seems likely that Koch's attitude was

---

[19] BPP 1896 (C. 7992) xlvi.Q.1033.

[20] Ibid, QQ.1364-1413.

[21] Worboys 2000.

[22] Sigurdsson 1945.

[23] Pritchard 1988.

[24] Collins and Grange 1983.

the result of his immersion in a centuries-old German controversy as to risk of disease in the food supply. Steamed tuberculous meat, for instance, continued to be sold in German cities in the early decades of the twentieth century in so-called Freibanken. Such meat was said to be safe and was not banned until 1941.[25] Similarly, the German habit of boiling milk meant that it was much rarer for bTB to spread by that route than in Britain.[26]

Koch showed courage in repeating his unpopular hypothesis in 1902, at the International Tuberculosis Conference in Berlin, in 1903 to the Brussels Congress on Tuberculosis, and again to the Washington Congress in 1908. The reaction of his audiences was by now less one of surprise than of outright hostility. At Brussels help was on hand because 'the German delegates closed ranks in the face of attack by the Belgians and French. Koch's views on bovine tuberculosis had become those of Imperial Germany'.[27] But at Washington his reception amounted to a public humiliation.[28] This irrevocably widened the cracks of polite scientific debate to chasms of vituperation.

As we hinted earlier, Koch was not a newcomer to controversy.[29] A premature announcement at the Tenth International Congress of Medicine at Berlin in 1890 that his 'tuberculin' was a cure for tuberculosis had proved to be an acute embarrassment.[30] It seems that on that occasion he was under pressure from the government to demonstrate the prowess of German science.[31] Koch had also quarrelled with Pasteur, accusing him of exaggeration and over-generalization. He was more of a lone empiricist than Pasteur and temperamentally he was incapable of the networking and proselytizing that made Pasteur into a household name in France, with a street named after him in every town. Koch even clashed with some of his German colleagues, and their lukewarm view of him is typified by Virchow who stated at the London congress that 'Professor Koch was not an infallible Pope, and the question was not by any means settled'.[32]

---

[25] Pritchard 1988.

[26] Cobbett 1917.

[27] Pattison 1981, 126.

[28] Rosenkrantz 1985, 158.

[29] Cobbett 1917; Rosenkrantz 1985.

[30] Koch 1890; Rosenkrantz 1985.

[31] Grange and Bishop 1982; Rosenkrantz 1985.

[32] *The Times* 27 July 1901, 7e.

The Times called Koch's 1901 speech 'a conspicuous example of the mischief that may be done by even a well-meaning departure from the principles of scientific caution and reticence'.[33] And Cobbett considered Koch's *ex cathedra* announcement to have been a disaster: 'It at once completely paralysed all the many efforts which were then being made in the interest of human public health to stamp out tuberculosis from among the herds of cattle'.[34] But on the other hand it did at least stimulate a surge in tuberculosis-related laboratory research in Britain, Germany, France and the United States by workers anxious to redress the balance.

The Royal Commission on Tuberculosis 1901-1911

After Koch's 1901 statement the first step on the long road to restabilizing the medico-sanitary consensus about the dangers of infected milk was made in 1902 by Ravenel, who was the first to isolate *M. bovis* as the cause of death in a child. His work was soon dwarfed in scale, however, by the power of state-sponsored research programmes in several European countries.[35] In Germany investigations were made by the Kaiserliche Gesundheitsamt (Imperial Board of Health) in Berlin, reporting in 1907, and in Britain a Royal Commission (RC3) was appointed in 1901 that lasted for ten years, with a brief to take evidence and conduct experiments rather than interview witnesses. As we will see in Chapter 7, although a Royal Commission (RC1) in the 1890s also involved experimental work, the renewed commitment in 1901 to intensive scientific investigation was with a view to settling the questions raised by Koch once and for all. Three temporary laboratories were established at Stansted in Essex staffed by pathologists Arthur Eastwood, Harold Hutchens and Louis Cobbett, joined by the bacteriologist brothers Stanley and Fred Griffith, on a project which lasted from 1902 until 1909.[36] They produced a series of detailed reports and were pioneers of state-funded research well before the Medical Research Committee was established in 1913.

The RC3's First Interim Report (1904) was little more than a holding

---

[33] *The Times* 5 September 1901, 7c.

[34] Cobbett 1917, 192.

[35] Ravenel 1902.

[36] For more on the at times troubled experimental work, see Waddington 2001, 2006.

statement but the Commissioners felt that they were already in a position to claim, in direct contradiction to Koch, that 'it would be most unwise to frame or modify legislative measures in accordance with the view that human and bovine tubercle bacilli are specifically different from each other, and that the disease caused by the one is a wholly different thing from the disease caused by the other.'[37] The Second Interim Report in 1907 was supplemented by four volumes of scientific results on investigations into the pathogenic effect of the different types of tubercle bacilli. The conclusion was now bolder:

> A very considerable amount of disease and loss of life, especially among infants and children, must be attributed to the consumption of cow's milk containing tubercle bacilli ....'[38]

The Commissioners were determined to press the point by concluding that administrative measures were required: 'Our results clearly point to the necessity of measures more stringent than those at present enforced being taken to prevent the sale or the consumption of such milk.'[39] Official backing came for this statement from the Board of Agriculture (BoA) in 1909. In their circular letter to Local Authorities of that year they declared that 'it must now be accepted as a fact that tuberculosis is transmissible by the agency of milk used for human consumption'.[40]

In their Final Report in 1911 the RC3 asserted that 'a considerable amount of the tuberculosis of childhood is to be ascribed to infection with bacilli of the bovine type transmitted to children in meals consisting largely of the milk of the cow'.[41] After this definitive work it became increasingly difficult to deny the science, although there remained many who resisted the conclusion that the scientific results demanded action to reduce the risk to the milk-drinking public by the pasteurization of milk. Contrary to the policy paralysis that continued in the UK, the poof of the transmission of tuberculosis from cattle to humans provided by Ravenel (1902) and Park (1913) was sufficient to persuade US policy-

---

[37] BPP 1904 (Cd. 2092) xxxix.134.
[38] BPP 1907 (Cd. 3322) xxxviii.36-37.
[39] Ibid. 37.
[40] BPP 1911 (Cd. 5761) xlii.215.
[41] Ibid.

makers to act.[42] They did so swiftly with a programme seeking to eradicate bTB in the nation's herds, starting in 1917.

Veterinary versus medical knowledge and expertise

Reading the contemporary literature on Koch's 1901 statement, it is overwhelmingly apparent that the reaction came principally from practitioners of medicine and public health. But what of the veterinary contribution to the understanding of bTB as a zoonosis and to preventative measures by way of mitigation for human health? As we will see in this section, the answer is far from straightforward, as a result of the complex and fragmented nature of veterinary expertise.

Much has been made of the distinction between medical and veterinary expertise in the nineteenth century. The argument is often along the lines that veterinary knowledge was taken more seriously on the Continent than in the anglophone world.[43] To a degree this is supported by the early establishment of veterinary training in France, Germany and Italy and the contemporaneous literature there on what was often called bovine 'phthisis'. And yet in France veterinary training continued to be almost exclusively horse-related until the 1870s, when cattle at last became important as a focus of attention. It was only subsequently that qualified veterinarians, who had previously struggled in competition with their untrained 'empirical' rivals such as farriers, could claim their own exclusive expertise. Part of this was meat inspection, which was added to their responsibilities in France and a law on animal health passed there in 1881 gave vets a monopoly in dealing with contagious diseases. With the formation of a state veterinary laboratory at Alfort in 1901, French veterinary science had at last arrived as the generator of unique and economically valuable knowledge.[44] A similar timeline was visible in the United States. The previously low status of veterinarians there was changing by the 1880s with their proven ability to eliminate diseases such as contagious bovine pleuro-pneumonia from some states.[45]

In Britain the division of labour and knowledge between doctors

[42] Pritchard 1988.
[43] Forbes 1907; Pattison 1984; Hunter 2004.
[44] Hubscher 1999; Berdah 2012.
[45] See Rosenkrantz 1985.

and vets that emerged in mid-nineteenth century was neither straightforward nor amicable.[46] It was a professional boundary dispute and a chasm of mutual disrespect between veterinary and medical practitioners that is a good example of what Latour calls the ontological purification of knowledge between humans and non-humans.[47] The moderns of the age sought to establish a distinction between nature and culture that had a direct reflection in the animal/human divide. Knowledge and action concerning animals was considered innately inferior, or more correctly one should say that specialist practitioners of veterinary science were thought inferior and unfit even to act as directors of their own educational institutions. Medical men intervened in matters concerned with animal anatomy and epidemiology, sometimes even advising governments on policy formation with regard to animal health.[48]

An important opportunity internationally for veterinary knowledge to come to the fore was the rapid extension of trade in animals and animal products in the nineteenth century. The demand was concentrated in the expanding metropolitan centres and was facilitated by improvements in transport both on land and at sea. The transport of live animals by rail and ship increased the potential for the spread of disease, including epizootics such as rinderpest, panzootics like pleuro-pneumonia, and slower spreading but also devastating zoonoses, for example bTB.[49] The veterinary reaction was multifaceted, depending not only upon the type of disease but also upon the nature of state involvement. There were four principal approaches from the mid-nineteenth century.[50] The first was inoculation as prophylaxis, as practised with sheeppox. The second involved the control of movement, such as the various restrictions and bans on live imports of European cattle into the UK under the Contagious Diseases Acts (1879, 1884 and 1897).[51] Third, there was slaughter, either in the extreme form used for the stamping out of cattle plague, or the more considered inspection and slaughter used for

---

[46] Nor was it in the United States. See Rosenkrantz 1985.

[47] Latour 1993.

[48] The imbalance of power and influence between the medical and veterinary professions is laid bare by Anne Hardy. She argues that poor meat hygiene was one consequence. Hardy 2010, 2015.

[49] Fisher 1986; Woods 2013.

[50] Koolmees et al. 1999.

[51] Perren 1978.

bTB in many countries from the early twentieth century.[52] The use of veterinary pharmaceuticals was the fourth approach, with a growing industry benefiting from the farmers' wish to protect the value of their stock.[53] In the case of bTB there was tuberculin from the 1890s as the principal diagnostic agent and various cattle vaccines, especially BCG from 1928.

Worboys demonstrates that the 1865/66 rinderpest epidemic was something of a turning point in Britain.[54] There was friction between medically-inspired theorising about aetiology, epidemiology, prophylaxis and therapy on the one hand, and on the other a veterinary approach which was more concerned with administrative measures such as inspection, diagnosis, and the control of cattle movement based on what amounted to an 'importation theory' of disease spread.[55] But it was the expertise of vets such as John Gamgee and the officers of the newly formed Veterinary Department of the Privy Council that came to the public attention and at last attitudes began slowly to change.

Despite these various successes for veterinary expertise, even as late as the 1890s it was claimed that the medical profession was disinterested in the developments in veterinary science. The *Veterinary Record* complained that 'English medical journals only quote from foreign papers, and carefully ignore all the work published in English veterinary periodicals, with the result that medical men are unacquainted with what is going on at home'.[56]

The Veterinary Surgeons Act (1881) gave vets statutory recognition but at this time most veterinary science was empirical, with knowledge focused in texts on individual species, rather than taking a general approach to the anatomical features or diseases shared by the various domesticated species. In the 1880s and 1890s this began to change as comparative pathology and veterinary bacteriology emerged at the research frontier, dominated by a small élite of academic vets such as John McFadyean, who could hold their own in any scientific forum.[57] The hybrid veterinary-

---

[52] Woods 2004a.

[53] Perren 1989.

[54] Worboys 1991.

[55] Worboys 1991, 314-17; 1992.

[56] *Veterinary Record* 7, 1894/5, 229.

[57] Pattison 1981.

medical literature they generated, for instance as published in the *Journal of Comparative Pathology and Therapeutics,* helped in understanding the process by which cattle pass their tuberculosis to each other in cramped cowsheds through respiratory means, and in assessing the risk of infection getting into their milk. Nevertheless in the UK responsibility for the public health in relation to meat and milk inspection by the 1880s was firmly in the grip of MOsH and not veterinarians. The latter had missed an historic opportunity for the advancement of their professional status during the public health fervour of the 1870s, although there was some compensation for them in an increased number of local authority positions for veterinarians under the Contagious Diseases Act (1878).[58]

British veterinary science was not given full University status until the formation of the School of Veterinary Science at Liverpool in 1905. Even the Royal Veterinary College (RVC) under the distinguished leadership of McFadyean struggled for enough funds to keep its scientific research credible. The RVC had very poor laboratory facilities and this was a handicap in generating the quasi objects (statistics, books, experiments, research networks) which are crucial in building influence and consensus.[59] This did change to a certain extent, however, in the early twentieth century in response to the 1901 controversy about Koch's statement. In 1905 public funds were at last made available for veterinary research, although the bulk of government commitment was to the extensive experiments of the RC3. Then in emergency wartime conditions, in 1917, the government was forced to create its own Central Veterinary Laboratory.[60]

The search for a clear-cut and higher status veterinary identity was not helped by the tension which seems to have emerged at the end of the nineteenth century between the laboratory science of animal diseases and the 'learning by doing' that was favoured by the veterinary profession generally, particularly by those vets involved in work with administrative or policy implications.[61] The latter group included many unqualified practitioners who tended to side with their clients against the imprimatur of the Veterinary Department or local authorities, and saw animal

---

[58] Woods and Matthews 2010.

[59] Pattison 1984.

[60] The decision had been made in 1914. Pattison 1984.

[61] Fisher 1993b; Woods 2013.

disease in the economic light of reduced productivity rather than as an issue that could be solved in a laboratory or even in a slaughterhouse. Understandably, having seen the scale of the problem of cattle disease at first hand, they were reluctant to support sweeping measures which might undermine their own living.

There were different epistemological foundations to these various views.[62] The medical and academic veterinary opinion was very much in the realm of laboratory-based experimental knowledge, a predictive approach to the epidemiology of cattle disease and assumptions about the value of state-imposed solutions concerning slaughter and restrictions over the movement of stock. The practical veterinarians and farmers lived in an unpredictable world where spatial and temporal variations of circumstances invalidated monolithic, inflexible rules and regulations, and indicated instead the desirability of modest and realistic incremental change.

Worboys notes that the veterinary bacteriology side of this debate had its problems.[63] A case study might be the career of Emanuel Klein, a Professor at the Brown Animal Sanitary Institution, who made at least three high-profile blunders in his diagnosis of animal disease. In 1875 he claimed to have identified the organism responsible for sheeppox; in 1877/78 he found a bacillus causing swine fever; and in 1886 he discovered a new variant of scarlet fever spread in cow's milk called 'Hendon' disease. All of these proved to be wrong. The vilification which followed served only to confirm the prejudices of practical veterinarians against their laboratory-based colleagues. This problematization of scientific knowledge was the basis for a rift between pure science and practical farming that was narrowed again only when applied science in the form of agricultural technology was able to demonstrate its benefits through increased productivity in the twentieth century.

Nor did the academic and practical vets always agree measures to protect the public health; and the picture was further clouded when a third type of veterinary surgeon emerged at the turn of the century. These were the individuals employed by local authorities to inspect cattle. The job involved travelling around the hinterlands of the large cities checking for diseased animals in order to prevent their milk and meat entering the

---

[62] Wynne 1996.
[63] Worboys 1992.

human food chain. A few vets were also hired as meat inspectors. Such individuals, whose numbers grew steadily in the first four decades of the twentieth century, acted as a wing of the local state and of course had a different set of values and objectives from their fellows. At first their official designation was Inspector of Nuisances or Sanitary Inspector, because the profession of Veterinary Inspector was not officially recognised until the Milk and Dairy Order of 1926. In 1938 the employment of public service vets was transferred from Local Authorities to the MAF and the centralized inspection of all dairy herds was enforced.

This late intervention by the British state was unusual by European standards. It is worth noting here the point on expertise that Freidson makes, that in the UK and USA professions were generated from the collective efforts of individuals, whereas on the Continent of Europe the state had a greater role in organizing both training and employment.[64] This helps to explain why filters and exclusions were so important within and between professions in the struggle to establish a body of knowledge that could be used as a lever to extract a degree of social status.[65]

Returning to the contestation between the veterinary and medical viewpoints, there was an interesting spat in 1890 about meat inspection in Liverpool. That year Thomas Walley, Professor of Veterinary Medicine at the Edinburgh Royal (Dick) Veterinary College had published the first edition of his *A Practical Guide to Meat Inspection*, which went on to be a popular text book that in time merited five editions. He claimed that his enquiries in Liverpool, Birmingham and Newcastle had shown that public health officials there had declined to implement the part of the Nuisances Removal Act for England (Amendment) Act (1863) that dealt with the seizure of diseased and unwholesome meat because they 'did not feel themselves competent, nor was it a part of their duty to exercise such a function'.[66] Walley repeated this accusation in speeches around the country, drawing the wrath and denial of Dr Edward Hope, the MOH (Medical Officer of Health) of Liverpool. Hope commented in the *Liverpool Courier* that 'our system of meat inspection is as good and thorough as it could possibly be'. He employed inspectors 'who

---

[64] Freidson 2001.

[65] For a thorough account of the emergence and performance of veterinary expertise, see Armstrong 2011.

[66] Walley 1890, 172.

have had long practical experience as butchers and slaughterers in the public abattoirs, and they must have a thorough acquaintance with meat of all kinds before they are allowed to undertake inspectorial duties'. On behalf of the veterinary profession, John McFadyean poured scorn on Hope's view.

> What delightful naiveté is exhibited in Dr Hope's statement as to what instruction is required in the case of candidates for appointments as meat inspectors … It is utterly absurd to appoint to this duty men who never had a veterinary training, or to set up as a court of appeal for cases of disputed seizure a board composed of butchers.[67]

McFadyean conducted a running battle with the medical profession from his editor's chair at the *Journal of Comparative Pathology and Therapeutics*. He was strongly critical of one Medical Officer who suggested that experienced butchers would make the best meat inspectors and he savaged another who argued that any MOH could diagnose cattle disease without the help of a vet.[68] From the other side, Henry Armstrong, the MOH of Newcastle for forty years, was equally dismissive of any independent role for veterinary expertise in the administration of the food system:

> The opinion of the veterinary surgeon as regards the diseases of animals … is often of the greatest value to the Medical Officer of Health. But there the function of the Veterinary Surgeon in public health work ends. It is for the Medical Officer of Health to say what is and what is not fit for human food.[69]

Such confrontational certainty was unlikely, however, in rural areas. Here the position of Medical Officers was delicate. Many were employed on a part-time basis by local authorities which resented the legal requirement to appoint a MOH in the first place. The councillors there were often farmers, with a vested interest in the status quo, and it is hardly surprising that resources for intervention in the food supply were scarce. There was even contempt expressed by some farmers and vets for MOH inspections.[70] Dr Christopher Addison later observed in the House of Commons that it was only the full-time Medical Officers with larger

---

[67] Ibid. 159-61.
[68] McFadyean 1896; 1897; 1900a.
[69] Armstrong 1900, 41.
[70] Wilson 1896/7.

authorities who were likely to feel secure enough to implement milk legislation in the way intended by Parliament.[71]

Another example of a dispute is the bitter little exchange between William Savage, a county MOH, and his veterinary protagonists, in the 1931 volume of the *Veterinary Record*. Savage's point was that even the most conscientious and skilled veterinary inspection could pick up only open cases of tuberculosis in cattle, and that sub-clinical cases escaped unrecognised.[72] It was quite possible for cows to have *M. bovis* in their milk but appear outwardly healthy and in this way at least twenty-five per cent of the culprits were not detected.[73] He opposed routine veterinary inspection as the best solution to the problem of bovine tuberculosis on these grounds and also because there were only very weak administrative powers within which to operate. He cited a number of obstacles:

- Farmers were not [in 1931] obliged to permit routine inspection of their cattle, nor even bring them in from the fields, unless there were good grounds to suspect the presence of a specific disease in the herd.

- Farmers were not bound to disclose changes in their herd or what became of tuberculous animals.

- Notification of disease was only required of the farmers when an animal showed gross symptoms of tuberculosis. Often they waited until the end of the lactation when the value of the beast had fallen below that of the compensation offered for slaughter.

- Even when tuberculosis was found, a dairyman could not be forced to change his methods and the disease was therefore likely to recur.

- Udder tuberculosis was detectable most readily just after milking but vets could not only operate at those times of day.

T. Eaton Jones, the Chief Veterinary Officer (CVO) of Liverpool, was highly critical of Savage, claiming that his city's inspectors had detected more diseased cows than had been identified through the microscopic investigation of milk.[74] Between 1925 and 1930 they had found sixty-eight cases of udder tuberculosis by routine inspection, the bacteriologists twenty-one by bulk sampling, and only thirty-eight animals had been

---

[71] HC Deb 1914 vol 63 cc 246-51.

[72] Savage 1929a, repeated in Savage 1938.

[73] Francis 1958; Wilson 1942; BPP 1933-4 (Cmd. 4591) ix.427.

[74] Eaton Jones 1931.

officially notified by their owners. Even the journal's editor could not resist intervening in an editorial that dismissed Savage's view.[75]

Savage's test was whether veterinary methods had 'merit as a means of reducing bovine tuberculosis'. He could see no evidence that they did and remarked that 'veterinary inspection at its best under practical conditions can only hope to remove the comparatively gross cases of infective animals'.[76]

In the absence of any surgical or drug-related cure for tuberculosis, Savage and like-minded doctors and sanitarians preferred three types of alternative action. The regulation of the conditions of production was a favourite, especially improving the physical infrastructure of buildings and insisting on minimum standards of cleanliness. This type of sanitary intervention had a long pedigree in the control of working class housing in large industrial cities where it was thought to have contributed to a reduction in a number of diseases including pulmonary tuberculosis. Another was the use of microscopes and guinea pigs in the bacteriological detection of infected milk, very much in the tradition of the positivist, exploratory science which held sway in the late nineteenth century. A third was the adoption of technologies which could eliminate *M. bovis* from milk by the action of heat treatment. Pasteurization became the watchword of this group from the 1920s onwards.

Opponents, usually from the farming and veterinary worlds, supported by smaller dairy traders, saw these measures as intrusive. There were doubts about the true extent of the disease and its real impact upon humans and, on the basis of what these antagonists took to be a vague hypothesis, they did not feel that it was worth threatening rural livelihoods by the increased costs of production that would inevitably flow from a slaughter policy or forced investment in new buildings. Preferable were the veterinary inspection of livestock and associated controls such as Tuberculosis Orders, and voluntary measures such as the vaccination of cattle or the segregation of diseased from health stock. Graded milk was another possibility, with the consumer enjoying a similar freedom to choose their level of protection. Grafted on, with much reluctance at first by farmers, was the National Clean Milk Campaign which used a sanitary smoke-screen to oppose slaughter and pasteurization.

---

[75] Anon. 1931a.
[76] Savage 1929b, 494.

Dairy and meat trades

As we have seen, the position that Koch took in London in 1901 was seriously undermined by the publications of the RC3 and by the overwhelmingly contrary consensus expressed at Washington in 1908 and other conferences. And yet constant repetition seems to have given Koch's statement some weight in the popular media and among certain interest groups. There were also the seeds of doubt sown in the minds of the legislators, especially those seeking the votes of farmers, and the dairy and meat trades. This is one reason for the extended inaction which followed.

The farming and food trading interests of course seized upon Koch's idea as a heaven-sent opportunity. The editor of the *Cowkeeper and Dairyman's Journal,* for instance, not a disinterested bystander, could hardly contain his relief: 'the dairy trade and all consumers of milk have cause to be thankful that the investigations of the great Professor Koch ... have led him to make the great and astounding statement that there is practically no fear of contagion from the consumption of milk'.[77] Yet in almost the same breath he admitted that 'farmers themselves are inclined to disagree with his [Koch's] conclusions, but they are not unhopeful that one result of his assertion may be the imposition by local authorities of conditions somewhat less severe than those which at present prevail in many towns ...'.[78] The *Meat Trades' Journal and Cattle Salesman's Gazette* was also clear on the value of the weapon that Koch had presented to them:

> We have every right to make the fullest possible use of Professor Koch's remarkable statement, with all that it implies to meat traders and meat consumers, because it was publicly made before the greatest assembly of scientists that ever met in London, and made with the full knowledge that its utterance would rouse the most hostile criticism.[79]

A *Times* editorial deplored this use of Koch by the food trades and others who:

> ... at once jump to the conclusion that Professor Koch has disproved that which, at the very utmost, he has only rendered uncertain; and are prepared at once to abandon all the harmless and not very troublesome precautions which the current belief had suggested for adoption. They

---

[77] *Cowkeeper and Dairyman's Journal* August 1901, 739-40.

[78] Ibid. 748.

[79] *Meat Trades' Journal and Cattle Salesman's Gazette* 14, no. 693, 322.

are ready to throw all their intellectual possessions into the furnace of an unintelligent scepticism, and to fall down before the calf which Professor Koch has set up for their adoption.[80]

Even in the mid-twentieth century there were farmers who felt empowered by Koch to reject public health interventions as faddist. As late as the end of the Second World War, 'the average farmer looked with grave suspicion on the ... interest displayed both by the medical and veterinary profession in milk production'.[81]

Conclusion

The *Mycobacterium bovis* was badly behaved. It slipped through a narrow gap in the reasoning of one of the greatest laboratory scientists who ever lived. Frankly it made a fool of him; he was not in control as he clearly expected to be. Trying to make sense of this and subsequent developments in the science of tuberculosis, Speake has argued that the ontological certainty that we associate with the germ theory of disease is in fact the result of claims-making by bacteriologists.[82] In the late nineteenth and early twentieth centuries it was by no means easy to make causal connexions between the presence of bacteria and a particular health outcome. According to this logic we might ask why so few people caught bTB when we know that germs were present in a substantial portion of raw milk and meat supplies. According to Speake,

> Germ theory ... could not explain the randomness of infections, determine the virulence of different strains of TB, and was incapable of determining the degrees of interactivity between different bacteria within bodies.[83]

This was in effect what Koch was pointing out, if somewhat ponderously. The 'known' risks associated with the consumption of raw milk were embedded in an ideational regime that reduced uncertainty by using technologies such as pasteurization that in reality were a scattergun approach that destroyed good bacteria along with the pathogenic ones.

---

[80] *The Times* 5 September 1901, 7c.
[81] C. Higgs, a dairy farmer, in Anon. 1944-45, 257.
[82] Speake 2011.
[83] Ibid. 531.

Laboratories and processing factories were institutional contexts for the assembly of intelligibility but, as Koch and many other workers in this area of science found, definitive results that could be useful as a solid base for action in the world were hard to come by.

Ultimately Koch's contribution to bTB was as a contrarian and so, through controversy, to stimulate a great debate about a disease that for decades had been infecting millions of milk drinkers in Europe and North America, especially young children. The academic, administrative and popular media interest that unfolded might not otherwise have been generated without Koch. Our task now is to understand why in Britain it took another half century for policy to become sufficiently aggressive and for funds to be made available for herds to be cleared of the disease and for milk to be heat treated to protect the consumer.

CHAPTER 3.

BOVINE TUBERCULOSIS: THE HUMAN IMPACT

Introduction

The Human Microbiome Project has discovered that healthy human bodies are host to trillions of microbiota; some of these are more welcome than others but many are indispensible for efficient organ function. In a sense we are the sum of our microorganisms. Human and animal bodies are assemblages of mammalian and bacterial cells, and some of the latter when shared are potentially deadly for both. At a metaphysical level this challenges our notion of the individual and we can certainly see that the open ecological profile of tuberculosis provides a strong link across what are otherwise thought of as separate species.[1]

In the last chapter the emphasis was on competitive centres of knowledge creation about the microbiota that concerns us, *M. bovis*. Now we will consider, first, the emergence of clinical understandings of bTB through its presence and effect at the various bodily sites of infection. Second, the chapter will attempt a number of estimates of the overall mortality from the disease in the British Isles from 1850, and we will also break these death calculations down by age and by the body site of bTB infection. A cartographic depiction of the impact of mortality then follows to illustrate the spatial pattern of the human impact at the county scale. An important calling point for all of these elements of the chapter is the career of Stanley Griffith, a little known but important researcher who devoted his life's work to the study of *M. bovis* in human subjects.

Bovine tuberculosis in the human body

Over the last two centuries bTB infection in humans has probably mostly been caused by the consumption of raw (unpasteurized) milk

---

[1] Schneider and Winslow 2014.

and in a smaller number of cases by undercooked, infected meat. In addition, the spread of bTB from person to person is theoretically possible because *M. bovis* can affect the lungs and follow the same path of airborne infection as *M. tuberculosis*.[2] The cattle-to-human route is also a risk where slaughterhouse workers breathe in infected aerosols when cutting out diseased meat or where stockmen and milkers spend time in the fug of the cowshed.[3]

Within two months of a bTB challenge via ingestion, the disease usually progresses with 'fever, sore throat, swelling of the tonsils and cervical lymph nodes, and vague stomach symptoms, sometimes including enlargement of the mesenteric lymph nodes'.[4] *M. bovis* then spreads to various sites in the body. Among the first glands to be affected are the upper cervical and retropharyngeal lymph nodes.[5] In the nineteenth century the associated abscesses and ulcers were thought to be characteristic of 'scrofula' in children (Figure 2.1).

By contrast the inhalation of *M. tuberculosis* yields different symptoms in humans, involving coughing, expectoration, tiredness, fever and pain in the chest.[6] In the nineteenth century respiratory tuberculosis, consumption and phthisis may have had separate clinical understandings but in practice the words were frequently used interchangeably.[7] Nevertheless it was generally recognised from an early date that primary lung foci were qualitatively different from tuberculosis manifesting itself at other sites.

When was the human toll from bTB first apparent? Scrofula is the early modern clinical term most associated with the disease, along with 'struma'.[8] Strong evidence came early on, in the 1840s, when data on the clinical examination of 133,721 children in charity schools, workhouses and factories around the UK was collected and published by Benjamin

---

[2] Schonfield et al. 1982; Hardie and Watson 1992.

[3] Sigurdsson 1945; Thoen et al. 2006.

[4] Pritchard 1988, 372-73.

[5] Wright 1908.

[6] Ponnuswamy 2014.

[7] Hardy 1988.

[8] For nineteenth century understandings of scrofula, see Lomax 1977. Strictly speaking struma is a swollen thyroid but the term was also used in the context of cervical tuberculosis.

Phillips.[9] He found that 33,271 had presented with 'certain marks of scrofula', by which was meant enlarged glands recognisable to the touch, and 4,127 (3.1 per cent) of these had the visible skin lesions of cervical lymphadenitis. As will be explained later in this chapter, it is reasonable to assume that seventy-five per cent of these scrofula cases would have been caused by *M. bovis*, and using this as an indicator we can speculate that 2.3 per cent of the children in Phillips' sample were suffering from bTB under a narrow definition.[10]

In addition, Phillips discussed enquiries that had been made in certain London schools among a total of 1,017 pupils. On the days of survey there were 102 absentees, fourteen of whom were said to have been absent due to 'scrofulous suffering'. Scaling up, this would have added a further 1.4 per cent, making a total of at least 3.7 per cent of all school children who could be said to have been scrofulous. Although there is no way of testing the quality of these data, there is a strong hint here of extensive mid-nineteenth century morbidity from non-pulmonary tuberculosis, a portion of which would have been of bovine origin.

Phillips was an example of the enthusiasts of the early Victorian statistical movement, gathering data from miscellaneous sources, though without any visible quality control. This approach was almost immediately replaced by state-inspired mortality statistics compiled on a systematic basis by what we might call the 'information state'.

The information state

The importance of facticity and statistics in the biopolitics of public health in nineteenth century Britain is well rehearsed.[11] An important element was the state as gatherer and analyst of information on the life cycle of the citizen, to the extent that the information state was increasingly constituted through the guardianship of data of ever-increasing accuracy and comprehensiveness.[12] According to Hacking, statistics 'may think of itself as providing only information, but it is

---

[9] Phillips 1846.

[10] Smith 1988.

[11] Foucault 1991; Dean 1999.

[12] Higgs 2004a.

itself part of the technology of power in a modern state,' providing an element of its legitimacy.[13] But Louckx and Vanderstraeten also see vital statistics the other way around, as 'state-istics', with society itself re-imagined in order to provide information efficiently to the state, in our case with doctors instructed on the diagnosis of disease in order to 'improve' the quality of medical data, such as records of mortality.[14] In this Foucaultian vein we may see public health statistics as a base stratum of governance just as in the private sector they also played a part in the development of life insurance, one of the earliest and most fundamental risk calculations to emerge in modern liberal economies.

Statistics not only provided a coping mechanism for the complexity of the new order that was emerging in Victorian Britain, their collection also addressed some of the associated fears of the age.[15] In the hands of both their generators and their critics they became political and therefore 'polyvocal resources'.[16] Societal order and trust came to draw upon both public and private investments in laboratories, statistical bureaux, maps, directories, censuses and insurance life tables. To study this period of data accumulation is therefore to try to understand the organization of particles of knowledge into objective, consensual facts. This production process was based upon cultural assumptions and contingent circumstances that require historical analysis if we are fully to appreciate the epistemological filters through which truths were generated.

Some interpreters of this newly numericised life became 'experts' and were ceded status in recognition of their special skills. When gathered in institutions dedicated to measurement, archiving and publication, these experts became miners of a seam of energy that has kept the lights of government on ever since. Collecting and curating vital statistics about the events of life and deaths is an important example of this expertise.

The visibility of citizens to the nation state was increased in the 1830s with the systematizing of mortality data in Britain. With civil

---

[13] Hacking 1991, 181.

[14] Louckx and Vanderstraeten 2014.

[15] Legg 2005.

[16] Rose 1991, 684.

registration in the hands of the General Register Office (GRO), and the recording and processing of information steadily growing with the hiring of new clerical and specialist staff, it was possible to publish annual summaries and reports of considerable breadth and sophistication. Death registration was only a small part of the duties of the GRO but the enthusiasm and innovative minds of superintendants of statistics William Farr, and his successors William Ogle and John Tatham, made it into an artefact of increasing significance.

Higgs sees the introduction of the cause of death recorded on death certificates from 1837 as a turning point in understandings of mortality.[17] Rather than the eighteenth century interpretation of illness as a function of a range of factors such as temperature, diet, stress, and exhaustion, there was now to be a single 'cause'.[18] This facilitated thinking of disease in terms of pathogens, which could then be mitigated physically by specific sanitary reforms rather than requiring deep-seated and holistic social change, with all of the political implications going with that. This was a technical and environmental short-cut that would have visible results in those same mortality records. The database did its job and arguing against sanitary theory became increasingly difficult as death rates for the principal diseases fell across the board. Interestingly, the germ theory that gradually replaced the sanitary paradigm was equally well served by death certification, which could now record ever finer sub-divisions of causality as new diseases and their pathogens were identified.

The efforts of Farr and his successors are important from our point of view. Their disease classifications - nosologies - gradually became more detailed and more subtle in their differentiation of tuberculosis by bodily site (Table 3.1). There was no recognition of bTB as such, but inferences can be drawn about the lung disease versus the non-pulmonary and we will follow a version of this approach in our calculations in this chapter.

---

[17] Higgs 2004a. For more on the origins, structure and interpretational problems of death registration, see Eyler 1979; Luckin 1980; Szreter 1991; Hardy 1994; Higgs 1996a, 1996b, 2004b; Williams 1996; Mooney 2009.
[18] Hamlin 1985.

Table 3.1 Nosological differentiation of tuberculosis in the reports of the GRO for England and Wales

Bodily site	Comments
Cervical	Scrofula not initially associated the lymphatic system. Seen instead as 'sporadic disease of uncertain seat' or as a residual category of 'other forms of TB' until 1900.
Abdominal	From the outset classified as *tabes mesenterica*, supplemented from 1901 with the more specific tubercular peritonitis. Tabes was eventually dropped in 1921.
Central nervous system	At first described as dropsy of the brain but later more specifically acute hydrocephalus and later still tuberculous meningitis and cerebral tuberculoma.
Bones and joints	Includes white swelling. Not an important separate category until 1911.
Genito-urinary	From 1921 but relatively rare diagnosis.
Skin	From 1858 *lupus vulgaris*. In nineteenth century sometimes confusion with skin cancer. Scrofuloderma another term used.
Respiratory/phthisis	The main category of recorded TB, known as phthisis or consumption. But *M. bovis* a small percentage of pulmonary cases.
Other	From 1901 disseminated TB, 1906 general TB, 1921 'other' TB.

Note: Followed in general terms by Scotland and Ireland.

From 1838 the early nosological account of tuberculosis was in effect fourfold: tuberculosis of the respiratory, central nervous, and digestive systems, with a residual category of 'sporadic disease of uncertain seat', known as scrofula, establishing in the minds of many observers a distinction between pulmonary and non-pulmonary tuberculosis.[19] From our point of view this was a key division, not only of bodily sites but also by implication of aetiology. In the first half of the twentieth century a universal trope of tuberculosis discourse was the assumption that non-pulmonary disease was caused by *M. bovis* and the pulmonary version by *M. tuberculosis*. Although in the most general terms this is correct, it is far too imprecise to stand as a reliable indicator of the burden of mortality in the UK as a whole, as we will see below.[20]

Among the other types of non-pulmonary TB, a common complication was infection, by the haematological route, of the central nervous system; this was the so-called tuberculous meningitis, mainly in the young.[21] The Registrar General's nosological terminology for this was 'hydrocephalus' until 1881 when the commonality of acute hydrocephalus and tuberculous meningitis was at last recognised.[22] Also

---

[19] Scrofula in this classification was therefore less precise than the definition we gave above.

[20] Clarke 1952.

[21] McCarthy 1908. For current understandings of TB of the central nervous system, see Thwaites 2014.

[22] This change was made 'in deference to the revised classification of the Royal

frequent in infancy was the disseminated form, miliary tuberculosis, which was usually fatal until the advent of streptomycin in 1948. Both children and adults were also susceptible to tuberculosis of the bones and joints,[23] but genito-urinary TB was concentrated in ages over fifteen.[24]

A source of potential error in calculating the impact of *M. bovis* is that in the nineteenth century there were fashions in diagnosis, and diagnostic depth varied according to region and the age and social status of the subject.[25] At first, in the period of voluntary registration of the cause of death up to 1874, there was also some resistance to the precision increasingly required by the Registrar General, with a continuation among some practitioners beyond the mid-nineteenth century of formerly common but vague categories such as 'decline'.

The GRO data have many other problems associated with them. In the early decades, for instance, there was a general undercertification of disease and this was a particular issue for tuberculosis because of its socially sensitive nature and the potential stigma of a diagnosis.[26] For our purposes this is particularly serious because there was not, nor could there have been, any direct identification of tuberculosis of bovine origin. Indeed scholars of tuberculosis as a whole have plenty of uncertainties to contend with, let alone looking at sub-categories of the disease. At this point it is worth contemplating further the limitations of the Registrar General mortality data for imputing the involvement of bovine tuberculosis. We will look at mis-diagnosis, under-reporting, and over-reporting.

College of Physicians'. *Supplement to Fifty-Fifth Annual Report of the Registrar-General*, PP 1895 (C.7769) xxiii(1).33.

[23] Berry 1908.

[24] Some forms of tuberculosis can be initiated by small invasions of mycobacteria. This is true of tuberculosis of the bones and joints which is disseminated in the bloodstream.

[25] Mooney 2009.

[26] Hardy 1993. See also Hardy 1994 for a general discussion of changing disease classification systems.

Still's problem

In his published thoughts about childhood tuberculosis, George Still, a physician at King's College Hospital, London, was particularly unforgiving in his assessment of the Registrar General's returns. Because the GRO data were based on death certificates, few of which were backed by a post mortem examination of the body, he claimed that 'they are of very little use in a scientific investigation, and may lead to entirely erroneous conclusions'.[27] This was because 'tuberculosis is by no means always easy to diagnose clinically in children'. One issue was the tendency in infants under two years for the generalization of disease, clouding identification of the primary focus.

There was a wide recognition among physicians of what we might call 'Still's problem' and, as a result, from the 1870s, they started publishing reports of post mortems and surgical cases in order to establish a more accurate view of the pathology of tuberculosis. These can be divided into two categories.

First, there was discussion of the proportion of hospital patients who died from tuberculosis, especially in children's hospitals, which was much greater than for the population as a whole. Commentators recognised the problems of representativeness with this observation, since these were acute cases and for children often weighted towards the disadvantaged end of the social spectrum. Yet they nevertheless concluded that in a broad sense tuberculosis was under-represented in the Registrar General's cause of death statistics.

The point here is not the precise percentage of tuberculosis cases in hospitals but the general observation that mortality from the disease was much higher in that acute category than the 7.5 per cent of deaths under ten years for the population as a whole in the decade 1891-1900. In retrospect this may seem like a statement of the obvious but to contemporaries it represented a clinically-based refinement of what were regarded as crude GRO estimates.

Second, both post mortems and surgical cases were said to give a more accurate indication of the bodily impact of tuberculosis by identifying its distribution in the various organs. This compared with the Registrar General's data compiled from diagnosis by palpation,

---

[27] Still 1899, 455.

symptoms, the identification of external lesions, or in some cases by guesswork where there had been no attending physician. Most clinicians agreed that visual inspection inside bodies was the most reliable indicator of disease, later supplemented by histological and bacteriological work on tissue and other samples, and from the 1920s by radiological imaging.[28] By way of example at the Royal Edinburgh Hospital for Sick Children, of the tuberculosis deaths, 83.7 per cent (1886-1902) had lymph glands that were tuberculous to the naked eye.[29] The abdominal glands were affected in 54.4 per cent (1886-1902) and 45.0 per cent of cases, mediastinal (thoracic) in 69.2 per cent (1886-1902) of cases, and both together in 39.9 per cent (1886-1902). The compiler of these data, Shennan, refused to impute any bovine aetiology but looking at seventy-two surgical cases (1911-13) of cervical gland tuberculosis at the same hospital, Sir Harold Stiles found ninety per cent to be of bovine origin.[30] At this hospital (1898-1908) there were 15,320 in-patients, 3.6 per cent with abdominal TB and 2.0 per cent with tuberculous meningitis.[31]

There may be some difficulty in distinguishing between primary and secondary infection but those reporting post mortems did at least show an awareness that this was a problem. Of main interest to physicians at the time was the balance between abdominal and thoracic sites, and also whether tuberculosis was the cause of death.

Overall, this post mortem and surgical research claimed, first, that tuberculosis was under-reported and, second, that much of the non-pulmonary version of the disease was abdominal in origin, the implication being of a link to bTB acquired through infected milk or meat. On the first point Cobbett mused that it 'seems certain that many deaths from tuberculosis get assigned to other causes', and 'it is probable that the error was still larger in the past, for it is reasonable to suppose that the progress of medical science and education has greatly increased the accuracy of diagnosis'. Particularly with regard to children, he argued that 'in the past the number of deaths from tuberculosis which were

---

[28] Brown and Sampson 1926.
[29] Shennan 1914.
[30] Stiles 1913.
[31] Thomson and Fordyce 1908.

assigned to some other cause must have outnumbered those which were wrongly assigned to the cause'.[32]

Thirty years earlier Sims Woodhead had observed that of 6,000 to 7,000 children examined at the Evelina Hospital, Edinburgh, only forty-six cases of consumption of the bowels had been diagnosed, leading him to speculate that 'only one-fifth of the real number are stated in the diagnosis charts to be suffering from abdominal tubercle'. He recommended that the Registrar General's recorded number of 'tabes mesenterica' cases 'might safely be multiplied by five to give the actual number of cases in which the mesenteric glands were affected'.[33]

But there was also a problem of over-reporting. Arthur Newsholme, in the most senior public health post as Principal Medical Officer of the LGB, asked 'are the statistics relating to tuberculosis trustworthy?' A good question. He commented that

> there remains ... in the national returns considerable understatement
> of the mortality from tuberculosis in early life, which is not completely
> counterbalanced by the return of many deaths as 'tabes mesenterica', in
> which there is no tuberculosis. There is no evidence that recent statistics
> of tuberculosis in early life are not fairly comparable with those of past
> years, and there is some evidence to the contrary.[34]

Newsholme was sceptical about tabes mesenterica and so was George Still, the critic we met earlier. Still regarded a diagnosis of tabes as 'slovenly', often being used 'to indicate almost any form of abdominal tuberculosis' and sometimes including 'the wasting of an ill-fed infant'.[35] Adding to this, Donkin acidly remarked that 'all kinds of intestinal and other disorders are constantly styled tabes mesenterica by those who fail to cure them.'[36] It was Farr who had originally given tabes credence in his nosologies from 1839, as did Greenhow in 1858 but, according to Gairdner, there was no equivalent diagnosis on the Continent.[37]

In Carr's opinion tabes mesenterica was normally thought of as covering tuberculous peritonitis, tuberculous enteritis (ulceration of the

---

[32] Cobbett 1917, 12.
[33] Sims Woodhead 1888, 52.
[34] Newsholme 1910, 23-24.
[35] Still 1901, 114.
[36] Donkin 1899.
[37] Farr 1885; Greenhow 1858; Gairdner and Coats 1888.

bowel) and caseation of the mesenteric glands.[38] Yet it was generally agreed that tuberculous peritonitis was rare in children under two and that the diagnosis of the others by palpation was uncertain.[39] In sum, for Newsholme tabes mesenterica was a diagnosis that should be applied

> only when it is clear that the patient has tuberculous disease of the abdominal lymphatic glands. Unfortunately it is often used in death certificates when the patient has died from a slow wasting disease accompanied or not by abdominal symptoms such as diarrhoea ... many of the deaths returned as tabes mesenterica would be found to be due to causes other than tuberculosis were all death certificates verified by autopsies.[40]

Ashby and Wright declared that 'mesenteric disease is much more frequently diagnosed than discovered post mortem'.[41] Marasmus, wasting often due to undernutrition, was thought to be a more accurate diagnosis in many cases than tabes mesenterica.[42] At this time, Sir Richard Thorne Thorne, in a decided understatement, commented that tabes mesenterica as a cause of death was 'by no means a precise and definite one'. But this was double-edged because he thought that

> whilst the wasting of a chronic infantile diarrhoea may be erroneously certified as tabes mesenterica, I have no doubt that the emaciation and other symptoms associated with fatal tabes mesenterica are not unfrequently entered erroneously in the death register under terms such as 'diarrhoea' and 'wasting'. Such errors probably balance each other.[43]

By the turn of the twentieth century tabes mesenterica was fading from the GRO's statistics. It did not disappear from published causes of death until 1921.

What is the conclusion to this under-reporting versus over-reporting controversy? Anne Hardy cannot countenance any reliance on respiratory tuberculosis mortality statistics before the 1870s, with further continuing issues for geographical analysis when deaths in hospitals, workhouses and sanatoria were not re-allocated to the place

---

[38] Carr 1898.
[39] Coutts 1908.
[40] Newsholme 1910, 29, 32.
[41] Ashby and Wright 1889, 109.
[42] Carr 1898.
[43] Thorne Thorne 1899, 30.

of residence.[44] But by about 1900 she thinks that 'registered tuberculosis mortality approximated to reality,' in England at least. Linda Bryder, however, shows that even the new system of registering tuberculosis morbidity from 1911 was fraught with problems of diagnosis that were eased but certainly not eliminated by technical interventions such as laboratory tests and then radiography.[45]

Given the complexity and uncertainty of attributing an aetiology of bTB to any individual case, it must have come as a relief to all concerned when bacteriological investigation became possible. We will see in Chapter 8 that it was available for detecting *M. bovis* in milk from the 1890s, and here we will pursue the equivalent developments for human samples, starting with the work of Stanley Griffith.

Stanley Griffith

Arthur Stanley Griffith (1875-1941) was a bacteriologist who came to prominence when working for the third Royal Commission on Tuberculosis from 1903 to 1909. His principal contribution was in the laboratory-based differentiation of *M. bovis* from *M. tuberculosis* in samples of sputum and tissue. Griffith subsequently continued this work at the University of Cambridge. Only a few low-key obituaries are available as a summary of his career but a picture emerges of a quiet and conscientious bench scientist who was the master of his chosen, narrow specialism. In retrospect we can add that through collaborations and by example of his technique, Griffith inspired a generation of bacteriologists to seek the origins of non-pulmonary tuberculosis and to type the mycobacteria found at various bodily sites.

The method developed by Griffith and his collaborators was painstaking and complex.[46] A sample of sputum or of tissue taken during surgery or autopsy was first injected into a guinea pig and after a number of weeks a culture was obtained from the animal's spleen, grown on coagulated calf serum, potato or egg media and then transferred to glycerin agar or glycerin broth.[47] The mycobacteria were then filtered

---

[44] Hardy 1994.
[45] Bryder 1996.
[46] Collins and Grange 1983.
[47] Sigurdsson 1945.

and injected into rabbits. This species was used because *M. bovis* kills them in thirty to sixty days but *M. tuberculosis* does not.[48]

A refinement of this method was possible from the early 1930s when Löwenstein and Jensen improved a solid egg-based medium for growing the mycobacteria and so made typing cheaper, quicker and more efficient. Later it was discovered that pyruvate, when added to the culture medium, enhances the growth of *M. bovis*, whereas glycerol inhibits it. It was therefore now possible to distinguish the colony types of *M. bovis* from *M. tuberculosis* but the process took eight weeks.

In his career Griffith published the results of several thousand typings, both pulmonary and non-pulmonary, most of which seem to have been his own work. Without him and the Medical Research Council (MRC) funding that supported his laboratory, it is fair to say that our understanding of the human pathology of bTB would be poorer. His death in 1941 was followed by a very different era in which, because TB in general came under greater control, large scale typing was no longer judged to be necessary.

Griffith's work is crucial to our story. His investigations yielded data that show the highest probability of *M. bovis* infection in the human body was at the abdominal and cervical sites, with consequences also for the central nervous system, bones and joints, the lungs, skin and genito-urinary organs. We will begin by analysing the emerging understandings of the pathogenesis in the late nineteenth and early twentieth centuries and conclude with a calculation of morbidity and mortality.

Table 3.2 shows the percentage of *M. bovis* identified at various sites by Griffith and a number of other researchers using mainly sputum and also some tissue samples.[49] As expected, the proportion of respiratory tuberculosis of bovine origin was low but the abdominal and cervical percentages were high. Over all the 9,676 cases examined in the first half of the twentieth century the average incidence of *M. bovis* infection was 14.7 per cent of the tuberculosis observed. Comparing this figure with other countries (Table 3.3) over the same fifty year period, we can see that Britain seems to have had proportionately a greater burden

---

[48] Thoen et al. 2006.

[49] Note that the rows do not necessarily sum because some workers reported without differentiating by age of the subject. Their results are included in the 'all ages' column.

of bovine infection in humans than anywhere else. The percentage of respiratory disease was low, as expected, at three percent attributed to *M. bovis* but, because the number of respiratory cases overall was more than the non-pulmonary, this was the principal site of *M. bovis* infection. We will develop this point further below.

Table 3.2 Bacteriological typing of human TB in Britain, 1901-50, showing the percentage of disease attributable to *M. bovis*

	0-4 years		5-14 years		≥15 years		All ages	
	Cases	%	Cases	%	Cases	%	Cases	%
Respiratory	93	2.2	89	5.6	1,470	2.9	5,372	3.2
Central nervous system	487	23.4	298	16.1	249	10.8	1245	19.8
Abdominal	14	64.3	8	87.5	12	50.0	34	64.7
Bones & joints	222	40.1	479	21.5	628	8.6	1,377	18.9
Genito-urinary	0	-	18	55.6	212	20.3	234	23.1
Skin	30	66.7	58	48.3	28	14.3	193	51.3
Cervical	168	78.6	268	70.9	189	37.6	651	62.5
Other	311	29.9	104	22.1	77	11.7	570	28.4
Total	1,325	34.6	1,322	31.3	2,865	9.0	9,676	14.7

Sources: The 56 sources are listed online.

Table 3.3 Bacteriological typing of human TB, 1901-50, showing percentage of *M. bovis*

	Britain	Denmark	Germany	USA	Other
Respiratory	3.2	5.3	4.3	0.0	2.1
Central nervous system	19.8	23.3	-	6.5	4.3
Abdominal	64.7	-	-	-	2.5
Bones & joints	18.9	-	4.9	27.7	3.3
Genito-urinary	23.1	-	14.3	6.3	2.0
Skin	51.3	19.2	23.3	80.0	11.1
Cervical	62.5	46.2	28.9	36.6	20.1
Other	28.4	19.2	8.0	8.8	7.8
Total	14.7	12.0	10.0	11.7	3.5

Sources: Table 3.2; Gervois 1937; Sigurdsson 1945.

One of the most interesting aspects of these bacteriological results from the first half of the twentieth century is that there was regional variation hidden behind the data in Table 3.2. This is exposed in Wilson's wartime analysis of 994 non-respiratory samples in England (Table 3.4), in which the North Midland and North West regions stand out as above average. It is also possible to look, in crude terms at least, at those respiratory cases of tuberculosis attributed to *M. bovis* (Table 3.5), again all in the first half of the twentieth century. Here Scotland stands out as having much higher rate of bTB infection than other regions.

Table 3.4 Bovine tuberculosis in English non-respiratory samples, 1943-45

Region	Samples	Bovine (%)
North East	119	11.8
North West	163	34.4
North Midlands	185	43.2
South Midlands	97	20.6
East	128	31.3
South East	95	13.7
South West	59	28.8
London and Middlesex	63	12.7
Others	85	15.3
All	994	26.3

Source: Wilson et al. 1952.
Note: The samples here were somewhat different from most of those used in compiling Table 3.2. They were from living subjects, hospital and sanatoria patients diagnosed as having non-pulmonary tuberculosis and were mainly of pus and some lymph node tissue.

Table 3.5 Regional variations in respiratory tuberculosis of bovine origin, mostly sputum samples

Locations	Sources	Cases	bovine (%)
Edinburgh, Glasgow, Lanark	Griffith 1914, 1916b; Wang 1916	102	2.0
North Eastern Scotland	Griffith and Smith 1940	540	9.1
Aberdeen	Griffith and Smith 1940	432	4.4
Midlands and South Scotland	Griffith and Munro 1944	515	6.0
Eastern Scotland	Griffith and Munro 1944	1165	5.0
North of England	Cumming et al. 1933 (all cases under 16 years)	391	3.1
North of England	Cumming 1935	888	1.5
English Midlands	Cutbill and Lynn 1944	2,010	2.3
English Midlands	Griffith and Menton 1936	230	0.8
South of England	Bulloch 1911	23	0.0
South of England	Griffith 1911, 1914, 1916a	151	1.3
South of England	Griffith 1930, 1937	509	0.4
South of England	Kayne et al. 1939	100	1.0
South of England	Cumming 1935	195	0.5
Wales	Cumming 1935	203	2.0
Republic of Ireland	Cumming 1935	320	0.0
Northern Ireland	Reilly 1950	1,060	0.1

Note: The full references are available online.

Human mortality in the British Isles from *M. bovis*

From the mid-nineteenth century the Registrars General for England and Wales and for Scotland and Ireland published annual mortality data that was broken down according to their pre-conceived nosologies. As we saw earlier, there are no official data on bTB from this source because there was no differentiation of individual deaths due to *M. bovis* or *M. tuberculosis*. We are forced therefore to make indirect estimates of bTB deaths if we want to use whole population data. It is possible, however, to make estimates of bTB mortality (Table 3.6) using the following methodology.

Table 3.6 Estimate 'A' of bovine tuberculosis deaths in England, Wales and Scotland, 1848-1960

Years	1	2	3	4	5	6	7	Total
1848-59	14725	25881	39870	387	0	30	14530	95422
1860-69	15505	22818	46943	642	0	218	15562	101688
1870-79	15354	23728	57552	545	0	318	15102	112598
1880-89	14091	21060	57412	0	0	379	21381	114322
1890-99	12989	19782	49935	0	0	374	26918	109999
1900-09	11944	17348	37430	0	0	413	26168	93303
1910-19	9815	14446	27688	1893	0	315	15083	69240
1920-29	8812	9065	14009	1818	522	433	10672	45331
1930-39	7035	6157	6581	1179	602	279	6253	28086
1940-49	6073	5232	4272	900	675	230	3542	20925
1950-60	2430	1009	795	289	397	47	857	5823
1848-1960	118774	166525	342488	7653	2196	3036	156067	796738
%	14.9	20.9	43.0	1.0	0.3	0.4	19.6	

Key: 1. Respiratory; 2. Central nervous system; 3. Abdominal; 4. Bones and joints; 5. Genito-urinary; 6. Skin; 7. Cervical and other sites.
Sources of data: Annual Reports and Statistical Review of the Registrars General of England and Wales, and Scotland.
Note: No Scottish data before 1855.

First, we will take Table 3.2, based on the work of Stanley Griffith and others, to be the basis for calculating bTB deaths for the period 1900-1950 and - with caution - also for the additional periods 1848-99 and 1951-60. Some elaboration is possible because the Griffith publications usually include an age breakdown of samples tested according to three age groups: 0-4, 5-14, and ≥15 years. This age differentiation is important because bTB at the abdominal site was most prevalent in those young children fed with cow's milk.

Next, for each county the number of tuberculosis deaths recorded by the GRO against each bodily site can be multiplied by the percentages in Table 3.2, taken in effect as probabilities that each death was due to a *M. bovis* infection. The output, Table 3.6, must be treated with caution because it depends upon the science behind Table 3.2 being reliable. On the whole the present author believes this to be a reasonable assumption. The work of Griffith and his collaborators was relentless in its accumulation of the world's largest database of bacteriologically typed tuberculosis samples, and as far as we can tell it seems to have been accurate within the technological limitations of the day.

Table 3.6 amounts to a summary of bTB deaths in the period 1848-1960. If we add the 20,000 or so estimated deaths in the island of Ireland in the period of civil registration from 1864, the toll for the British Isles is over 800,000, making it by far the largest, the most sustained, and the most deadly food-borne zoonosis in British history. No estimate is offered here of the additional morbidity that went with bTB infection in this period but it was undoubtedly substantial.[50]

It is important to make clear that these dramatic numbers must be accompanied by several weighty warnings. First, as we have made clear above, there are diagnostic and nosological uncertainties, particularly in the second half of the nineteenth century when, according to Table 3.6, bTB mortality was at its peak. Stripping out the most doubtful diagnoses, such as tabes mesenterica, would reduce the headline figure for abdominal tuberculosis, for instance. Our instinct is that the figure of 816,525 (Estimate A) for the British Isles is therefore an upper limit. A lower limit (Estimate B), reducing the abdominal estimate by half for the period 1848 to 1924, would be 645,281.

Second, on a technical point about the Registrars General data, it is worth noting that for England and Wales it would have been possible to start our series in 1837, although the early years are not normally thought to be consistently reliable. The equivalent series for Scotland starts in 1855 and in Ireland 1864, so there is an element of mismatch at the outset. In addition, although the respective annual reports generally used the same nosology, there were differences in the way sub-types of tuberculosis were grouped for publication. There were also differences through time, such as bone joint disease not being separately listed for some years, and the 'other' category changing.

Third, the estimates have been modelled using the bacteriological typing of Griffith and others in the first half of the twentieth century. Not all of these workers recorded the age of their subjects and their data has been excluded because Table 3.6 has been built by applying age-specific typing estimates to age-specific mortality data at the various bodily sites of disease.

Fourth, no bacteriological differentiation of *M. bovis* and *M. tuberculosis* at the various sites is available for the nineteenth century. The admittedly heroic assumption has been made here that estimates for 1848-99 can be made on the same basis as for 1900-60. The potential

---

[50] An appendix will be published separately online including more detail on the methodology of estimation; the changing GRO nosologies of tuberculosis; the nature of the datasets for Scotland and Ireland (Northern Ireland and the RoI); and the calculation of a countywise breakdown of bTB mortality for the decade 1891-1900.

problem with this is if there was a shift in relative terms as to the principal sites of infection. We have no reason to believe that the *M. bovis* contribution to pulmonary tuberculosis will have changed. But, as has been pointed out, there were certainly shifting fashions in diagnosis and this means that the further back one goes, the less the structure of the data resembles the world of Griffith. There is also some evidence that more cow's milk was being fed to infants towards the end of the century, which will have increased the risk of abdominal disease.

Taking this analysis one step further, it is interesting to analyse the geographical patterns observable in the available data. Unfortunately the publication by the Registrars General of regional mortality data with a full nosological breakdown was somewhat patchy. From our point of view the optimum period to have this would have been for the decade or so up to the First World War, before pasteurization began commercially common in London and a few other large cities (see Chapter 5), thus revolutionising the risk of exposure to infection. In the pre-pasteurization period the fullest nationwide GRO dataset available with a breakdown countywise is a little further back, in the decade 1891-1900. This has been used in the compilation of Figure 3.1, employing the same approach that was outlined above for Table 3.6. In the map death rates are the basis for comparing counties.

Figure 3.1 is remarkable because it shows a concentration of human *M. bovis* deaths in three regions: (a) the Central Belt of Scotland, (b) London, and (c) a large group of English counties stretching from the North Midlands, through the North West to the North East. The spatial pattern of these regions and the other parts of England, Wales and Scotland is well organized and demands an explanation. The most viable hypothesis seems to be in terms of exposure to risk. We can show that cows were more diseased in some milk-producing regions than others. If we know where the milk from each region was consumed, we have a chance of estimating heightened risk, in general terms at least.[51] Some milk was moved over long distances to supply the needs of consumers in large cities, such as London, which might otherwise appear to be an outlier.

Maps for the 1920s onwards could be drawn but the spread of

---

[51] This is similar to a statistically significant positive correlation in Swedish counties between bTB in cattle and humans in 1935-40. Sjögren and Sutherland 1975.

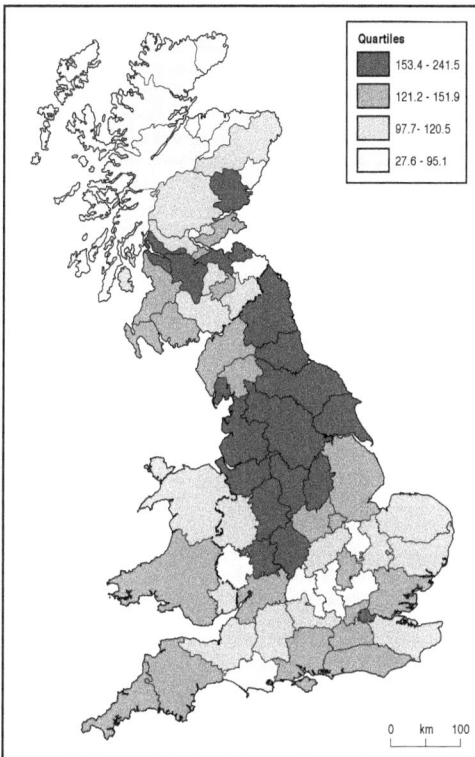

Fig 3.1
Estimated bTB death rate, age 0-4,
per 100,000 living, 1891-1900
(Source: See text)

pasteurization, at first in big cities after the First World War, later in smaller cities and towns, and really only after the Second World War in rural areas, created different patterns. This positive trend for consumers living in towns and cities can clearly be glimpsed in Table 3.7 using nationwide data compiled by Lethem of the GRO.

Table 3.7 Death rates from abdominal tuberculosis per million children 0-5 years in each category

	1921	1931	1938	1944
London administrative county	136	24	12	6
Combined County Boroughs	437	157	63	35
Combined Urban Districts	366	134	77	42
Combined Rural Districts	252	92	63	60

Source: Lethem 1946, 82.
Note: Abdominal tuberculosis in this age group was chosen because, according to Lethem, 'abdominal tuberculosis in growing children is almost always of bovine origin'.

Modern-day *M. bovis* in humans

Following a voluntary start to tuberculosis notification in Brighton in 1899, this became a further source of data as notification implied the official recognition and recording of serious morbidity. Notification became compulsory in all Poor Law institutions in 1908 and was extended to the whole population by the National Insurance Act (1911). At first the emphasis was upon pulmonary tuberculosis but by the time the scheme was operational in 1913, non-pulmonary disease was also included. In 1913 there were 80,788 notifications of pulmonary tuberculosis and 36,351 of non-pulmonary, a ratio of just over 2:1. Gradually these numbers fell, to 37,879 and 12,810 respectively in 1938. The shortages of medical resources during and immediately after the war saw a rise to a peak in 1949 of 44,480 cases of the lung disease but non-pulmonary tuberculosis continued to fall due mainly to the gradual spread of pasteurization. As a result, the ratio between the two types of disease increased as much as 8.6 in 1959 before falling back to about 3:1 again by the 1970s. On the whole historians of tuberculosis are not enthusiastic about the quality of the notification data and we will not pursue them further here. As a probably more reliable alternative, Figure 3.2 graphs estimated bTB mortality derived from the Registrar General's data, with its interesting hinge point at the turn of the century when bTB ceased its rise as a proportion of tuberculosis deaths overall.

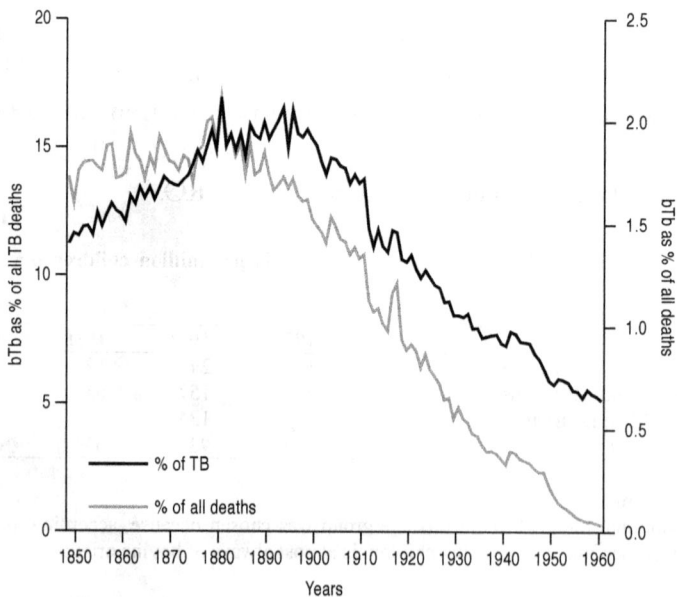

Fig 3.2 BTB as an estimated proportion of all tuberculosis deaths and all deaths in Great Britain, 1848-1960 (Source: Registrar General of England and Wales, *Annual Reports* and *Statistical Review*, Registrar General of Scotland, *Annual Reports*)

After the Second World War three developments were responsible for a significant fall in tuberculosis morbidity and mortality. The widespread use of BCG from 1953 was a major step forward in disease prevention in Britain, although as a vaccine it was not as effective in other countries. Second, the advent of streptomycin in 1948 was a threshold in drug therapy. Both of these developments were important for all forms of tuberculosis; the third, pasteurization adopted nationwide in the 1950s, was specific to *M. bovis*. We could also add improved x-ray facilities in a postwar era of mass miniature radiography, and by then overall the picture was much brighter in terms of preventative, diagnostic and therapeutic systems.[52]

Because of these developments, the typing of tuberculosis strains was never again a clinical priority, irrespective of the expertise acquired by the bacteriological followers of Griffith. Candidly, identification of the *M. tuberculosis* complex is enough for most clinicians, without drilling down to sub-types, because treatments in humans were identical, at least until it was shown that *M. bovis* is resistant to the drug pyrazinamide.[53] Even now molecular techniques are expensive, as are trained staff capable of conducting assays.[54] Modern differentiation is by biochemical, drug susceptibility and supplemental tests or by various molecular techniques.[55]

There are postwar mortality data for bTB based upon bacteriological analyses but their usefulness is debatable. In 1980 the provision of accurate figures of *M. bovis* infections was described as 'impossible' by the Public Health Laboratory Service of Great Britain. This was because the services for tuberculosis bacteriology were not centralised and the regional laboratories varied as to whether they made a distinction between *M. bovis* and *M. tuberculosis*. Nor were the data collated systematically even in those centres which took an interest.[56]

We know that there is bTB morbidity and occasional mortality today but the numbers are thankfully small. There are several reasons for

---

[52] Hardy 2003c.

[53] Hardie and Watson 1992; Grange and Yates 1994; Drobniewski et al. 2003.

[54] Thoen et al. 2010.

[55] Collins and Grange 1987; Pritchard 1988; Grange and Yates 1994; Gormley et al. 2014; Perez-Lago et al. 2014.

[56] TNA: MAF 257/12.

continued caution though. If a taste for unpasteurized milk develops, as seems possible given the publicity this product gets for its claimed health-giving properties, then the risk will rise, especially in an era when the disease is not under satisfactory control in cattle. This pales into insignificance, though, by comparison with the threat from drug-resistant tuberculosis. At the moment bTB is spreading amongst hard-to-reach and hard-to-treat vulnerable groups such as drug users and sufferers from HIV/AIDS. A perfect storm would ensue if this spread to the general populations of developed countries where overuse has diminished the effectiveness of antibiotics.

Surveillance data published by the Health Protection Agency of Public Health England show that people aged 65 and over account for the majority of human *M. bovis* cases, probably mostly reactivations of infections latent since the pre-pasteurization era. In the younger age groups the majority of cases are in those born overseas, again in circumstances where milk control was lax.[57] The numbers are historically very small at present, the average annual notifications of bTB for each country in the UK for 1999-2014 being as follows: England 20.2, Wales 1.5, Scotland 3.4, and Northern Ireland 1.7.

Conclusion

In this chapter we set out to look at knowledge of bTB in human bodies through infections and various body sites and to quantify the human health consequences of the cattle-bTB-human assemblage. This socionatural association proved to be deadly for over half a million people and disrupted the lives of many more. The patterns were far from straightforward, however.

Mortality from tuberculosis overall fell steadily in the nineteenth and twentieth centuries. While there is debate about the causes and correlates of this macro-scale trend, it seems likely that the respiratory version was radically reduced in response to the environmental improvements of the late nineteenth century, especially in housing conditions, for the probability of catching 'phthisis' had been exacerbated before that by overcrowded and ill-ventilated accommodation. On the other hand, as the use of cows' milk increased in the second half of the century, *M.*

---

[57] Ormerod 2014.

bovis infections became *more* common, especially amongst infants who had been taken from the breast. The British taste for raw milk made this problem worse than it would have been had the boiling of drinking milk been as common as on the Continent.[58] There were fears about the reduced nutritive value of boiled milk and heating was rejected as a practice by many mothers because it was thought to be a cause of constipation in their babies.[59] Later, the use of powdered milk, which had been heated during manufacture, and of pasteurized liquid milk were to help in the gradual elimination of *M. bovis* infection.

---

[58] Thorne-Thorne 1899; Smith 1988.
[59] Roberts 1973.

CHAPTER 4.

THE EVOLVING VETERINARY SCIENCE OF BOVINE TUBERCULOSIS

> The epidemiology of bovine TB is highly complex and many of the processes driving the current epidemic are not fully identified and/or observed. Hence, bovine TB is largely 'an unobserved epidemic'.[1]

Introduction

We saw in Chapter 3 that understanding the aetiology and pathogenesis of bTB in humans has been far from straightforward. The present chapter will argue that historically this has also been the case for cattle, with several aspects of the disease and its control still uncertain, even today. We will take the science as far as the 1970s, at which point it became obvious that the newly discovered presence of a wildlife reservoir of disease in the British Isles, particularly badgers and deer, would be controversial. The bTB problem then moved into the public domain, well beyond specialist scientific debate. Later, in Chapters 12-14, we will bring the veterinary science up to date in order to provide a context for the discussion of modern control measures and their failure to eliminate bTB from the UK's national cattle herd.

Our argument in this chapter will be that the gradually incremental but contested evolution of veterinary knowledge partly helps to explain the pitifully slow eradication response by successive administrations in London, Edinburgh and Dublin/Belfast. Without such an understanding of the evolution of science policy and its conversation with vested interests, it would be all too easy to slip into the comfortable position of being wise after the event, in this case complex events. Chapters 7-11 will present a political and administrative history of bTB that will complement and build upon our story here.

---

[1] Skuce et al. 2011, 37.

Pathogenesis in cattle

In many respects bTB came to be anatomically better understood in cattle in the nineteenth and early twentieth centuries than in human bodies because of the easy access for viewing carcase lesions in the abattoir by research veterinarians, public health doctors and inspectors. It was the last group who published most data concerning the sites of visible disease, through observation of large numbers of slaughtered cattle. As a result, it is possible to observe a changing emphasis in the literature through time as the average infected beast moved from being extensively diseased to the present situation where it is not uncommon for reactors to the tuberculin test (TT) to have no visible lesions at all on slaughter. This shift has in turn affected theories of epidemiology and pathogenesis.

Table 4.1 Evidence of bTB infection in cattle

- in sputum - if the lungs diseased
- in faeces - if sputum from diseased lungs is swallowed
- in urine - if the kidneys affected
- skin - a swelling as an immune reaction to a tuberculin challenge
- in blood - gamma-interferon assay
- udder - veterinary inspection for induration
- in milk - guinea pig testing
- tissue lesions - abattoir inspections
- advanced bTB - loss of weight, reduced milk yield, chronic cough

In the late nineteenth century George Fleming and others believed that airborne transmission was the key to bTB in cattle but at the turn of the twentieth century von Behring and Calmette, arguing from experience with human subjects, insisted on a primacy of intestinal infection, which they claimed could then spread to the lungs via the mucous membrane of the alimentary tract.[2] But today most researchers once again see the respiratory tract and associated lymph nodes – tracheobronchial and mediastinal – as most at risk, followed by the cranial lymph nodes - retropharyngeal, submandibular and parotid.[3] Most lesions (in number though not always in size) are found in the dorso-caudal apex of the lungs, close to the pleural surface, so at the far end of the longest direct route into the lungs.[4]

---

[2] Fleming 1875; Stamp 1948.
[3] Goodchild and Clifton Hadley 2001; Domingo et al. 2014.
[4] Cassidy 2006.

Even small numbers of mycobacteria in aerosol form can lead to an immunological response, followed by pathology.[5] This is not altogether to rule out the other route - the ingestion of infected milk, grass, water or nasal mucous - but the number of mycobacteria required to create an infection via that pathway is 100-1000 times greater than by aerosol.[6] It is important to note that in the first half of the twentieth century abattoir records *did* show animals with lesions in their alimentary and abdominal lymph nodes but this may have been because pastures contaminated with *M. bovis* were more common then than they are today.[7]

Among modern-day infected cattle, about twenty per cent excrete *M. bovis* and most of these have the lesions in their lungs and lymph nodes that are required for further onward infection. These lesions are sometimes too small for routine abattoir detection but they do progress if the disease is not detected.[8] Abattoir records today show sixty per cent of primary complexes in the lymph tissues of the thoracic cavity whereas Tables 4.2 and 4.3 show a more prominent role for the intestines and the lungs in the first half of the twentieth century.[9] In the case of Edinburgh in 1946, the lungs were implicated in eighty-five per cent of animals. These infections were often linked to other sites, suggesting that progressive disease was not uncommon at that time. The frequency of disease in the lungs in the past is not because the pathogenesis of the disease has changed but because in the era of tighter control since 1950 fewer animals have had a chance to develop full-blown lung tuberculosis.[10] We are nowadays simply looking at an earlier stage of the disease. In the late nineteenth and early twentieth centuries it was not uncommon for infected cattle to progress through all of the phases of the disease to the final one of generalized tuberculosis, by which time it was no longer possible to identify the primary lesion.[11] By then the animal may have been suffering from emaciation, fever, induration of the udder, and a persistent cough.[12] In the present era these symptoms

---

[5] Neill et al. 2001; Neill et al. 2005; Dean et al. 2005.

[6] Sigurdsson 1945 says millions; Dean et al. 2005.

[7] McFadyean 1910; Phillips et al. 2003.

[8] Skuce et al. 2011.

[9] Stamp 1944; Stamp 1948; Stamp and Wilson 1946; Neill et al. 1994; Whipple et al. 1996.

[10] Neill et al. 2005.

[11] Sigurdsson 1945.

[12] Menzies and Neill 2000; Westergaard 2007.

remain as common in parts of South Asia and Africa as they were in Europe and North America one hundred years ago.[13]

Table 4.2 Abattoir records of bovine body parts destroyed because of TB

	Edinburgh 1908-25	Liverpool 1921*	Bury 1923-26	Birmingham 1925*	Ayr 1924-48*	West Ham 1926-32*
Heads	7,930	132	74	1,019	-	-
Lungs	10,029	621	186	1,890	10,633	2,377
Pleura	1,820	-	103	-	-	112
Stomachs	-	58	44	1,473	-	93
Intestines	-	70	10	-	-	51
Omenta	-	-	-	-	-	81
Mesenteries	-	-	45	-	-	59
Peritoneum	228	-	51	-	-	112
Bowels	3,666	-	-	1,472	9,233	-
Hearts	30	17	22	1,147	-	102
Spleens	1,721	21	37	1,454	-	103
Livers	3,262	163	136	1,488	-	302
Kidneys	-	29	30	926	-	30
Pancreas	-	-	-	-	-	55
Udders	489	20	5	602	-	30
Uterus	-	-	1	-	-	-
Lymph glands	186	-	-	-	-	-
Other	359	-	-	-	-	48

Note: * cows only.
Sources: MOH Annual Reports; Trotter 1904; Watts and Robertson 1950; TNA: CAB 58/190.

Table 4.3 Sites of TB lesions in Edinburgh cows, 1946

	Cows	%
Head	277	9.2
Lungs and lung glands	1,103	36.8
Head and lungs	283	9.4
Intestine	110	3.7
Intestine and head	27	0.9
Intestine, liver and head	20	0.6
Intestine and lungs	384	12.8
Head, intestine and lungs	297	9.9
Lungs and liver	76	2.6
Head, lungs and liver	29	1.0
Lungs, liver and intestine	113	3.8
Head, lungs, intestine and liver	265	8.8
Liver	16	0.5

Source: Stamp and Wilson 1946.

In the 1950s Francis estimated that about ninety per cent of infections in British cattle were respiratory and ten per cent alimentary, proportions that were confirmed in Denmark by Plum.[14] When cattle cough or sneeze they spray minute droplets in aerosol form that can stay airborne, as can mycobacteria attached to fomites such as small

---

[13] Verma 2006; Zinsstag et al. 2006.
[14] Francis 1947; Francis 1958, 18; Francis 1972a, 51; Grange and Collins 1997.

(<10μm) dust particles.[15] It seems that ninety-four per cent of *M. bovis* can survive ten minutes of being suspended in the air, and their half-life of viability is ninety minutes.[16] Attached to dust, there will be only a few per particle but they can survive for three to eight days and in cattle sputum for thirty to forty days.[17] As a result, cattle-to-cattle transmission is a high risk in crowded cattle sheds with poor airspace management, and maybe also head-to-head at farm boundaries. Nineteenth century dairymen thought that a warm environment encouraged a higher milk yield but in their unventilated cowsheds there would have been a greatly increased probability of such droplets being inhaled directly.[18]

Once the infection has taken hold, lesions appear after about fourteen days, as grey translucent nodules that later with necrosis become pale yellow in colour and develop a caseous core.[19] These may then become whitish to yellowish nodules of fibrous tissue, 'tubercles', often still small and difficult to detect. These granulomas are the body's way of localizing the infection and allowing the inflammatory and immune mechanisms to destroy the mycobacteria.[20] Later some of this caseous material becomes calcified, forming nodules that encourage the description of bTB as 'the grapes', 'angle-berries' or 'pearl disease'.

The presence of lesions in the airways facilitates the spread of *M. bovis* by aerosol. It used to be thought that such 'open' lesions were rare but this misapprehension was probably because in the slaughterhouse many of the small lesions present are only found in the lymph nodes, especially in the lungs, and it is these that are sectioned and closely inspected.[21] On the contrary, later research suggests that even animals in the early stage of infection begin shedding mycobacteria and become infectious to others.[22] The RC1 in 1895 had thought this unlikely and

---

[15] Langmuir 1961; Youmans 1979; Pritchard 1988; Phillips et al. 2003.
[16] Gannon et al. 2007.
[17] Sigurdsson 1945.
[18] BPP, 1896 (C. 7992) xlvi.QQ.1508-9.
[19] Thornton 1962; Cassidy et al. 1998; Pollock et al. 2006.
[20] Thoen and Barletta 2014.
[21] Menzies and Neill 2000.
[22] Ibid.

influential figures such as Arthur Newsholme agreed with them.[23] But views began to change in the 1920s.[24]

In infected humans it is safe to say that only cases with direct smear positive sputa are a risk to their immediate contacts but in cattle the situation is different. The primary focus may remain localized or progress slowly but the healing which often occurs in humans is less common in cattle, which have more secondary complexes.[25] As a result, all tuberculin-positive cattle are seen as 'open' cases.[26] Nevertheless, some latency *is* possible and this has major implications for testing.[27] If the disease reactivates in perhaps just one animal per herd it may well contribute to the large number of herd breakdowns for which there appears to be no attributable source.[28]

Infection in the bovine body gradually builds. This is possible by contiguity diffusion from one organ to its neighbour but also via the lymphatic system and the haematological route to the liver, kidneys, meninges, serous cavities and, most important for human health, to the udder.[29] By the time there are visible symptoms, such as emaciation, a chronic cough or a diseased udder, both the carcase and milk are potentially dangerous for human consumption. Miliary tuberculosis may be one consequence, with numerous millet-sized tubercles forming throughout the cow's organs such as lungs, kidneys, liver and spleen.[30]

In the late nineteenth and early twentieth centuries there was a lot of discussion about the risk of tuberculous cows producing diseased milk.[31] The widely accepted view in the 1930s and 1940s was that about 0.5 per cent of such cows were a hazard to milk drinkers.[32] Later evidence suggested that the reality was closer to four per cent of tuberculin reactors that excrete bacilli in their milk, although only

---

[23] BPP 1895 (C. 7703) xxxv.631; Newsholme 1908.
[24] Jordan 1933.
[25] Neill et al. 1994.
[26] O'Reilly and Daborn 1995.
[27] Pollock and Neill 2002; Olea-Popelka et al. 2008; Skuce et al. 2011.
[28] Neill et al. 2005.
[29] Thornton 1949; Francis 1958; Neill et al. 1994; Whipple et al. 1996.
[30] Thornton 1962.
[31] See Chapter 8.
[32] Hopkins Committee 1934; Wilson 1942.

twenty-five per cent of these showed any udder lesions.[33] At a stroke this latter evidence undermined one of the principal control measures that for decades had relied upon the skill of inspecting veterinarians to eliminate tuberculous animals by examination of the udder.[34] Their work may not have achieved this result but it did generate a great deal of data that are summarised in Table 4.4. An interesting and valuable aspect of the tabulation is the regional variation displayed. This hints at many more cases of advanced disease in cows kept in cities such as Bradford, Salford, Leeds and Liverpool, and also at a lower level in counties including Cheshire, Durham, Essex, and Middlesex, but very

Table 4.4 Evidence of bovine udder tuberculosis in the early twentieth century UK

Location	Cows	TB udder (%)	Location	Cows	TB udder (%)
Aberdeen 1926-27	19,966	0.14	Lincolnshire, Holland	-	0.05
Bedfordshire	-	0.06	Lincolnshire, Kesteven	-	0.04
Berkshire	-	0.04	Lincolnshire, Lindsey	-	0.07
Birmingham 1900-5, 1917-19, 1923, 1925	14,445	0.14	Liverpool 1901-37	171,960 city 47,820 country	0.42 1.19
Blackburn 1902-12, 1920	-	0.6-2.9	Manchester 1900, 1903-11, 1921	92,073 city 24,851 country	0.02 0.81
Bradford 1910-11, 1915, 1918-19	16,212	2.10	Middlesex	-	0.55
Buckinghamshire	-	0.06	Monmouth	-	0.03
Cambridgeshire	-	0.07	Newcastle 1908-25	9,223	0.54
Cheshire	-	0.24	Norfolk	-	0.04
Cornwall	-	0.01	Northamptonshire	-	0.02
Cumberland 1927-30	39,641	0.10	Northumberland	-	0.06
Derbyshire	-	0.16	Oxfordshire	-	0.04
Devon	-	0.01	Peterborough	-	0.23
Dorset	-	0.03	Salford 1921	91	3.30
Dumbarton, 1926-27	9,449	0.01	Sheffield 1901-14, 1921-29	Country City	0.59-4.84 0.14-1.10
Durham	-	0.57	Shropshire	-	0.10
Edinburgh 1900-1912	37,256	0.31	Somerset	-	0.03
Edinburgh 1926-27	7,709	0.30	Staffordshire	-	0.29
Ely	-	0.03	Suffolk	-	0.03
Essex	-	0.39	Surrey	-	0.29
Fife, 1927	12,355	0.11	Sussex, East	-	0.13
Gloucester 1927-31	327,434	0.06	Sussex, West	-	0.03
Hampshire	-	0.11	Warwickshire	-	0.12
Hertfordshire	-	0.09	Westmorland	-	0.01
Huntingdonshire	-	0.06	Wigtown 1926	3,668	0.14
Isle of Wight	-	0.03	Wiltshire	-	0.17
Kent	-	0.03	Worcestershire	-	0.03
Lanarkshire 1910-29	438,924	0.11	Yorkshire, East Riding	-	0.06
Lancashire	-	0.18	Yorkshire, North Riding	-	0.10
Leeds 1901, 1914	4,500	0.93	Yorkshire, West Riding 1928-30	256,988	0.13
Leicestershire	-	0.07			

Note: date 1931 unless otherwise stated.
Sources: Medical Officer of Health Annual Reports; People's League of Health 1932a; Savage, 1929a; Lloyd 1902; TNA: MH 56/100.

---

[33] Kaplan et al. 1962.

[34] See Chapter 10.

low rates in Cornwall and Devon. While a coherent spatial epidemiology does not immediately present itself in this table, there could be said to be a difference between cities and their immediate densely stocked hinterlands on the one hand and the more distant countryside with fewer animals per unit area on the other.

Diagnostics: the Tuberculin Test

Our story so far is that knowing bTB in the nineteenth and early twentieth centuries was a matter of visibility: lesions in an opened carcase or physical changes in the udder. An important alternative for live animals came in 1890 with Koch's discovery of tuberculin. This was a filtrate of mycobacteria killed by heat but, rather than providing a cure for human tuberculosis as originally intended, it proved to be better suited as a means of testing animals suspected of having the disease. This is because infected cattle are allergic to proteins in the tuberculin and produce antibodies as a reaction. These circulate and can then be detected, a process of 'bringing into being' invisible microbiota that has been called 'enpresenting'.[35]

A major issue for the credibility of the skin test is that the majority of reactors look perfectly healthy and under such circumstances farmers have always found it difficult to accept the need for slaughter, with its attendant inconvenience and loss of income.[36] BTB as mediated by the TT is not knowable to them. This is important because it marks a fork in the history of this disease. The empirical ontology of the abattoir has always been easy to believe in but from 1890 onwards it was proposed to condemn cattle on the basis of a diagnosis emerging through the deployment of testing equipment. In the sense understood by the practical farmer, the disease did not exist until the veterinarian said it did. This ontology of emergence is an altogether different way of seeing the world.[37] But more than that, different practices produce different realities. While most observers can recognise a gross lesion in a carcase, the various skin and blood tests produce a surprising degree

---

[35] Van Loon 2002.

[36] Myers 1977.

[37] Law and Lien 2013.

of variation according to the technology employed, the injection site and the operator.

(a) The tuberculin

As a test for cattle disease, tuberculin was pioneered by Gutmann in Russia and by Bang in Denmark, both in 1891, and it then spread quickly across the Continent.[38] In Britain, McFadyean at the RVC manufactured tens of thousands of tuberculin doses, but the unit cost was very high at £13 per animal, at a time when the average cow was worth less than that.[39]

From the outset there were technical problems with the tuberculin itself. The use of different methods in the various manufacturing laboratories resulted in varied strengths of preparation, a fact that was not helped by there being sixteen different brands on the market in Britain alone by the early 1930s.[40] In addition, Koch's so-called Old Tuberculin could not be purified because the active tuberculo-proteins had become mixed with proteins in the growth medium.[41] The resulting false positives during testing were an embarrassment and the inconsistencies arising persuaded the British authorities to undertake the mass production of tuberculin themselves.

Attempts at purifying tuberculin were pioneered in the US by Florence Seibert in the 1920s.[42] Then in 1940 the British government selected a tuberculin produced by the US Bureau of Animal Industry, which caused difficulties for three reasons. First, it had been made from human strains and was much stronger than anything previously used in the UK. It was a purified protein derivative (PPD) originating from mycobacteria grown on a synthetic medium and standardized using chemical and biological techniques. Second, it was designed for the US standard Single Intradermal Test (SIT) administered at the caudal fold, not a site used in the UK. This so-called Weybridge tuberculin was gradually phased in but, third, it was soon found that it lacked specificity under British conditions and its greater potency led

---

[38] Sessions 1905; Francis 1958.

[39] In 1911 an official estimate of average value was £12. TNA: MH 80/4.

[40] Rabagliati 1932.

[41] De Vine 1924; Newton 1924.

[42] Doig et al. 1938.

to a fourfold increase in the number of reactors detected.[43] Some of these additional breakdowns were caused by the avian strain used in the double intradermal test (DIT) but anyway the dose was too high for local conditions and in 1942 it was reduced to prevent false positives.[44]

Eventually, in April 1943, despite the problems, it was decided that UK skin testing should move entirely to the PPD.[45] This continued for decades until 1975 when at last there was a switch from this human-based PPD to a bovine strain.[46] This was to be AN5, which had been isolated as long ago as 1948 and since then had been grown on because of its suitable characteristics for manufacturing purposes.[47] As hoped, the change led to an improved specificity of the test. It has been suggested that in future it would be helpful to replace this tuberculin with a *M. bovis*-specific purified antigen in order to minimize the problem of non-specific sensitisation to skin tests.[48] Despite a great deal of research, it is clear that today's tuberculin has yet to be perfected. The potency still varies to the extent that the diagnosis of bTB may be less reliable with some batches than with others.[49]

(b) The injection site and testing protocol

The choreography of the TT has changed over the years. A number of different approaches to the testing of cattle have been tried in order to get the most precise and reliable result. In the 1890s the injection was subcutaneous, with the veterinarian looking for a febrile response, a rise in temperature of 2.7-3.6°C, peaking between the twelfth and twenty-first hours. At one stage it was thought necessary to take the tested animals' rectal temperature every two or three hours.[50] This inevitably put practical limits on what could be achieved by a single vet.[51]

In the UK the subcutaneous method was quickly overtaken by the

---

[43] Ministry of Agriculture and Fisheries (1949) *Report of proceedings under the Diseases of Animals Acts, 1938 to 1947* London: HMSO.

[44] TNA: MAF 35/486; *Farmers Weekly* 22 May 1942.

[45] Green 1946; Anon. 1947a; Monaghan 1994.

[46] Lesslie et al. 1975.

[47] Paterson 1948; De la Rua-Domenech et al. 2006; Hewinson et al. 2006.

[48] De la Rua-Domenech et al. 2006.

[49] O'Reilly and Daborn 1995; Schiller et al. 2010.

[50] Delépine 1900, 1201.

[51] Parker 1917; Francis 1947.

intradermal, which also became the standard in America from 1920, using the caudal fold at the base of the tail as the injection site. Various European countries soon followed suit, although most preferred the side of the neck as more sensitive for a reaction - a swelling. With the intradermal method there was a significant saving of time and therefore of expense, leading to its widespread adoption. It was, however, susceptible to an unscrupulous minority of farmers in Europe and North America who soon learned that surreptitiously dosing an animal with tuberculin shortly before a test would make it unlikely to react and so avoid the possibility of slaughter.[52] Alternatively after an unsuccessful test, some farmers sold their reactors on to unsuspecting purchasers.[53]

In 1921 the Tuberculin Committee of the MRC recommended re-tests at six-monthly intervals by the combined subcutaneous and ophthalmic methods and three additional temperature measurements.[54] Very soon, though, it was realised that the intradermal test was superior and in 1925 the committee changed its recommendation to the DIT.[55] This was intradermal because it was easier to administer than the subcutaneous, and double to minimize the number of uncertain cases.

The DIT was the official test in the UK from 1928 to 1947. It used the first injection of tuberculin for 'sensitising' the animal and 48 hours later a second, diagnostic, injection was made. PPD tuberculin was not really suitable for the DIT and so from 1942 there were field experiments with a comparative test, also with two injections, but now one with mammalian tuberculin and the other avian.[56] The reason for two injections was that cattle in the UK and some other countries are frequently exposed to non-tuberculous mycobacteria in the environment. Without a comparison it was felt that these environmental mycobacteria would create a lot of false positives. There were teething problems at first with standards of interpretation about how much more œdema at the mammalian site than the avian constituted a reactor.

---

[52] In Britain this in theory was not illegal at first because tuberculin was not a controlled drug in the Therapeutic Substances Act (1925). Roadhouse and Henderson 1941; Palmer and Waters 2011.

[53] Edgar 1898/99.

[54] Ministry of Health, *On the state of the public health ... 1923* London: HMSO; Buxton and MacNalty 1928.

[55] MRC 1925; Buxton 1927.

[56] Ritchie, in Anon. 1945-46.

An experiment on 10,000 cattle in 1946 was set up to see whether the UK should also switch from the DIT to the Single Intradermal Cervical Test (SICT), and this did indeed happen in June 1947.[57] Part of the cost benefit analysis was that only two farm visits by the veterinarian were needed instead of three.

(c) Tuberculin Test results

The sheer scale of the problem in the British herd quickly became evident when John McFadyean in 1900 reported that a total of 11,151 cattle had by then been tuberculin tested, of which 2,716 (24.4 per cent) had reacted and another 145 were unconfirmed.[58] Interestingly, all eighty-one tests in the Channel Islands had been negative and only seven per cent of the 1,175 tests in the counties of Cornwall, Devon, Dorset, and Somerset were positive. However, of 1,238 cattle tested in Sussex and Hampshire, fifty per cent reacted, and Queen Victoria's own pedigree herd at Windsor had been found to be riddled with tuberculosis.[59] McFadyean was understandably puzzled by such geographical variation.

The situation in Europe (Table 4.5) was also one of extreme variability, from only a few tuberculin reactors in Bulgaria, Finland and Portugal to high rates of infection in the increasingly intensive and industrialised agriculture of Austria-Hungary, Germany and parts of France.

The private and public programmes of testing that started in the early twentieth century in Britain revealed an extent of disease that everyone found alarming. Cows supplying Birmingham's milk were the first to be tested on a large scale, and from 1907 to 1927 no less than 40.4 per cent of the 2,136 inspected were found to be reactors.[60] This was more than the thirty per cent estimated by John McFadyean in 1921 and the 24.2 per cent of 3,229 first tests in the country as a whole in 1924-5.[61] The number of farmers coming forward to have their herds tested was low, however, despite the Birmingham corporation offering

---

[57] TNA: MAF 56/400.
[58] McFadyean 1900b; Bishop 1908.
[59] McFadyean 1899a.
[60] Savage 1929a, 38.
[61] Anon. 1895a; McFadyean 1921; National Milk Conference Committee 1926.

Table 4.5 Europe: reactors to the tuberculin test

	Cattle tested	% TB
Austria, 1897	2,,314	39.8
Moravia, 1893-95	4256	36-48
Belgium, 1896	19,004	48.8
Bulgaria, 1939	35,000	2.1
Denmark, 1893-1904	404,651	24.0
1909-22	96,771	10.5
1938	5,574	21.9
Finland, 1897-1912	118,358	6.5
France, 1903	-	15-50
1921	-	15.7
1926	67,000	25.9
Paris, cowsheds, 1905	1,351	41.8*
1910	1,683	39.6
1916	971	29.8*
Seine	11,901	34.0*
Germany, 1937	3,351	49.0
W. Germany, 1952	-	59.0
Bavaria, 1895	5,402	37.2
Bavaria, 1896	2,596	41.9
Prussia, 1937	306,653	31.3
Saxony, 1891-1904	3,083	68.0
Hungary, 1902-07	22,923	20.4
1910-13	-	10-13
1930-31	-	28-35
Italy, 1903	-	30*
Norway, 1895-1918	50,493	7.2
Portugal, Lisbon, 1903		30*
Portugal, 1938	20,879	2.8
Sweden, 1897-1908	306,372	30.7
1909-28	69,272	23.8
Switzerland, 1894	212	41.0
1930	-	40.0

Note: * cows only.
Sources: Salmon 1906; Hutyra and Marek 1912; Ernst 1914; Francis 1947; Meyn 1952.

free tuberculin and free veterinary inspections.[62] That city's forty per cent was matched or exceeded in later estimates by the MH, the MAF, the MRC and the People's League of Health (PLH) and forty per cent became deeply grooved as the most quoted figure for the average level of infection in the British dairy herd in the 1930s.[63]

Not all of those who were part of this conversation realised that only a small proportion of the tuberculin reactors were capable of discharging the mycobacteria dangerous to human health; it was about one per cent according to the PLH.[64] And there were reasons to think

---

[62] *Cowkeeper and Dairyman's Journal* February 1910, 197; Savage 1928; Waddington 2004.

[63] Savage 1929a, 179; Ministry of Health 1931; People's League of Health 1932a. However, Hamill 1933 and 1934 estimated fifty per cent.

[64] People's League of Health 1934.

the forty per cent figure was on the high side.[65] When it was used by the Hopkins Committee in 1934, they were referring to cows rather than to all cattle, and moreover to mature dairy cows, not heifers. The percentages for other classes of cattle were almost certainly lower, much lower in the case of grass-fed beef and store cattle. Later estimates of average cow infection were thirty-five per cent in 1949 and thirty per cent in 1950.[66]

Following the establishment of the National Veterinary Service in 1937/8, the MAF decided to make a large survey in order to gauge the scale of the problem they faced. The TT was administered in 1938-9 to 364,286 cattle in 12,300 closed herds. The results showed a 12.98 per cent positive reaction on average, with 56.67 per cent of herds having no reactors, 23.55 per cent less than 10 per cent of the herd positive, and 19.77 per cent with more than ten per cent positive. According to Ritchie, best estimates based on this survey were that there were twenty per cent of reactors in England, 7.5 per cent in Wales, and 23.1 per cent in Scotland. He put the average for Britain as a whole at seventeen to eighteen per cent for all cattle and thirty to thirty-five for cows.[67] This survey did not seek statistical representativeness in that it concentrated on self-contained herds, which bred their own replacements.[68] The true figure would therefore have been higher overall. Nevertheless the survey confirmed the previously suspected pockets of bTB in the North West and South East of England and in the east of Scotland (Figure 4.1).[69] This was a worrying outcome because the major conurbations of Liverpool, Manchester, London, Glasgow and Edinburgh relied on these source regions for their daily milk supply. There were no calls for eradication to be concentrated in these regions, however, because in open herds the disease was possibly coming with young stock bought every year from the breeding regions.

---

[65] Montgomerie 1937; Francis 1947.
[66] Savage 1949; TNA: MH 35/785.
[67] Ritchie in Anon. 1945-46.
[68] MAFF 1965.
[69] According to Francis 1947, the figure for Cheshire was likely to have been sixty to eighty per cent.

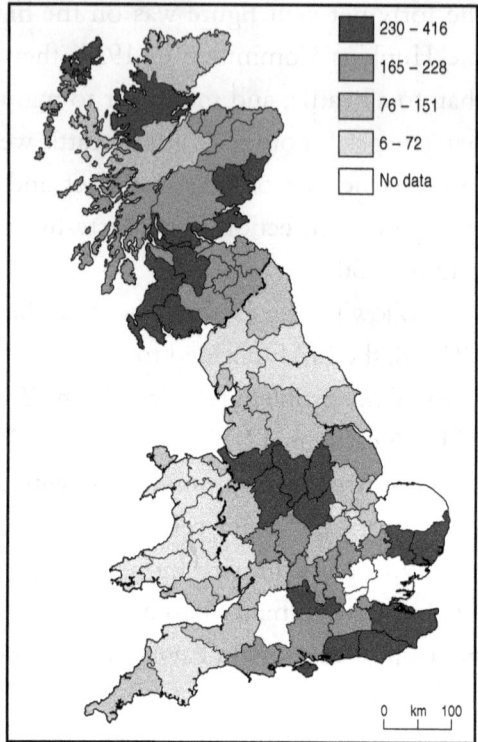

230 – 416
165 – 228
76 – 151
6 – 72
No data

Fig 4.1
The percentage of cattle in each county
or group of counties that reacted
positively to the tuberculin test in the
1938-39 survey
(Source: Francis 1947)

0   km   100

Vaccines

Once Koch had isolated the tubercle bacillus it was inevitable that attempts would be made to find a vaccine against tuberculosis. In Germany in the first decade of the twentieth century Von Behring's method was to vaccinate calves but his bovovaccine at best gave only partially positive results and the injection had to be repeated after two years.[70] Some of the early experiments with live *M. bovis* injected into cows were a failure because the animals produced mycobacteria in their milk.[71] By far the best known and most successful vaccine for both humans and cattle was BCG, an attenuated strain which emerged from laborious experiments between 1908 and 1921. Various trials with cattle were then undertaken but the Lübeck disaster in 1929, in which children died after vaccination, brought the whole approach into question and the field results for livestock were anyway disappointing. The veterinary use of BCG seems to have faded in the 1950s only to be resurrected experimentally in the last few years.

---

[70] Robertson 1909; Linton 2005.
[71] Francis 1947.

Conclusion

This chapter has looked at the early science of bTB in cattle. One important take-home point is that the disease has been a moving target. In the early twentieth century there was abundant abattoir evidence of it being a lung disease but today the centre of gravity of primary lesions is lymphatic. This is an important indicator, not of a change in pathogenesis, but rather a shift in the stage of disease that presents at slaughter. In short, bTB in cattle now tends to be a recent infection rather than advanced disease.

A second important conclusion is that throughout the twentieth century bTB proved to be exceptionally difficult to pick up through tuberculin testing. This was partly due to technical issues with the tuberculin and with the testing protocol, and we will add to this in Chapter 14, where it will be argued that there is a relatively high proportion of infected cattle that at various times are anergic and which therefore have to be found by other means. The history of testing right down to the present day has therefore been one of limited success. Such technical indeterminacy is frustrating for all concerned and it has proved to be one of the greatest weaknesses in the drive against *M. bovis*.

Veterinary knowledge has grown and been restructured by the difficulties of dealing with bTB. Tongue in cheek we might even say that veterinarians have been taught a thing or two by the mycobacterium but never quite enough to eliminate it. *M. bovis* has been their shadowy foe and also their master. In Britain there has been such a major and long-running problem that the veterinary profession itself would be different without its path dependence on bTB.

CHAPTER 5.

THE PASTEURIZATION OF BRITAIN: HOW HOT FOR HOW LONG?

Introduction

The pasteurization proposition is twofold: to kill pathogenic organisms such as *M. bovis* and to improve keeping quality.[1] But to the late James Steele it was much more than a technological solution to the bacterial load of milk. He claimed that 'pasteurization is one of public health's triumphs over the ignorance and superstition of past ages'.[2] Indeed the subject of pasteurization has attracted hyperbole at both the positive and negative ends of the rhetorical spectrum for over 100 years now. Our plan in this chapter is first to lay out the technical changes that have taken place, and in the next chapter there will follow a socio-political interpretation of the multi-faceted and long-lasting opposition to the heat treatment of milk.

The notion of heating liquids was not new. Scheele had used it to preserve vinegar in the 1780s and Pasteur famously applied the same idea to wine in the 1860s and to beer in 1870.[3] He surmised that poor keeping quality was due to contamination from the atmosphere and then set out to prove that heat could destroy the bacteria responsible for fermentation. The added value of these bacteriological insights was incalculable, as was Pasteur's shift of emphasis away from boiling to lower temperatures (50-60°C) that did not change the taste of the fluids that he was experimenting with.

The adoption of heating technologies did not necessarily prove that germ theory was correct but it did demonstrate the power of Pasteur's ideational regime as actionable.[4] In the 1870s Fjord in Copenhagen was among the first then to apply it to milk.[5] His success meant that the

---

[1] Cronshaw 1947.
[2] Steele 2000, 175.
[3] Davis 1950.
[4] Speake 2011.
[5] Frederiksen 1919; Westhoff 1978.

large-scale heat treatment of milk spread in Germany and Denmark in the early 1880s, but it was the latter country that seems to have been the first to encourage pasteurization with a view to protecting the consumer from bTB.[6] A law passed in 1898 prescribed that skim milk and buttermilk destined for use as food for calves and pigs had to be heated to 80°C, as had any cream to be used in making butter for export.[7] The rationale was that eliminating disease from foodstuffs was vital for the Danish economy, which at this time was dependent upon agricultural exports. Pasteurization therefore minimized the risk of reputational damage.

The idea of pasteurizing milk in bottles was furthered in Germany by von Soxhlet in 1886.[8] This German and Danish technology was imported into the USA in the early 1890s and it was in New York City that a pro-pasteurization anglophone discourse first found its feet.[9] By far the best known proponent was Nathan Straus, who claimed that his network of milk depots was saving lives by providing germ-free milk at a subsidised price.[10] His efforts appealed to the late Victorian sensibility of philanthropy but he also had a personal motive because his two year old daughter had died of an infection contracted, he thought, from contaminated milk.

Pasteurization was also the answer to a difficult question for milk dealers in large American cities. As populations grew in the rapid urbanization of the 1880s and 1890s, the demand for perishable foods of all types increased, even for relatively expensive products such as milk. But the very same urban growth was responsible for the displacement of farmers from the peri-urban area, with the effect that milk either had to come from the diminishing number of cowsheds left within the city boundary or from pastures further afield. The urban cowkeepers were eventually put out of business by rising costs and sanitary regulation, for instance the notorious swill dairies in New York where animal welfare was poor, so this left the market open to milk brought by road or rail. In hot weather the logistical challenge was for dealers to prevent spoilage

---

[6] Aikman 1895; Hill 1943.

[7] Jensen 1909; Rosenau 1912.

[8] Gerber and Wieske 1903.

[9] Harvey and Hill 1967; Holsinger et al. 1997.

[10] MacNutt 1917; Parker 1917; Moore 1921; North 1922.

and heat treatment was the solution of choice for many of them from the mid-1890s, starting in New York and Baltimore.[11] Because of the distances and summer temperatures, some milk was heated more than once before it eventually reached the consumer. This treatment was done surreptitiously in the early years because dealers were unsure how consumers would react if they knew that their milk had been pasteurized and anyway their motivation was mainly to add a day or two to the shelf life of what was often a poor quality product.[12]

A key point about the heat treatment of milk is finding the right balance between temperature and holding period. If the process is too hot for too long the destruction of bacteria may be achieved but other constituents may be damaged, for instance enzymes, vitamins and minerals, along with organoleptic properties such as odour, flavour and colour, and physical properties like the cream line and viscosity. There are potentially an infinite number of temperature/time combinations (Figure 5.1) but in practice these were historically

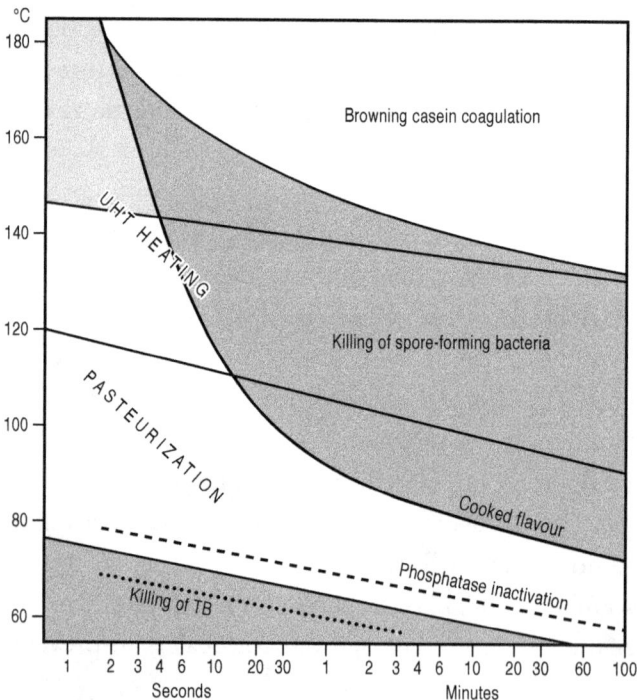

Fig 5.1 Diagram of bacterial death points (Source: after Hall and Trout 1968)

---

[11] Parker 1917.

[12] Ayers 1916; Hall and Trout 1968.

limited by the technologies available and by the perceived risk from the bacteria commonly carried in milk.[13] Moderate heat will kill most microorganisms in milk that are of potential harm to humans: coliforms, salmonella, listeria, campylobacter, brucellosis, scarlet fever, diphtheria, typhoid fever and paratyphoid.[14] Higher temperatures are really only required for *M. bovis* and *Coxiella burnetii* but precision was beyond the early heat treatment plants, which were crude and unreliable. At first not all machines in Britain even had the ability to record the temperature of the milk they were processing.[15]

Returning to Denmark, in the 1890s Copenhagen's Health Commission found that their pasteurization equipment was neither efficient or effective. In 1899 twenty-three of their 389 samples of pasteurized milk failed the Storch test, indicating that they had not been heated to 80°C as prescribed for the 'flash' method then in vogue. This flash pasteurization technique was therefore refined from 1900 to 1905 in what came to be known as the 'Danish heater'. Milk was taken to a high temperature for thirty to sixty seconds by steam in the wall of a jacketed cylinder. The milk was then immediately cooled. In other designs the milk was pumped between cylindrical surfaces or through tubes that were heated by water or steam.[16] A disadvantage flash pasteurization was the loss of the cream line, a problem in the perception of many consumers.

In these early machines it proved difficult to ensure that all of the milk in a batch was heated equally and a survey published in 1914 found that forty-three per cent of flash pasteurizers in America were not being used at the specified temperature.[17] It is not surprising then that several outbreaks of milk-related infectious disease were traced to suppliers using this technology.[18] The flash method was eventually banned in the UK for drinking milk in 1923.

The city of Chicago was the first in America, in 1908, to impose compulsory pasteurization, followed by New York in 1910.[19] The

---

[13] Kay et al. 1953.

[14] Atkins 1992.

[15] Gofton 1931; Myers 1940.

[16] Kilbourne 1916.

[17] Ayers 1914.

[18] Hall and Trout 1968.

[19] Hall and Trout 1968.

following year the US National Milk Standards Committee argued for a regulated minimum time-temperature combination, 62.8°C for 30 minutes. This did not stick, however, and the next fifteen years saw many different temperature/time combinations adopted in American cities. The 'Endicott experiments' (1921-23) attempted to find an optimum solution, coordinated by Dr Charles North in six different laboratories with a view to providing the most comprehensive information to date on bacterial thermal death times. The industry's record was found to be woeful, with many machines not being properly insulated, having poorly calibrated thermometers, leaky valves, poor design of milk flow, and insufficient attention to the timing of holding periods.[20] But it was not until the 1927 follow-up publication of North and Park that a scientific consensus began to emerge. They suggested a temperature of 61.1°C held for a minimum of 30 minutes, which conveniently was the standard that had already been used by New York City and fifteen other large American cities for more than a decade.

Meanwhile the British in their Milk (Special Designations) Order (1923) required even more heat, in the band 62.8 to 65.6°C for the same time period, 30 minutes, with the batch then immediately cooled to 12.8°C. But there is nothing sacrosanct about these temperature/time standards and they were constantly reviewed as engineering and micro-biological knowledge progressed.

Following the widespread condemnation of flash pasteurization in the 1910s and 1920s, the alternative 'low temperature long time' (LTLT) technique was widely adopted. The original concept was again first developed in Denmark but it was twice as expensive per gallon processed as the flash method and was not used on a large scale until further refinements by Charles North in the USA in 1907.[21] North's design made possible the successful installation of a large facility that used temperatures of 60-66°C, held for thirty to forty-five minutes.[22] This was the 'holding' method that became popular around the world because it was considered more efficient in killing pathogens and did not change the taste of the final product as much as high temperature treatment.

---

[20] Westhoff 1978.

[21] TNA: CAB 27/230.

[22] Kilbourne 1916; Roadhouse and Henderson 1941.

The third major type of pasteurization was the High Temperature, Short Time (HTST) method, which was used first in 1923 but not added to the US Public Health Service Milk Ordinance and Code until 1933. The specification was 71.7°C for fifteen seconds. In the UK this technology was not allowed officially until the Milk (Special Designations) Regulations (1941) and then only because existing equipment was struggling to cope with demand. By the end of the war it was clear that HTST was superseding the holder method and its continued use was assured by the Milk (Special Designation) Regulations (1946).[23] There were some who regarded HTST as a retrograde step but its key advantage was that it allowed a quicker turnover of milk.[24] The machinery was also less bulky than the holder plant but as efficient.[25]

Savage, the aptly named, waspish commentator on dairy matters, was dismissive of the quality of pasteurized milk in the 1920s and 1930s. He reminded his medical audience in a 1931 journal article, for instance, that there was no obligation on UK milk dealers to declare whether the product had been heat-treated or how many times.[26]

In the period 1945-1965 only one out of 1,759 samples of pasteurized milk tested in the UK was found to contain live *M. bovis*.[27] But there were still plenty of examples in the 1950s of milk samples failing the phosphatase test, meaning that they had not been properly heated.[28] Although the risk was greatly reduced by the HTST process, it was not eliminated and there have been occasional alerts. As recently as 1998, for instance, there was a public health scare about *Mycobacterium avium subspecies paratuberculosis* - an alleged cause of Crohn's Disease - surviving pasteurization. As a result, the big British supermarkets decided to require their suppliers to increase the heating period from fifteen to twenty-five seconds at 72.5°C.[29]

The fourth type of heat treatment is in-bottle sterilization, which holds the temperature at 110°C for sixty minutes or 120°C for six

---

[23] Mattick 1944.

[24] Enock 1943.

[25] Society of Dairy Technology 1953.

[26] Savage 1931a.

[27] Wright 1967.

[28] Smith 1959.

[29] *Guardian* 12 August 1998, 4.

minutes.[30] At first this had a poor taste before the invention of the homogenizer in 1904 but the advantage was that sterilized milk could be stored for months and did not need regular daily deliveries.[31] It was most popular with working people whose houses often lacked storage for food.

Our fifth and final technology is Ultra Heat Treatment (UHT), which was developed out of HTST. It uses 285°C for fifteen seconds or 300°C for half a second.[32] UHT milk was introduced to the USA in 1948 but did not gain national recognition there until 1981. It has an extended shelf life of six to nine months, making it popular in countries such as France, Belgium, Spain and Portugal, but it has almost no traction amongst consumers in the British or American markets, where fresh milk is preferred.

The pasteurized milk supply

There was little heat treatment in Britain until the turn of the twentieth century because the industry was comfortable with its use of chemical preservatives.[33] With such additives coming increasingly under official scrutiny and public displeasure, pasteurization began to replace them in London from 1903.[34] By 1911 twenty per cent of that city's milk supply was heat treated in one way or another, increasing steadily to sixty per cent in 1922 and ninety-five per cent by 1932.[35] For the country as a whole only 1.5 per cent of the milk supply generally was pasteurized in 1926 but there was a lot of regional variation, as demonstrated in Table 5.1.[36] The majority of retail milk was still unpasteurized in 1939 and that remained true in many small towns and rural areas well into the 1950s.[37]

In Britain the driver for the speed of adoption of pasteurization was undoubtedly dairy company profitability far more than any public

---

[30] Lane 1933.

[31] Jenkins 1970.

[32] Lampert 1965.

[33] Hill 1943.

[34] Mackenzie 1899; Hope 1901; P.P. 1919 (Cmd 483) xxv.666.

[35] Tustin 1929; Seligman 1932; Wright 1933; Wilson 1942; Smith 1950.

[36] HC Deb 25 February 1926 vol 192 c698.

[37] Munro 1945.

Table 5.1 Milk pasteurization in big cities, 1933

	Total milk consumption (Galls)	Pasteurized under licence (galls)	Holder used but not licensed (galls)	Flash method (galls)	Percentage of supply pasteurized
Glasgow	65,000	9,500	38,600	8,790	87.5
Birmingham	55,000	13,750	-	2,750	30.0
Liverpool	45,790	6,193	7,597	150	30.4
Manchester	50,000	37,500	2,500	500	81.0
Sheffield	24,149	6,704	-	-	27.8
Leeds	22,000	5,700	900	1,500	36.8
Edinburgh	24,378	191	15,023	-	62.4
Bristol	18,680	8,657	900	900	56.0
Total	304,997	88,195	65,520	-	50.4

Source: Wright 1933, 3.

health concern. Just as in America, it was introduced as a means of delaying the souring process and thus increasing the product's shelf life.[38] McFadyean's apparently cynical interpretation was actually not far from the truth:

> If it had not been essential for the dairy trade of today (a series of large combines collecting milk of various ages over a wide area) to find some system whereby they could ensure delivery to the consumer in a sweet condition, it would appear doubtful that general pasteurization of milk would ever have come to the fore.[39]

Nevertheless public health monitoring of pasteurized milk did lead to technological developments that eventually brought this sector of the industry under control. The new methods were based on the realization that enzymes are eliminated from milk at specific temperatures. The first was discovered in 1881 and we now know of seventy in cow's milk.[40] Storch's test (1899) focused on peridoxase, one of the more heat resistant enzymes, and catalase was also investigated early on. But it was not until 1934 that Kay and Graham found phosphatase to be the best candidate because the conditions for its destruction by heat were very similar to those for *M. bovis*.[41] Phosphatase disappears at 71°C for fifteen seconds and *M. bovis* is killed at 70°C over the same period. The so-called phosphatase test therefore became vital in checking that pasteurization machinery was working properly.

[38] Macewen 1910; Shaw 1919.

[39] MacFadyen 1938, 148-9.

[40] Fox and Kelly 2006.

[41] Davis 1950.

Adoption of the test was slow in the UK, with many local authorities delaying to 1940, but Table 5.2 shows for the example city of Leicester that attention to the quality of pasteurization did eventually improve matters.

Table 5.2 The proportion of pasteurized milks in Leicester failing the phosphatase test

	samples	% unsatisfactory
1937	343	62.97
1938	1,811	10.77
1939	2,288	3.54
1940	1,749	3.95
1941	1,525	5.31
1942	1,173	3.67

Source: McHugh 1943, 113.

Sanitation discourse and clean milk[42]

Although in 1908 J.W. Green made one of the first claims that pasteurization would leave dirty production untouched, his statement was embedded in decades of discourse arising out of Victorian commentaries on sanitation.[43] In the previous ten years or so this particular framing had been deepened by visual evidence from mechanical milk separators which, in addition to dividing the cream from the skim milk, had produced a residue known as 'separator slime'. Now there was a measurable manifestation of the dirt in milk, and it was usually the farmer who was blamed, not just for dirty cowsheds and unwashed milkers' hands but also for a type of moral failing. Ben Davies picked up on this in his comment that 'if you are decent you cannot help producing clean milk'.[44]

The National Clean Milk Society (NCMS) was a major proponent of the need for certification. It was founded in 1915 by Wilfred Buckley and Waldorf Astor both of whom thought this would be the best route to a tuberculosis-free milk supply.[45] For them the use of pasteurization would have been an admission of defeat; clean certified milk was the best interim solution until the whole supply could be cleaned up.

The NCMS was involved in a wide range of activities. It sponsored

---

[42] This section draws upon Atkins 2010a.

[43] Green 1908.

[44] TNA: CAB 58/186.

[45] Buckley 1922.

a number of National Milk Conferences in the 1920s, at which the issues were formally debated, and it held meetings all over the country on the best methods of keeping milk clean in its journey from cow to customer.

The 'clean milk' argument was that farmers would have no incentive to produce clean milk if they knew the germs would be killed later when it was pasteurized.[46] Dirty and ramshackle byres would not be improved, the herd would stay riddled with a variety of diseases, including bTB, and the sale of stale milk would be sanctioned.

It was not until the Milk and Dairies (Amendment) Act (1922) and its accompanying Order that full and specific provision was made for certified milk. This included detailed definitions of graded milk, the introduction of bacteriological counts, and also a definition of pasteurized milk for the first time (Table 5.3). Despite this legislative activity, the government did not actually expect graded milk to become popular. The grades devised addressed the bTB problem either by heat treatment, by the veterinary inspection of cattle, or by tuberculin testing.

Table 5.3 Designated milks in the UK, 1923

- Certified – cows had to pass a tuberculin test and have a veterinary examination every six months. Bottled on farm but pasteurization not allowed. Not more than 30,000 bacteria per cc; no B. coli in 0.1 cc.
- Grade A (TT) – cows had to pass a tuberculin test and have a veterinary examination every six months. Pasteurization not allowed. Not more than 200,000 bacteria per cc; no B. coli in 0.1 cc.
- Grade A – Inspected every 3 months by vet and certified free of clinical tuberculosis. Pasteurization not allowed. Not more than 200,000 bacteria per cc; no B. coli in 0.1 cc.
- Grade A (Pasteurized) – Inspected every 3 months by vet and certified free of clinical tuberculosis. 145-150°F (62.8-65.6°C) for at least 30 minutes, then cooled to 55°F (12.8°C); apparatus to be approved. Not more than 30,000 bacteria per cc; no B. coli in 0.1 cc.
- Pasteurized – No veterinary examination necessary. Heating as for Grade A (Pasteurized). Not more than 100,000 bacteria per cc.

Source: Atkins 2010.

In 1924 only 1,400,000 gallons of Certified milk were produced in 1924 and 1,200,000 gallons of Grade A (TT). In 1926 graded milk still accounted for less than one per cent of consumption and in 1933 it was

---

[46] Green 1908.

produced by less than one per cent of the nation's cows.[47] One reason was that clean and designated milks had premium retail prices.[48]

It was not until the introduction in 1935 by the Milk Marketing Board (MMB) of a 1d producer premium per gallon that the situation was revolutionised by a supply-side surge. This was the introduction of Accredited Milk by the MAF.[49] To qualify for the Accredited roll, farmers had to submit their herds to six-monthly veterinary inspections and agree to the removal of any tuberculous cattle. In addition, their milk was tested at least three times a year and had to have less than 200,000 bacteria per c.c., and B. coli absent in 1/100 c.c.. Note that *M. bovis* was not included and confusingly was instead dealt with by a separate grade known as Attested milk.

In 1949 the Milk (Special Designations) Act and Orders insisted for the first time that all milk had to be graded. By 1954 there were only three categories: Tuberculin Tested raw milk, which came from herds attested free from tuberculosis; Pasteurized milk, which had to be sold in bottles; and Sterilized milk. Soon after the national herd was declared free from tuberculosis in 1960, there was no further need for the TT designation (from 1964), but technical advances enabled a new one of UHT in 1965.

To recapitulate, clean milk in the account above was not the same as milk free of bTB. The pious hopes of the NCMS that freeing milk of dirt and improving its bacteriological quality would also control diseases such as bTB proved to be wide of the mark. Incentivising farmers required a variety of cues and no market mechanism has ever been enough to clear the dairy herd of tuberculosis. That needed a ruthless area-based eradication strategy in the 1950s.

Medical argument: the example of the British Medical Association publicity case

Medical intervention in the pasteurized versus clean milk debate had profound implications, not least because the doctors appeared at first not to speak with a single voice.

---

[47] Newman 1926, Harvey and Hill 1936.

[48] Dixey 1937.

[49] See Chapter 10.

The quality of pasteurized milk in the capital was so low in 1908 that the Central Hospital Council for London decided that no hospital should take commercially treated supplies.[50] It was about this time that Great Ormond Street Hospital for Sick Children decided to pasteurize its own milk.[51] But probably the strongest point of resistance to pasteurization was the Infants' Hospital run by Drs Robert Mond and Ralph Vincent. They used only raw milk because, as Mond commented, 'it had been said that the man who heated good milk was a fool and the man who heated bad milk was a knave'.[52] His views were extreme, claiming that boiling or pasteurizing milk was 'responsible for the killing of a large number of babies'.[53] Vincent was also outspoken.[54] He argued 'that the risk of children contracting tuberculosis from the ordinary milk supply is so slight as to afford no justification for the "sterilizing" processes that have been so rigorously advocated in recent years'.[55] Vincent published his last paper in 1914 and died in 1922 but his anti-pasteurization views were still being quoted by the National Federation of Milk Producer-Retailers in 1933.[56]

As the technology of heat treatment improved, more doctors were won over to the possibility of eliminating some key infectious diseases, such as bTB in humans. By the 1930s and 40s the argument was not settled and one can occasionally detect the exasperation this caused in editorials in medical journals:

> Pasteurization is one of those subjects that tend to generate more heat than light. It is a great pity that medical men who oppose pasteurization support their case by misstatements of fact, or by ignoring those facts which are available to anyone who will take the trouble to spend an hour or two in a medical library. It is a pity, because their misstatements and ill-informed views are given much prominence in a press often

---

[50] *The Times* 10 February 1908, 10d; 19 September 1913, 4c.
[51] People's League of Health 1932b.
[52] *The Dairyman, The Cowkeeper and Dairyman's Journal* May 1923, 440.
[53] Mond 1914.
[54] *The Times* 24 September 1912, 8f, and 30 September, 4c.
[55] Vincent 1911.
[56] Letter to the Editor, *Manchester Guardian* 9 January 1933, 16, c.2-3: 'An American incident'.

enough, unfortunately, more anxious to please certain interests than to get at the truth of the matter.[57]

The continued opposition, although certainly in a small minority by 1930, gave a loophole to the policy-makers. Thus Earl de la Warr, then Parliamentary Secretary to the Ministry of Agriculture, in 1931 issued a call for unanimity before the state could be expected to intervene:

> The medical profession ... would also help the government if they would make up their minds as to what they really felt about milk. Before the medical profession come down on the farming industry for not taking certain steps about milk, they should really make up their minds what they wanted the farmers to do.[58]

From the early 1930s, however, a highly motivated group of eminent doctors and research scientists were actively involved in calling for pasteurization. Graham Selby Wilson, Professor of Bacteriology and the London School of Hygiene, and Viscount Dawson of Penn, the King's physician, seem to have been the coordinators. In particular they wrote letters to the *Lancet*, the *British Medical Journal* and *The Times*, and these were so widely quoted in the literature of the day that they certainly seem to have made the desired impact.[59] By 1933 the government's own advisers on medical policy were willing to state that 'it is clear that the only way of ensuring a safe general milk supply is pasteurization'.[60] Wilson's book in 1942 was also a major landmark, and was published in the same year as a MRC report warning of the increase of tuberculosis during the War.

Conclusion

Hooker argues that immunization and pasteurization were two of the earliest practices of preventative medicine explicitly based on the notion of risk reduction.[61] They became necessary following the failure of the sanitary model to deliver protection at the population level, and can be seen as a logical stage in governmentality. But, as this chapter has shown, the heat treatment of milk was slow to deliver on

---

[57] Anon. 1943a.
[58] Anon. 1931b, 387-88.
[59] Dawson of Penn et al. 1930; *The Times* 6 March 1934.
[60] Hamill 1933, 1497. Hamill was Deputy Chief Medical Officer.
[61] Hooker 2001.

its promises. At the technological level it cannot be said to have been reliable for the first four decades of its existence, probably into the 1930s. Finding designs that brought together the necessary elements, such as holding periods and accurate temperature measurement was an issue, but the socio-technical context was perhaps even more significant, depending upon the achievement of consensus about what constituted the criteria for safe treatment. For the majority of consumers in the UK, however, this Simondian individuation towards an affordable and reliable pasteurization plant was meaningless. It was not until the 1950s that killing the bacteria in milk was attempted for the milk supply in all regions and not until the 1960s that it was finally achieved. We will investigate some of the social and political obstacles to this roll-out in the next chapter.

Together Chapters 5 and 6 demonstrate the half century and more of uncertainty that was associated with the hardware and socially-embedded aspects of pasteurization. As the common milk supply remained heavily infected throughout this period, *M. bovis* had an extended opportunity to find its way past the lax controls in the UK food system. Its zoonotic possibility spaces, outside of London and a few other large cities, also expanded as the number of liquid milk consumers increased in the 1930s and 1940s.

CHAPTER 6:

ANTI-PASTEURIZATION DISCOURSES: RESISTANCE AND MODERNITY[1]

Probably no subject outside religion and politics has been the cause of more prolonged and bitter controversies than the proposal compulsorily to pasteurize all milk.[2]

Introduction

In governance research there is discussion of protests organized by social movements to counter the oppressive tendencies of the neo-liberal state, and there has also been work on everyday resistance, both intentional and unintentional, in the senses discussed by Scott and de Certeau.[3] Rose suggests that the latter may helpfully be theorised as reactive to a dominant discourse.[4] He deploys a Nietzschean dialectical approach to conceptualise spaces that are other to the normative and sees their long-term coherence as arising out of performativity. Speake shows that the resistance to milk pasteurization can, similarly, be seen through Rose's notion of an ideational regime. He focuses on the uncertainty surrounding germ theory and argues that pasteurization does nothing to solve that since it does not discriminate between pathogenic and non-pathogenic forms of bacteria. Instead the heating process is, for Speake, a form of obfuscation that 'strengthened the rationality for laboratory work, legitimising an empiricist, reductionist, monocausal approach to scientific theorising'.[5]

The present chapter, while recognizing the central role taken by processing technologies in the twentieth century, picks up this point about spaces other to the dominant discourse. It suggests that resistances to pasteurization in the UK were multiple and that they

---

[1] This chapter draws extensively upon Atkins 2000a.
[2] Davis 1950, 528.
[3] Scott 1985; de Certeau 1984.
[4] Rose 2002.
[5] Speake 2011, 530-31.

possessed sufficient aggregate power to delay the universal adoption of heat treatment and sow seeds of doubt in consumers' minds. The phenomenon was diffuse, however, lacking a core narrative. Evidence of an anti-pasteurization advocacy coalition in even a broad sense is absent and instead a series of separate positions emerged adducing discursive threads that in turn were nutritional, economic, environmental, cultural, spiritual, or political (Table 6.1). The only coherence to this amorphous

Table 6.1 The main pre-Second World War arguments against pasteurization

Sanitation
- Pasteurization may be used to mask low-quality or stale milk
- Pasteurization is an excuse for the sale of dirty milk and discourages the efforts to produce clean milk

Nutrition
- Pasteurized milk has a cooked flavour and is less palatable
- Pasteurization diminishes the nutritive value of milk - reduces vitamins (e.g. vitamin C) and minerals (e.g. calcium) made unavailable
- Pasteurization destroys beneficent enzymes, antibodies, and hormones.
- Pasteurization takes the 'life' out of milk
- Children and invalids thrive better on raw milk
- Cooked milk is likely to be constipating

Physical and Bacteriological Quality
- Pasteurization reduces the cream line
- Cheese is better when made with unpasteurized milk
- Pasteurization destroys the healthy lactic acid bacteria in milk, and pasteurized milk goes putrid instead of sour
- Pasteurization favours the growth of bacteria in the milk
- Pasteurization kills the bacilli in milk and leaves them to decompose when exposed to the air
- Pasteurization destroys nature's danger signal. It destroys the lactic-acid-producing bacteria and rather than turning sour normally, pasteurized milk turns putrid

Public Health and Safety
- Pasteurization is often inefficient and imperfectly pasteurized milk is worse than raw milk
- Toxins present as result of disease-bacterial action are not destroyed by pasteurization
- Pasteurization fails to destroy bacterial toxins in milk. With 'infected milk from udder infection the bacilli may be protected in particles of purulent or mucoid matter'
- Pasteurized milk may diminish resistance to disease
- Pasteurization, by eliminating tuberculosis of bovine origin in early life, leads to an increase in pulmonary tuberculosis in adults
- Pasteurization is unnecessary, because raw milk does not give rise to tuberculosis
- The death-rate from tuberculosis is lower in rural areas where all milk is raw
- Pasteurization would reduce the incentive to eradicate disease in cattle
- Pasteurization affects the disease resisting property of milk
- Pasteurized milk interferes with the proper development of the teeth and predisposes to dental caries
- Pasteurization produces scurvy and rickets
- Pasteurization reduces the fertility of animals fed on it and might lower the human birth-rate. 'The shadow of depopulation and national decline is looming in the near future'
- Pasteurization would lead to an increase in infant mortality
- The medical profession is not unanimous in support of pasteurization
- Pasteurization is not advocated by the Pasteur Institute

Economics
- Pasteurization will increase the price of milk
- Small dealers will have to buy pasteurizing apparatus or go out of business
- In rural communities the quantities of milk sold are so small that pasteurization is impractical and, anyway, milk goes directly and promptly from producer to consumer
- There are always some people who demand raw milk

Sources: Kenwood 1926; Menton 1930; League of Nations 1937; Sutherland 1938; Picton 1938; Wilson 1942; Hall and Trout 1968.

and complex whole was its embeddedness in the evolving modernity of early twentieth century Britain. This in itself tells us a lot about the way food systems by this time had come to stand in for wider truths.

There was a growing consensus among doctors in the 1930s in favour of the heat treatment of milk as a public health measure, but from 1900 to about 1930 the field was held by the anti-pasteurization campaigners. This loose grouping of interests was able to forestall or dilute all of the legislation that came forward. This was achieved by skilful parliamentary manoeuvring and a fortuitous combination of events that saw Westminster's attention focused first on the Great War and then later on a series of other major political issues. It was not until the Milk and Dairies Act came into operation in 1925, followed by the Milk and Dairies Order in 1926, that the pro-pasteurization activists began to regroup, using the need to eliminate bTB as one of their main arguments.

Nutrition

Immediately after the First World War, just when pasteurization was spreading in large cities such as London and Glasgow, science presented the anti-lobby with their best argument. This was the so-called 'newer knowledge of nutrition' and it confirmed the presence in milk and other foods of the micro-nutrients which came to be known as 'accessory food factors' or vitamins. Hopkins had worked on this topic from 1906 to 1912 but it was the further research of Eijkman, Funk, McCollum, Drummond and Mellanby that established the detailed implications, and by 1920 vitamins were becoming widely known as an important source of the building blocks of bodily healthfulness.[6] After this, milk drinkers gradually became aware of the micro-nutrients they were consuming, and concerns were raised about the possibly negative effect that pasteurization might have upon vitamins, along with trace elements, enzymes, antibodies, and hormones.[7]

This new perspective was added to existing culturally embedded views that were extensions of positive thoughts about mothers nourishing their babies and the cleansing whiteness of milk. The vitamin concept

[6] Hopkins 1912, 1913, 1919 and 1920; McCollum 1957.
[7] Plimmer and Plimmer 1922, 1925.

reinforced a mythology about milk being nature's most complete and balanced food, although after the age of six months this is far from the truth of course, with only vitamin B_{12} coming close to supplying in a glass of milk the recommended daily allowance required by the body for a particular nutrient.[8] Indeed, a large portion of the world's adult population lacks the intestinal enzyme lactase and therefore cannot even metabolise the sugar in milk, leading to stomach cramps and other side effects.

Doubts surrounding the nutritional impact of pasteurization upon milk were key to the debates about its suitability as a means of processing. The facts were so unclear until the late 1930s that we can characterise the argument in retrospect as one of mutually assured uncertainty. Already in 1909 Janet Lane-Claypon had claimed in print that heating milk had no negative impact on the nutrition of rats but these results were not considered to be decisive and subsequent confirmatory work over the next thirty years divided into two streams. The first was the laboratory research and animal feeding projects of the National Institute for Research in Dairying (NIRD) at Reading and the second was a number of experiments in school feeding.

The chief motivation of the Reading School was their belief in the need to produce clean milk. This and their early work on the constituents of milk led them to question the efficacy of the process and the results of pasteurization. In 1922 Williams and Mattick, for instance, brought out an anti-pasteurization paper in the popular magazine *Modern Farming*.[9] They deployed three arguments. First, they predicted that pasteurized milk would become a food of the poor, who would never be able to afford high quality raw milk, and who would therefore be deprived of its health-giving properties. This was because the pasteurization process at their time of writing was being used by the large dairy companies as a means of extending the shelf life of their cheap, and generally low quality, standard bulk milk. Second, there was the frequently heard charge of vitamin loss, and 'an infinity of other changes of which we have as yet no knowledge' because science had yet to scope all of the healthy properties of raw milk. Finally, they asserted that 'claims which have been made in this country that pasteurized milk has greatly reduced

---

[8] Claeys et al. 2013.
[9] Williams and Mattick 1922.

mortality from a disease such as epidemic diarrhoea are now proving to be fallacious.'[10] This infuriated readers from the other side of the argument, such as Ben Davies of United Dairies, who wrote in protest demanding the right to put the contrary view. His published comments were characteristically forthright:

> Every great cause has 'to run the gauntlet' when it is assailed in turn by every foe. Indifference, contempt, ridicule, prejudice, ignorance, as well as the prompting of rival interests all seek to bar the way. But in vain! Truth is great and will prevail ... So far from opposing it, dairy farmers should regard pasteurization as their great safeguard ...[11]

There were many animal-feeding experiments in the 1920s and 1930s in Britain and America. Overall the Reading work on pasteurization in this period was later summed up by John Golding, in his evidence to the Hopkins Committee, as having shown that pasteurization destroys certain of the enzymes and antibodies, 'the nutritive significance of which is at present not known'.[12] They also found lower weights and loss of hair (B vitamin deficiency) among rats fed on pasteurized milk.[13] Likewise there were negative results from American researchers in the 1920s, who found in their experiments that rats and children did not thrive on pasteurized milk.[14]

In 1931 the MRC was asked to initiate research on pasteurization.[15] Voices raised now included the MH and a question was asked in the House of Commons.[16] But Sir Walter Fletcher, as Secretary of the MRC, was resistant. Instead the following year he published under the MRC imprint a literature review of work to that date on vitamins in nutrition. This report includes a carefully worded statement that evidence of a deleterious effect of careful pasteurization upon milk's nutritive properties was 'not decisive' and concluded that 'it is in any case at present advisable to pasteurize the ordinary milk supply to prevent the

---

[10] Ibid.

[11] Davies 1923, 12.

[12] TNA: CAB 58/185.

[13] Mattick and Golding 1931, 1936.

[14] Daniels and Loughlin 1920; Daniels and Stearns 1924.

[15] See Chapter 5 for 1923 requests to the MRC for research on milk pasteurization.

[16] TNA: FD 1/1355.

spread of milk-borne diseases'.[17] This was a holding statement until definitive experimental results were published.

The second stream of work was with children. In the 1920s there were several attempts to establish the value of milk on the growth of school children, but the survey work of the most prominent study, by the Scottish Board of Health, drew criticism from statisticians for poor experimental design.[18] Then from 1934 to 1937 a comparison was undertaken of the nutritive value of raw and pasteurized milk on 8,435 school children sponsored by the MH and the MMB.[19] Waldorf Astor, as Chairman of the Milk in Schools Advisory Committee of the MMB, had originally suggested this project as a means of monitoring the nutritional impact of the Milk in Schools Scheme (MISS) and the research plan was devised by John Boyd Orr, one of the committee members.[20] From the outset there was a concern that the scientific planning of the survey should allow for a better sampling frame than had been available before.[21] This experiment was planned to be definitive.

The field research started in February 1935, with children in each school randomly divided into four feeding groups: biscuits only; one-third of a pint of pasteurized milk; two-thirds of a pint of pasteurized milk; and two-thirds of a pint of raw milk per day. 6,097 children were present at all four medical examinations and only their data were used in the final report.[22] Overall the results showed no significant difference in the nutritional outcomes of the children fed on raw and pasteurized milk.

Returning to Reading, the Milk Nutrition Committee also sponsored a series of feeding animal experiments on calves and rats at the NIRD and also at the Rowett Research Institute in Aberdeen. The results were published between 1937 and 1939 and demonstrated clearly that, although heat treatment reduced the vitamins B and C, these could be compensated for by supplementation (Table 6.2).[23] Once this was taken into account, there was no discernible difference between raw

---

[17] MRC 1932, 221.

[18] Corry Mann 1926; Leighton and McKinlay 1930; Pollock 2006.

[19] Milk Nutrition Committee 1937, 1938a, 1938b, 1939.

[20] TNA: MH 56/105.

[21] TNA: MH 56/105; JV/7/217.

[22] TNA: MH 56/525.

[23] Milk Nutrition Committee 1937-39.

and pasteurized milk for digestibility, growth and other nutritional considerations.

Table 6.2 The percentage loss of nutritional value when cow's milk is heat treated

	HTST Pasteurization	UHT
Vitamin A	0-5	0-5
Vitamin B_1 (thiamine)	0-10	0-10
Vitamin B_2 (riboflavin)	0	0-10
Vitamin B_3 (niacin)	0	0
Vitamin B_5 (pantothenic acid)	0-10	0-10
Vitamin B_6 (pyridoxine)	0-10	0-10
Vitamin B_7 (biotin)	0-10	0-10
Vitamin B_9 (folic acid)	0-10	30-50
Vitamin B_{12} (cyanocobalamin)	0-10	15-20
Vitamin C	10-25	30-100
Vitamin D	0-10	0-10
Vitamin E	0-10	0-10
Whey proteins	10	70
Lysine	1-2	4-13

Sources: Chapman et al. 1957; Hartman and Dryden 1965; Lampert 1965; Komorowski and Early 1992; Varnam 1994; Claeys et al. 2013.

Intriguingly the NIRD researchers were in effect contradicting the earlier work done in their own laboratories. In their 1937 paper Wilson, Minett and Carling, for instance, were explicitly dismissive of previous feeding experiments, arguing that 'none of them, in our view, definitely answers the main question at issue'.[24] The rapidly growing contemporary literature was thoroughly and impartially reviewed by Kon in the *Journal of Dairy Research*[25] and by the outbreak of war in 1939 the consensus was that, overall, 'no detrimental effect of any practical importance is brought about by holder pasteurization ... [the] fear that the nutritive quality of the milk was less than that of raw milk ... [was] entirely without scientific foundation'.[26]

This remains the received wisdom today, although our knowledge has grown. We now know, for instance, that the storage of milk in clear glass bottles leads to greater a vitamin loss than during heat treatment. About half of the riboflavin is lost in an hour, for instance.[27] Also, it seems that 'heating mainly modifies the functional properties of milk proteins (e.g. emulsifying and water binding properties, solubility), but has little effect on their digestibility and nutritional properties'.[28] Modern

---

[24] Wilson et al. 1937, 243.

[25] See also Kon 1972.

[26] Anon 1939, 1145.

[27] Schaafsma 1995.

[28] Claeys et al. 2013.

dairy chemistry textbooks underplay nutritional modification by heat treatment and stress instead physical changes such as the 'decrease in pH, precipitation of calcium phosphate, denaturation of whey proteins and interaction with casein, lactose isomerisation, Maillard browning and modifications to the casein micelle'.[29]

Commercial arguments from the milk trade

There was a variety of ideas about pasteurization from the milk trade, many of which were about hard-headed self interest. One might have thought that heat treatment would have been welcomed by all commercial operators because of its ability to keep milk 'fresh' for longer. But there was a hierarchy of enthusiasm. In 1933 Joseph Maggs, the Chairman and Managing Director of United Dairies, spoke for the larger companies, many of whom were already investing in the processing machinery and transport infrastructure:

> It is extraordinary that with such a safeguard as pasteurization available there should be any hesitation in enforcing its universal application. It is our view that the absolute guarantee of the healthfulness of the milk supply, however carefully produced, is to be found only in its pasteurization.[30]

Small and medium sized wholesalers and retailers were more wary of pasteurization. They opposed any machinery standard because of the investment required for upgrades and they preferred to do the processing themselves rather than see it concentrated in the hands of the larger dairy companies, with all of structural implications that would have had for their long-term prosperity. The London and Provincial Master Dairymen's Association, their representative group, was able to attract 600 of their members to a mass meeting in January 1923, so they were a voice to be reckoned with.[31] They also opposed the milk designation orders as imposing too much regulation.

In the industry's third tier were the producer-retailers, who dominated the market in rural areas, small towns and in some regions. In 1931 it was estimated that they delivered half of the nation's milk

---

[29] Tamime 2009, 168.

[30] *The Statist* 122, 1933, 635.

[31] *The Dairyman, The Cowkeeper and Dairyman's Journal* March 1923, 326.

supply and that most of their share was raw.[32] One point made was that farmers in financial difficulties were sometimes forced to retail their own milk but that this was time-consuming and many preferred to concentrate on their core business.[33] Any proposal for compulsory pasteurization would have borne down on the livelihoods of this group in particular. Most could not afford pasteurization equipment, let alone the running costs which were about 1.25-2d per gallon, thus cutting their retail margin.[34]

Thoroughgoing support for the producer-retailers came from the NFU, which recognised the strength of their grassroots voice and feared them as a potential rival if they ever organized separately. An example was the challenge to the Milk Marketing Scheme (MMS) that came from the producer-retailers in 1935/6.[35] Although the subsequent vote went overwhelmingly against the producer-retailers and in favour of the status quo, the NFU continued with its support, as it did subsequent to an unsuccessful legal challenge by the National Federation of Producer Retailers to the MMB in the High Court in 1937.[36]

The 'natural order'

As we will see, much of the ideological support for the anti-pasteurization cause came from the right wing, although both Matless and Whipple recognize that it is impossible to identify one ideological label because the 'reference points' for an ideal socio-political order included 'High Toryism, guild socialism, imperialism, [and] fascism'.[37] It is ironic then that those of this political persuasion should have found themselves supporting a producers' monopoly, the MMB, and seeking protection for small farmers from the market forces of a truly liberal order of free trade.

The inter-war period was characterised by complex cultural and ultimately political interpretations of environment, nature and landscape. These templates for judging the worth of modernization

---

[32] TNA: MH/56/88.

[33] Wright 1933.

[34] Anon. 1945a.

[35] *The Times* 18 May 1936, 20b; 27 July 1936, 19b.

[36] *The Times* 27 October 1936, 9d; 29 June 1937, 6a.

[37] Matless 1998; Whipple 2010.

and social change were mediated in a number of embodied ways that included views about the production of food and drink, its processing, marketing and consumption. In this section we will rehearse the five strands of this that together make a coherent story about a struggle to preserve an imagined world of order and quality in food systems.

(a) Neo-romanticism and anti-modernism

The environmentalism of the early twentieth century had clear roots in the dirt and disease-oriented hygienist discourse of the Victorian era. But it also had a new element of what Trentmann calls 'neo-romanticism', a bourgeois cultural movement that had offshoots in various countries.[38] The fresh air, hiking and healthy body ideas of the well-organized and highly popular German youth movements of the 1920s and 1930s had their parallels in Britain and inspired a broad-spectrum response across the class and political divides.[39] The Boy Scouts and Girl Guides, the Ramblers' Association, the Youth Hostel Association, the Order of Woodland Chivalry and the Kibbo Kift Kindred all represented in their own way a muscular interpretation of leisure in the open countryside, a new and institutionalised somatic experience of nature arising spontaneously out of civil society that amounted to an action-based lifestyle philosophy forging what for Matless is 'a particular landscaped version of English citizenship', a new set of identities which were mediated through the relationship between humans and nature.[40]

According to this logic pasteurization was wrong because it interfered artificially with nature and therefore challenged the position of humans in nature. Instead there should be a preventative and protective understanding of well-being. Breathing the fresh air of the countryside was appealing but in the 1920s and 30s there were other challenges to modernism that had an element of neo-romanticism.

A vital strand of neo-romanticism, was scepticism about modern farming methods such as the use of fertilizers and other agro-chemicals, the introduction of mechanized cultivation and machine milking, and the separation of the consumer from the farmer by corporate intermediaries

---

[38] Trentmann 1994.
[39] Jefferies 2011.
[40] Matless 1995.

such as large food companies or marketing boards. The anti-modern discourse here was subtle and complex, including themes as varied as the displacement of jobs in the countryside that forced migration to urban slums, the degradation of soil fertility leading to irreversible soil erosion, and opposition to the pasteurization of milk.[41]

Here we have the roots of the popularisation of organic farming by figures such as Lady Eve Balfour and Sir Albert Howard. They drew inspiration from the techniques of recycling organic matter but another input came from the theosophical teaching of Rudolf Steiner (1861-1925) on biodynamic farming.

Conford argues that organicism appealed to right wingers from the 1920s to the 1940s, whose interpretation of society through an organic analogy implied that functional hierarchies are somehow 'natural' and who saw ordinary people as 'biological stock'.[42] Rolf Gardiner and Lord Lymington, both from the hard right, were founder members of the Soil Association in 1945, the latter serving on its Council from 1947 to 1950.[43] Some of their fellow political travellers shared their ecological views, such as Jorian Jenks, agricultural policy adviser to Mosley's British Union of Fascists and a leading light in the Soil Association from 1947 to 1963.[44]

Lady Balfour, the founder in 1945 of the Soil Association, was especially critical of pasteurized milk, which she said was in the true interests only of the large dairy companies, who were enabled 'to sell milk several days old without the customer being aware of the fact', and of the dirty producers, 'for raw milk must be clean or it goes sour, only pasteurization enables the dirty milkers to get away with it'.[45] For her, 'pasteurization can never be a good thing in itself. It should be regarded even by its advocates as the lesser of two evils. The necessity for it, where it exists is a confession of failure. The aim should be to abandon the practice just as soon as the need for it - unhealthy cows and dirty methods - can be eliminated'. For most organicists pasteurization

---

[41] Lymington 1938.
[42] Conford 2005.
[43] Ibid.
[44] Moore-Colyer 2004.
[45] Balfour 1948, 210-11.

was criticized as a proof of the failure of modern farming.[46] It treated the symptoms and not the cause of the problem, which in their view was the over-intensification of production in conditions of dirt and disease, coupled with a disregard for the traditional principles of good husbandry.

(b) Vitalism and nature-mysticism

Another side of early twentieth-century environmentalism was its spiritual underpinning, what Matless calls nature-mysticism.[47] This entailed a reverence for the sublimity and wholeness of nature which extended from the transcendental contemplation of landscape to what nowadays would be called 'deep ecology'. D.H. Lawrence was an inspiration to many of his contemporaries with his self-confident Nietzschian individualism, and a strong bio-mysticism derived from Haeckel and Emerson.[48] Lawrence's philosophy was vitalistic, based upon a belief in the restless energy of the universe, and his novels stand for the preference of many of his contemporaries for the life force of the organic over the cold calculation of a mechanistic modern civilization.[49] In his favour Lawrence did not approve of domination and Trentmann argues that British neo-romanticism in general never became as extreme as the Continental versions which eventually lent support to fascism.

Lymington and Gardiner were fully aware of Steiner's work on spiritual science, including his contribution to biodynamic agriculture, and it is no surprise that their writings also had vitalistic overtones. Indeed, much of the anti-pasteurization rhetoric seems to have absorbed the notion of hidden energies and unknown qualities, to the extent that it was common to hear comments such as '[I] do not like sterilized or pasteurized milk, which [I] regard as dead milk'.[50] Even on a purely scientific basis it is (even today) possible to argue that heat treatment may degrade certain precious qualities that are unknown to science. Vitalists go

---

[46] Kerr 1924.

[47] Matless 1998.

[48] Bramwell 1989.

[49] Ebbatson 1980.

[50] Dr Kerr, Medical Officer of Newcastle in an after-dinner speech. *The Dairyman, The Cowkeeper and Dairyman's Journal* June 1924, 534-38.

further and claim that raw food contains living qualities that are above and beyond those of nourishing the body with calories, proteins, vitamins and minerals.[51] Enzymes were said to be among these.[52]

After all, milk is a complex substance whose organic chemistry is still not fully understood. It contains 100,000 types of molecular species, most of which have yet to be identified and studied.[53] Extending this point, there has long been an argument that the heating of foods may cause negative changes and that raw is therefore superior to cooked. One thinks here of John Harvey Kellogg (1852-1943) and his breakfast cereals and also Maximilian Bircher-Benner (1867-1939), who pioneered a balanced diet of raw vegetables and fruit.[54] The latter promoted raw food and carbohydrates over cooked food and animal protein, reasoning that they had a higher nutritive value than anything cooked. Although rarely discussed in this way, opposition to milk pasteurization is in practice a sub-set of food rawism.

Vitalists believe in a natural life force and see illnesses as embodied disturbances of this.[55] Cures are therefore best drawn from naturopathy, homeopathy and similar ideas. Interestingly the philosophical context was rarely evident when such ideas were expressed. In the early twentieth century it was possible to take for granted that 'some people are fond of using the phrase "the biological property of milk", and refer to milk as a "living fluid"'.[56]

Mother's milk is indeed the most vital of fluids, with its overtones of cleanliness (associated with its whiteness) and health-promotion. It was ironic that, as breast-feeding declined amongst certain groups of women in the early twentieth century, it was the substitute, cow's milk, that introduced the risk of bTB. Nor was it generally appreciated that the composition of the two milks is rather different, the latter lacking the species-specific immuno-globulins which give human milk its protective properties against infantile diarrhoea and certain other diseases (but not tuberculosis).

---

[51] Hills 1892.
[52] Lane-Claypon 1916.
[53] Singh and Bennett 2002.
[54] Meyer-Renschhausen and Wirz 1999.
[55] Bechtel and Richardson 1998.
[56] Davis 1950.

(c) Physical deterioration and eugenics

The depressed tone of much food literature at the turn of the twentieth century was influenced by a debate about the 'physical deterioration' of the nation, especially stemming from poor childhood nutrition and the debilitating effects of urban living. By way of example, recruits to the army were said to have been poor physical specimens who could not be expected to represent their country effectively in imperial conflicts such as that against the Boers in South Africa.[57] Such fears were later rekindled in the 1930s by Sir John Boyd Orr's finding that half of the population were undernourished.[58] Although politicians were keen to play such statistics down, there were many who saw the modernization of British society as a failure in terms of the living standards of a majority of the people.

Gradually the pessimism turned to thoughts of action and the eugenics movement of the 1920s and 1930s drew strength, not only from its enthusiasm for fresh air and exercise and from its obsession with notions of racial purity, but also from ideas about healthy and wholesome food.

It was the lot of milk to bear much of the ideological baggage about food and nutrition during this period. The eugenicists claimed that the vigour and fertility of the nation would be threatened by pasteurization, making milk into an unnatural substance.[59] In doing so they entrained any science showing that pasteurization modified the 'natural' constituents of milk. As we saw earlier, one example was the research at the NIRD, Reading, which seemed to show that rats fed on a diet of sterilized milk were unable to reproduce, and that those fed solely on pasteurized milk suffered from vitamin B deficiencies.[60] Sutherland claimed that, as a result of pasteurization, 'the shadow of depopulation and national decline is looming in the near future'.[61]

Writers as varied as Viscount Lymington and Sir George Stapledon were advocates of this view of deterioration.[62] For them whole foods,

---

[57] Dodd 1904; Gilbert 1965; Bayliss and Daniels 1988.
[58] Orr 1936.
[59] Sutherland 1938; Picton 1938.
[60] Mattick and Golding 1931, 1936.
[61] Sutherland 1938, 704.
[62] Lymington 1938, 1941.

including milk, unmodified by processing, were an essential part of national salvation, including milk, which if produced under the correct conditions would be free from disease and should not therefore require the intervention of pasteurization.

One final point should be raised on the theme of eugenics. It again relates to health at the macro-scale. The principle of inoculation was of course well understood in the early century but, despite many experiments and several false dawns, there was no reliable anti-tuberculosis vaccine for the human population.[63] It was therefore suggested by some commentators that milk with a small infective dose of mycobacteria might actually be beneficial in conferring some immunity on its regular consumers.[64] Any heat treatment which might kill these bacteria was therefore opposed as interfering with the only known practical mechanism of mass-inoculation.[65] In truth there *is* evidence that long-term exposure to bovine tuberculosis does indeed reduce morbidity and mortality (Marfan's Law) from the adult lung disease caused by *M. tuberculosis*, but the dose was of course uncontrollable and the risk therefore unknown. It seems that some parents deliberately fed milk to their young children in anticipation of such a benefit and they were indirectly encouraged in this by several eminent experts in the first half of the twentieth century who appeared to suggest that *M. bovis* was not seriously pathogenic in humans.[66]

The Manchester Referendum

Imagine the scene. It was a cold day in December, four days before Christmas 1932. The occasion was a Town's Meeting in Manchester's Town Hall in Albert Square, of the type occasionally held to discuss controversial issues associated with the Manchester Corporation Bills. But for this one 700-900 people filled the Great Hall. The *Manchester Guardian*'s reporter was clearly impressed by the theatre:

> The attendance which crowded into the large hall was unprecedented in its numbers. Not another person could have been accommodated and hundreds who wished to attend were unable to gain admission. The

---

[63] BCG was not commonly used in Britain until the 1950s.

[64] Lyle Cummins 1925.

[65] Bibby 1944.

[66] Cobbett 1917; Riviere 1917; Calmette 1936; Pritchard 1988.

meeting began at noon, and half an hour later qualified electors were pressing up the Town Hall stairways unwilling to believe they would be excluded. It was fully 2.30 pm when the meeting broke up and the intervening two and a half hours had been charged with excitement ... The trouble centred mainly round the proposal that all milk sold in Manchester shall be pasteurized.[67]

The meeting was described by the press as 'rowdy' and the pasteurization clause 'aroused stormy opposition, and it was with the greatest difficulty that the Lord Mayor could preserve sufficient order to permit of reasonable debate ... An elector, opposing the clause, declared it was all "scientific nonsense", adding that "pasteurization of milk and rendered it unfit for human consumption", a remark which had a mixed reception of boos and cheers'. [68] The crowd outside carried placards bearing the slogan 'pasteurized milk will kill your babies'.

The storm clouds had started gathering earlier in 1932, in January, when the MOH, Dr Veitch-Clark, had recommended that the local authority should make pasteurization compulsory throughout the city.[69] The Public Health Committee adopted this as policy and the full Council agreed, by fifty-five votes to thirty-seven.[70] About seventy to eighty per cent of the city's supply was already heat-treated and the councillors may well have thought that the issue was therefore unlikely to generate controversy.[71] They were wrong.

From 1899 Manchester's Milk Clauses had enabled the city authorities to trace any tuberculous sample back to the producer. But these powers were repealed on 1 September 1926, twelve months after the 1915 Act came into operation. After that they had to hope for action to be taken by the authorities where the milk was produced.[72] The Council was now trying to find a better solution. Part X of the Manchester Corporation Bill 1933 was devoted to the milk supply, insisting that only certified milk, Grade A (TT) milk, or pasteurized milk would be authorised for sale. The Council's case was that a high proportion of the non-

---

[67] *Manchester Guardian* 22 December 1932, 11, c.5.

[68] *Manchester Guardian* 22 December 1932, 11, cc 1-2.

[69] Public Health Committee, 7 December 1931.

[70] Against an amendment to delete the clause. *Manchester Guardian* 15 December 1932, 11, c.4.

[71] *Manchester Guardian* 7 January 1932, 12, c.1.

[72] TNA: MH/56/84.

pulmonary cases of tuberculosis notified in Manchester in the previous eighteen months was probably the result of consuming milk that, on testing, had been found to be carrying the disease (Table 6.3).

Table 6.3. The milk consumed by non-pulmonary tuberculosis cases notified in Manchester in 1931/2

Age in years	Cases	Tuberculous milk samples	Pure milk	Per cent consuming tuberculous milk
0-5	60	55	5	91.7
5-15	113	109	4	96.5
<15	141	135	6	95.7
All ages	314	299	15	95.2

Source: *Manchester Guardian* 20 December 1932, 11a

The local Ratepayers Council protested against the pasteurization clause on the grounds that the matter would be strongly contested in Parliament, and should be dealt with nationally, not at Manchester's expense.[73] Opposition to the clause came also from the NFU, the British Dairy Farmers' Association and their local branches, citizens groups and even some local Members of Parliament attempting to surf the wave of popular feeling. A factor was the likely negative effect upon producer-retailers, the kind of small farmer who would be unable to afford pasteurization machinery.[74] For historical reasons east Lancashire had many of these.

Especially active was John Newton, a County Councillor, member of Droylesden Urban District Council, and chairman of the Lancashire Diseases of Animals Committee. He later claimed credit for defeating the clause as a result of addressing a large number of meetings. Newton's populist stance was to reject the germ theory of disease and therefore any notion that milk was involved in the spread of tuberculosis. His arguments are summarised in Table 6.4.

The pasteurization clause in the Bill was rejected by a show of hands in the Town's Meeting so overwhelming that the Lord Mayor concluded that 'it is unnecessary to count, the resolution is obviously lost'.

Despite rejection of their proposals by the Town's Meeting, the Council decided to put the pasteurization issue to the wider franchise.[75] The Public Health Committee held a press conference at which their

---

[73] TNA: MH/56/85.

[74] *Manchester Guardian* 11 January 1932, 16, c.2.

[75] City of Manchester 1933.

Table 6.4. John Newton's arguments against pasteurization

- Those who wished to drink raw milk should not be prevented from doing so.
- Pasteurized milk was expensive.
- Large-scale handling led to the standardization of butter fat down to the legal minimum.
- The consumption of raw milk would lead to a decline in tuberculosis.
- The Royal Commission on Tuberculosis had 'only succeeded in producing their evidence by roundabout and unscientific means'.
- Milk is full of natural bacteria that are essential to life. Pasteurization would kill them, and milk would become 'a cemetery of dead bodies'.
- 'If you feed a child on pasteurized milk and nothing else it will die just as surely as if you give it poison'.
- Too much power would accrue to the wholesale trade.

Sources: Wynne 1928; Newton 1932.

Chairman, Councillor R.G. Edwards, made out their case. He was careful to note the endorsements of the Manchester Branch of the BMA and of the children's hospitals in the city. He also reminded the public that each case of tuberculosis which required sanatorium treatment cost the Corporation £15-16,000 a year, and so was a drain on the rates. Meanwhile the debate in the public prints continued and between December 1932 and May 1933 there were twenty-nine letters to the Editor of the Manchester Guardian about the pasteurization question, representing a wide range of opinion.

On 10 January 1933 a referendum was held on the Corporation Bill as a whole. Voters were asked to express their opinion of each of fifteen clauses, and fourteen were lost, including compulsory pasteurization by 29,637 votes to 15,004. One councillor called this a 'triumph for organised vested interests' because some wards had allegedly been flooded with leaflets once again using the catchphrase 'pasteurized milk will kill your babies'.

The Town's Meeting and the referendum had raised passions on both sides of the argument but the debate was not confined to Manchester. London and Glasgow were watching the situation in Manchester in the hope of emulating their stand on pasteurization but they were to be disappointed. The debate about pasteurized rumbled on for decades after this skirmish in Manchester. It was resolved in practice by the commercial logic of the dairy trade not by principled decisions by politicians.

Perhaps more interesting is society's seeming inability to deal with controversies of this kind. As Martin comments with regard to the clash about the fluoridation of water, very often such long-running disputes are characterised by non-engagement between the antagonists. They often ignore each other's positions, or cite the opponent selectively, and a stalemate ensues. Personal attacks on the integrity of individuals are common.[76]

Conclusion

In some European countries the debate and disagreement was curtailed. In the Netherlands, for instance, pasteurization was made compulsory in 1922 by Royal Decree.[77] Sweden followed in 1940.[78] In Britain the special conditions of the Second World War were a threshold and it was possible in 1945 to claim that 'the old debates on pasteurization were over'.[79] The balance of power had shifted decisively in the favour of those who advocated pasteurization and 'the "milk enthusiasts" had entered into their kingdom at long last'.[80] Gradually pasteurization spread in the 1950s from the large cities to the smaller towns and rural areas. Tuberculosis was becoming less of a threat and the Tuberculin Tested grade of milk was finally abolished in October 1964 as no longer necessary. For the five per cent of market milk that continued to be raw, the grade 'TT' was changed to 'Untreated'.

The postwar anti-pasteurization movement may have hoped to be left in peace as a niche market among consenting consumers aware of the risks they take, but they came under periodic attack from the 1950s to the 1990s. The pasteurization of milk was made compulsory in Scotland in 1983 and there were moves to extend this to England and Wales in 1989 and again in 1997-98 as a result of the international regulatory drive of the Codex Alimentarius Commission of the United Nations. The 1990s debate gained a great deal of publicity, mainly as a result of the activities of single-issue lobby groups such as the Campaign for Real Milk and particularly the Association of Unpasteurized Milk Producers and Consumers, founded in 1989. Several arguments were deployed, for

---

[76] Martin 1991.
[77] Swaving 1928.
[78] Francis 1958.
[79] Davies in Anon. 1945b, 340.
[80] Hammond 1956, 271-72.

instance about the loss of freedom of choice - less about objections to interference by the nanny state than the need to celebrate lifestyles where an individual's identity is drawn from conscious and informed decisions about risk-taking. Another is the point that there are far fewer cases today of contamination in raw milk than in eggs, poultry meat or even water. Technical, agronomic and regulatory advances mean that it is arguably possible now to produce a better quality unpasteurized milk than at any other time in history.

After a lengthy consultation process about the possible compulsory enforcement of milk pasteurization in England and Wales, the MAFF in January 1999 renewed its approval of 'green top' milk but at the same time increased the stringency of the hygiene tests it has to pass. This was no doubt intended as a means of squeezing the remaining producers by increasing their costs, but the debate continues because the issues underlying the state-inspired enforcement of food safety are so fundamental to the relationship between consumers and their food environment.

By 2014 the mood of UK regulators had begun to change. As a result of a movement that originated some years ago in Italy, the Food Standards Agency in Britain held a consultation on allowing unpasteurised milk to be sold from vending machines in shops. For some decades hitherto it has only been available by direct sale from a relatively small number of producers.

In other European countries the debate has continued, for instance in France where there is resistance from the producers and the consumers of raw milk cheeses and other dairy products. In America the interstate sale of unpasteurized milk was banned in 1987, but twenty-nine states permit raw milk to be sold off-farm and sometimes in grocery stores.[81] Taste, health and nutritional value continue to be cited by consumers as factors in choosing raw milk and the civil liberties argument plays well here as in other aspects of American politics.

It would be wrong to see pasteurization as an issue on its own. The 1920s and 1930s were particularly lively for dairy politics in the UK, with some bitter disputes about preferred directions of policy and regulation. Pasteurization, although important for many interest groups,

---

[81] Headrick et al. 1997; Weisbecker 2007.

was therefore just one discursive strand among many, and one that was intertwined - inextricably it seemed at the time - with others. There is a fuller history here still to write.

CHAPTER 7.

DISEASED MEAT AND BOVINE TUBERCULOSIS

Introduction

Chapters 7 to 11 will look at bTB policy in the UK in the period up to 1971. In addition to the standard sources such as newspaper and other media reports, the Hansard record of parliamentary proceedings, and official pronouncements and publications, we will call upon the unpublished archives of civil servants and ministers. One reason for this approach is that Martin Smith has argued that the policy-making literature, by concentrating on *observable* behaviour has given an incomplete picture.[1] Power is neither transparent nor easily measurable, not even in the documents of Whitehall departments held in the National Archives, but there at least we can see civil servants being candid in their discussions because they knew that they would be protected by a thirty year embargo on the release of the papers.[2]

These archives take us into the liminal intertextual world of the 'memo' or 'minute'. Following the successive handwritten comments one can see the twists and turns of opinion and advice which gradually takes on a collective form in which authorship is lost. The memoranda individuate and merge into an in-house consensus, the elements of which are present from the outset but the ritual of input, commentary, analysis, extension and technical expertise has to be played out. The outcome is not determined but there is a narrowing of possibilities as extreme views are excluded, often without ever being expressed.

Not so straightforward, but nonetheless providing useful insights, we will also use memoirs, biographies and official histories. By way of example, in his account of agricultural politics from a Whitehall perspective, long-term insider Harold Dale argued that before the initiation of the MAF in 1919 civil servants had a minimal capacity

---

[1] Smith 1993.
[2] Smith 1998.

to formulate their strategic vision. According to him, the predecessor body, the BoA (1889-1919), was largely hands-off with regard to active policy. They may well have seen themselves as representing the interests of farmers in Whitehall but they had little contact with the agricultural community.[3] He acknowledged an attention to infectious livestock disease forced by the Cattle Plague (1865-66) and pursued by the Veterinary Department of the Privy Council Office, formed in 1865. But was Dale right? No, according to the MAF's own official history.[4] Their claim is that there *was* a central strategic vision, particularly with regard to animal health, and that it was the government's vigilance that was responsible for various periods of restriction on the importation of live animals and the passing of a series of Contagious Diseases (Animals) Acts. With specific reference to bTB and meat, in this chapter we will add a number of dimensions of governance, the individual stories of which will then unfold in Chapters 8 and 9.

Diseased meat

It is generally supposed that by the mid-nineteenth century at least twenty to twenty-five per cent of the meat retailed in the UK was affected by diseases, including some such as tuberculosis that were dangerous to humans.[5] It is difficult to be more specific than that because of the sizeable unofficial trade in low quality and often diseased animals that was both unquantified and uninspected. We have to rely on the occasional flashes of insight to be found in the contemporary literature. For instance the veterinarian Charles Hunting reported that in 1847 he had conducted 3-4,000 post mortems of cows in London cowsheds and found over twenty per cent of them to be tuberculous.[6] A few decades later, in 1879, eighty per cent of the portions of meat sold wholesale in London's Smithfield market were said to have been from tubercular animals,[7]

---

[3] Dale 1939.

[4] Winnifrith 1962.

[5] Perren 1978, Chapter 4.

[6] NVA 1891.

[7] Carpenter 1879, 647.

and in 1881 an estimated ninety per cent of beasts inspected at the Metropolitan Cattle Market showed some symptoms of tuberculosis.[8]

There are two points to bear in mind before we accept such data at face value. First, the London slaughter figures refer to dairy cattle rather than to all animals. Many were from the city's cowsheds and it was suspected at the time that the infection of cows was heightened by the confined and intensive conditions in which they were kept.[9] Likewise in Glasgow twenty per cent of the 3,000 cows slaughtered between 1887 and 1889 had tuberculosis, but the figure for beef cattle killed there was much lower, at 0.45 per cent.[10]

For Britain as a whole, more representative, non-market data were gathered in 1892 when those animals suspected of suffering from a separate disease, pleuro-pneumonia, were slaughtered. Of these, 22.3 per cent of cows and nearly fifteen per cent of other cattle were found incidentally upon inspection to be tuberculous.[11] These approximate proportions of disease were then confirmed a decade later by the acknowledged experts Sheridan Delépine and John McFadyean, who suggested national averages for bTB of twenty to thirty-one per cent and thirty per cent respectively.[12]

Our second point to consider is that there were regional variations of disease incidence, with some cities - such as London, Liverpool and Manchester - suffering to a much greater extent than other parts of the country.[13] Table 7.1 shows that there were also variations in the exposure of consumers depending on where they lived. If they ate cow beef, as many did because it was cheaper, they ran less of a risk in Belfast and Blackburn than in Newcastle or Edinburgh. The logistics of the cattle trade played a part here because the large cities dominated the market for cows fattened after their useful life as milkers had ended. There was also the anonymity necessary for the widespread trade in low grade and diseased meat that eventually found its way into sausages and pies.[14] Eventually the railways made it possible to transport carcases or

---

[8] Behrend 1893. For more on diseased meat, see Waddington 2006.

[9] Atkins 1977.

[10] Anon. 1889a.

[11] [McFadyean] 1895b.

[12] Delépine 1899; McFadyean 1901.

[13] For more about regional variations in the incidence of tuberculosis, see Perren 1978.

[14] Waddington 2011.

Table 7.1 Cattle tuberculosis discovered at slaughter in the UK

Location of slaughter	Cattle slaughtered	TB (%)
Aberdeen, 1922-25	126,911	1.31
Ayr, 1924-48	40,111*	32.23
Belfast 1909-13, 1917, 1919, 1922-4	161,306*	15.00
Bellshill, Lanarkshire, 1904-08	2,179*	30.38
Birkenhead 1892-8, 1915, 1920	225,228	0.53
Blackburn, 1920	*	9.69
Bradford 1918-21	56,659	2.74
Bury 1911-25	52,292*	1.33
Croydon 1920	757	1.72
Dublin 1926	*	23.9
Co. Durham 1847	3-4,000*	20.00
Edinburgh 1890	27,769	0.65
Edinburgh 1919-30	30,000*	42.70
Edinburgh 1937	*	44.50
Glasgow 1887-9	3,000*	20.00
Glasgow 1889	52,000	0.45
Glasgow 1900, 1905, 1910, 1914, 1935, 1940, 1943	442,878	9.54
Halifax 1915	9,185	0.05
Liverpool 1895-6	4,321*	10.60
Liverpool 1913-16, 1918, 1920	95,950	1.02
Liverpool 1921-55	400,093*	21.82
London 1892	*	25.0
Edinburgh 1890	300	40.00
London (Metropolitan Cattle Market) 1881	*	90.00
London (Metropolitan Cattle Market) 1895-1901	500*	46.8
Ditto	1,238	4.69
London (Metropolitan Cattle Market 1929)	*	51.00
(City of London abattoirs) 1918-27	630*	33.33
Manchester 1895-6	367*	29.4
Newcastle 1917, 1919-25	158,700	0.68
Newcastle 1922-5	121*	78.0
Newcastle 1943	5,224*	47.5
Newcastle, Edinburgh, Cardiff 1946	*	42.38
Newcastle, Edinburgh, Belfast 1950	*	33.98
Northern Ireland 1949	600	33.50
Salford 1920	1,365	2.05
West Ham 1926-32	9,813*	59.51

Note: * cows only.

Sources: MOH Annual Reports; Creighton 1881a; RC1 1895; King 1901; Bibby 1911; Savage 1929a; Gofton 1925; Norris 1928; Francis 1947; Watts and Robertson 1950; Francis 1958.

even live animals quickly, and the larger meat markets then attracted an even higher portion of the national trade.

Table 7.2 shows similar patterns on the Continent. Again there is a large range, from high incidences of disease in northern European countries such as Denmark, Germany and Russia, to a lesser problem in Portugal and Yugoslavia. What we seem to have in both Britain and elsewhere is evidence of a disease that had two components in its spread. First there were clusters of bTB in the intensive pasture-based dairying zones and, second, infection followed the networks of trade, proving to be a problem especially for urban meat and milk supplies.

Table 7.2 Tuberculosis discovered at slaughter, Europe

Location of slaughter	Cattle slaughtered	TB (%)
Austria: Vienna, 1893-95	-	1.5
Copenhagen, 1888	-	16.3
Copenhagen, 1890-93	132,294	17.6
Copenhagen, 1895	-	29.7
Copenhagen, 1899	-	32.3
Denmark, 1924	150,000	30.0
France, 1914	-	10.0
Versailles, 1911	15,540*	11.1
Germany, 1904-07	-	17.9-21.2
Germany, 1917	*	28.4
Germany, 1924	*	30.8
Bavaria, 1895-97	200,000	5.0
Bavaria, 1898-1906	-	5.7-10.3
Berlin, 1890-93	142,874	15.1
Berlin, 1902	-	25.35
Kiel 1895-96, Leipzig 1897	19,144	47.5
Hungary, Budapest, 1899-1911	-	13.8-25.2
Italy, 1900	-	10-30
Luxembourg, 1910-18	-	23.4
Netherlands: Amsterdam and Rotterdam, 1896	-	4.0-4.2
Poland, 1938	-	8.0
Portugal: Lisbon, 1937	-	8.0
Prussia, 1895-97	800,000	12.0-14.0
Prussia, 1898-1906	-	16.1-23.4
Saxony, 1895-97	80,000	26.3
Russia: Moscow, 1894	-	7.2
Moscow, 1898-1908	-	30.5-37.6
Moscow, 1913 and 1926-29	398,549	38.6
Sweden, 1921-28	981,343	28.6
Switzerland, 1891-96	2,212	12.1
Yugoslavia, 1938	200,000	0.5

Note: * cows only.
Sources: RC1 1895; Legge and Sessions 1899; Salmon 1906; Hutyra and Marek 1912; Ernst 1914; TNA: CAB 58/186; Savage 1929a; Francis 1947.

Meat and the politics of bovine tuberculosis[15]

Regulatory performances with regard to diseased animals and their products remained largely at the local level until at least the First World War. The first thread of activity was in regard to the centuries-old problem of 'unsound' meat rotting due to poor hygiene or the absence of a suitable means of preservation. The common law was the usual remedy, particularly in nuisance and later in torts as that side of the law developed. In addition, there were ancient institutions such as the local courts leet - some of which had a carniter, or meat taster - and later the magistrates' courts, for challenges about meat quality.

These pre-modern local arrangements were at times overwhelmed by the sheer scale of the meat trade that grew in parallel with the rapid urbanization of Britain from the eighteenth century onwards. At mid

---

[15] This section draws upon Atkins 2004.

century the seizure of diseased meat was authorised by the Nuisances Removal Act (1846) and the Town Improvements Clauses Act (1847). Later, the Public Health Acts, 1867 in Scotland, 1875 in England and Wales (as amended in 1890), and 1891 for London, allowed for the inspection of meat and its seizure if unsound; but these powers were sparingly used and anyway their definition of 'disease' was that of the Contagious Diseases (Animals) Acts, which did not consider tuberculosis until the very end of the century.

In this early period vociferous local trade lobbies kept local MOsH off balance and were able to minimize the number of prosecutions.[16] Slaughtermen and butchers saw MOsH as ill-informed and it was certainly true that most of them were unfamiliar with the detail of meat inspection and even lacked textbooks for reference purposes.[17] Curiously government Ministers refused to acknowledge that any of this was a problem. It was Walter Long, Conservative MP and President of the LGB, for instance, who in 1904 declared that: 'the training which every registered practitioner must have received as a student is sufficient to render him competent to detect tuberculosis in a carcase'.[18] He did not consider it necessary to appoint specialist meat inspectors with veterinary knowledge as by this time was routinely the case in France.[19]

A second thread of meat politics in this period concerned epidemic disease amongst live animals on farms or in markets. The rinderpest in 1866 and subsequently diseases such as pleuro-pneumonia and foot and mouth were the subject of various types of compulsory slaughter policies, and much contestation arose as to whether farmers and cattle traders should be compensated and, if so, whether the funds were to come from local or central budgets.

Robert Koch's discovery of the tubercle bacillus announced in 1882 was a stimulus for political activity. An early skirmish came in 1883, when the Privy Council, pandering to trade prejudice, 'consulted' the Irish government about cattle tuberculosis, although there was no evidence at all that store cattle shipped from Ireland to Britain were any more infected than home-bred animals. In the same year the National

---

[16] Newsholme 1935.
[17] Brown 1901.
[18] HC Deb 12 July 1904 vol 137 c1359.
[19] Pattison 1984.

Veterinary Association (NVA) passed a resolution in favour of scheduling tuberculosis under the Contagious Diseases Act of 1878, and further approaches to the Privy Council on the same lines came in 1884 from the Yorkshire Confederation of Butchers' Associations and in 1885 from the town council of Hull.[20] Progress seemed possible in 1887 when Lord Cranbrook (President of the Council) and Lord Lothian (Secretary of State for Scotland) met with the Police Commissioners of Paisley, one of the most progressive local authorities with regard to animal disease, to discuss the possibility of Orders in Council to allow them to seize diseased carcases.[21]

Action did not follow immediately but a Departmental Committee (DC), which had already been planned to look at the problem of pleuro-pneumonia in cattle, was instructed to extend its brief to include tuberculosis. This enquiry was chaired by the well-known agricultural-ist, Jacob Wilson. There were 44 witnesses and the report in 1888 of this committee was a milestone in two ways.[22] Evidence was collected for the first time on the tuberculosis threat in the food supply and the committee recommended the scheduling of tuberculosis under the Contagious Diseases (Animals) Act. This suggestion was endorsed by the Veterinary Department of the Privy Council Office but controver-sially their decision was rejected by the successor body, the BoA, created in 1889.[23] They refused scheduling under the Act for six stated reasons: the problem of detecting tuberculosis in live animals; other diseases could be mistaken for tuberculosis; the threat to valuable pedigree herds if slaughter was indiscriminate; the valuation of cattle would be contentious; imported animals would have to be inspected, adding greatly to the burden of administration; and there was insufficient evidence that stockowners were willing to bear the loss and inconvenience of mass slaughter. But it seems certain that the potentially crippling cost of compulsory slaughter was the real inhibiting factor, because farmers would have received seventy-five per cent of the market value of each beast.[24] This issue of slaughter and who should pay went on to become

[20] Walley 1889; HC Deb 21 March 1890 vol 342 c1554.
[21] [McFadyean] 1888a; BPP 1898 (C8831) xlix. QQ.155-57.
[22] Wilson Committee 1888.
[23] BPP 1889 (C.5679) xxvii.10; BPP 1890 (C.5995) xxv.11.
[24] [McFadyean] 1895c.

a potent fuel of agricultural politics at the turn of the century and we will return to it later.[25]

Meanwhile, it was dead meat rather than live animals that was making the headlines. The so-called 'Glasgow case' in 1889 was symptomatic of the early sparring that took place between certain health-conscious local authorities and a profit-orientated meat trade that paid little or no attention to disease. It involved the Glasgow local authority successfully prosecuting a butcher and a meat wholesaler under Scottish legislation for illegally displaying diseased meat, thereby creating a modern precedent for attaching responsibility for quality (defined in terms of disease) to particular actors in the food system. As a result, the *Lancet* enthusiastically, if somewhat prematurely, pronounced the sale of tuberculous meat to be 'now illegal … even where disease is limited in distribution and the carcase otherwise apparently sound'.[26] The *Meat Trades Journal* claimed this case to be 'momentous in the extreme', and the *Sanitary Record* saw it as 'almost impossible to overestimate the importance of the decision given in Glasgow'.[27]

A heated debate was unleashed between the local state and the meat trade but the judgement also created friction between farmers and butchers. The latter wished to shift blame for unfit meat to the producers and discussed amongst themselves the possibility of requiring a warranty from their suppliers.[28] As we will see below, later in 1908 the fledgling NFU drew the initial impetus for its foundation from this breakdown in trust and from the perceived need to protect the interests of small-scale cattle farmers from an onslaught by the middlemen.

The associated discourse of trust, responsibility and regulation is a sub-set of a wider debate in the late nineteenth and early twentieth centuries that encompassed worries about the adulteration of foodstuffs and also the deterioration in food quality and healthiness that was said by some hygienists to have arisen from the success of increasingly intensive farming, linked to industrial processing and manufacturing.[29]

---

[25] BPP 1899 (C. 5679) xxvii.8-9.

[26] Anon. 1889b, 1314.

[27] *Meat Trades Journal and Cattle Salesman's Gazette*, 1 June, 1889, 12; *Sanitary Record* 1889.

[28] The legal status of warranty was an important legal issue. For a full discussion see Atkins 2010a, Chapter 8.

[29] French and Phillips 2000; Atkins 2010a.

The Glasgow Case

Q. I understand you first examined the carcase of the bullock?

A. Yes.

Q. Tell us what you found.

A. On the left side of the bullock the disease was pretty well defined and very red all over the lining of the animal, about six inches by eight, all rosy red nodules …

This was Peter Fyfe, a Glasgow Sanitary Inspector under questioning by Comrie Thomson, counsel for the local authority at the trial of Hugh Couper and Charles Moore for the illegal possession of diseased meat for sale as human food.[30] The case was brought under Section 26 of the Public Health (Scotland) Act, 1867, and was regarded by all concerned as a test case of both the will and the ability of the local state to impose the highest standards of meat inspection as appropriate according to current science.

The background was the extraordinary prevalence of diseased meat in the markets of large cities and a nonchalance about it bordering on complacency among most actors in the food chain.[31] In 1889, Dr George Goldie, MOH for Leeds, confirmed these fears when he claimed that 'I have no doubt that my town is largely fed on tuberculous meat'.[32] Amongst the general public, there was a suspicion that livestock owners and butchers were well aware of the problem but preferred concealment to costly remedial action. In the opinion of the Chief Veterinary Inspector for Manchester, 'it is perfectly easy to pass on to the public meat for consumption which is diseased'.[33] The problem was focused especially in small country slaughterhouses where 'tubered' meat was trimmed of all the visible evidence, for instance 'stripped' of the serous membranes, which often displayed tell-tale signs such as tuberculous nodules or 'grapes', before being sent on to poor city neighbourhoods for use in sausages.[34] The animals concerned were called 'mincers' because their meat ended up in sausages.

---

[30] Anon. 1889a, QQ. 27-28.

[31] For more on the Glasgow case and meat inspection generally, see Waddington 2006.

[32] Anon. 1889a, Q.3450.

[33] Holburn 1905.

[34] Simon 1863; *Annual Report of the Agricultural Department of the Privy Council Office on the*

Some cities employed specialist meat inspectors but on the whole these officials were modestly educated and many were even less *au fait* with disease symptoms than their employers.[35] It was not until 1899 that the Royal Sanitary Institute introduced a formal examination for meat inspectors, so very few were properly qualified at the turn of the century. A survey of meat inspectors in 1896 showed 191 employed by the London Boroughs and the City but only twenty-six in ten other English towns and cities and thirty-one in five Scottish urban areas. In Glasgow, policemen acted as inspectors until 1898 when they were replaced by qualified vets, and this professionalization of meat inspection was a trend that was found increasingly across Scotland and also on the continent.[36] Another survey in England in 1904 showed that, of 206 meat inspectors, only two were vets.[37] Those listed in London were mostly Sanitary Inspectors, whereas in the provinces they were Inspectors of Nuisances. Cities such as Liverpool and Manchester relied on former butchers, and the continuing absence of formal qualifications such as meat inspection certificates in the return suggests that most local authorities were still looking for practical rather than professional skills.[38]

The situation in provincial England and Wales was significantly behind that in other advanced countries, such as Belgium, France, Germany and Denmark, and it was certainly no match for the United States' meat inspection programme established in 1891 and formalized in the Federal Meat Inspection Act of 1906.[39] There is some justification therefore for Ostertag's arch comment that 'England, which is otherwise so well organized with regard to public sanitation and called the cradle of hygiene, is entirely without a regulated system of meat inspection'.[40] Part of the explanation for this may lie in the rivalry between the MOsH, who wished to retain their control over all aspects of public health inspection, and the veterinary surgeons, who, although they had all of the necessary practical experience to find evidence of disease in meat, were politically weak and lacked social status. The MOsH did not consider vets to be

---

Contagious Diseases Inspection and Transit of Animals … 1888, BPP 1889 (C. 5679) xxvii.9.
[35] BPP 1898 (C. 8824) xlix.343.
[36] Dunlop Young 1929.
[37] BPP 1904 (326) lxxxii.727.
[38] Waddington 2006.
[39] Roberts 1986.
[40] Dunlop Young 1929, 244.

competent to deal with matters affecting the public health.[41] But in reality their own administrative response was also inadequate because both they and their inspectors had a wide range of duties, and food was certainly not their top priority.[42]

In policy terms, the extensive debate about tuberculous meat and milk in the 1880s had little impact. This is evidenced particularly in the inability of lobbyists to have tuberculosis treated on a par with rinderpest, where a draconian policy of slaughter and movement restrictions had been tried, or pleuro-pneumonia, where restrictions on imported livestock were enforced with increasing stringency over time.[43] The point here is that threats to the profitability of this important industry had more effect on the minds of policy-makers than the, to them, more nebulous threat to human health.

The international scientific debate about diseased meat

As we saw in Chapter 2, gradually a consensus emerged in the 1880s that both infected milk and diseased meat were responsible for the development of the disease in humans.[44] A number of important International Congresses highlighted the problem of bTB. At the International Veterinary Congress in Brussels (1883), for instance, there was a campaign by Bouley to encourage the seizure of any whole carcase that contained even a small portion of diseased meat. Although passed by a majority of only one vote, this became a widely sanctioned policy, which was then re-endorsed at the subsequent congresses in Paris (1888, 1889), and London (1891).[45] At Paris in July 1888 Chauveau was President of the Congress for the Study of Tuberculosis in Man and Animals and he seems to have been determined that a full airing should be given to the work of Villemin, Cornil and others on tuberculosis as a zoonosis.[46] He achieved an overwhelming consensus, confirmed by a vote with only three dissenters, in favour of a resolution that 'there is reason to pursue, by every means, including the compensation of

[41] Koolmees et al. 1999.
[42] Creighton 1881b; Lydtin et al. 1883; Behrend 1893.
[43] Worboys 2000.
[44] For more on the scientific debate, see Waddington 2006.
[45] [McFadyean] 1888b; [McFadyean] 1891a; Arloing 1889; De Jong 1889.
[46] [McFadyean 1888b].

those interested, the general application of the principle of seizure and destruction of the entire flesh of tuberculous animals, whatever may be the gravity of the specific lesions found in these animals'. The following year, also in Paris, Chauveau and Nocard convened the Fifth International Congress of Veterinary Medicine, with 635 delegates, only four of whom disagreed with the collective statement that 'the flesh of tuberculous animals ... ought to be excluded from consumption by men or animals, no matter what may be the degree of tuberculosis and the apparent qualities of the flesh ...'.[47] The sentiment was similar in Paris in 1891, this time due to the 'vehement pleading' of Saturnin Arloing.[48]

The Paris Congresses were very significant. They influenced opinion in Britain to the extent that many experts changed their view from one of scepticism concerning the need for regulation of tuberculous meat, to one of firm conviction that whole carcases should be kept off the market even if only small amounts of diseased material were found. The Glasgow local authority was merely the highest profile example of such a Damascene conversion.

The tide in favour of restrictions on diseased meat was in full flood in July 1888 when the French government issued a decree.[49] They made bovine tuberculosis a notifiable disease and insisted that the entire carcase should be condemned wherever the tubercular lesions were not confined to the visceral organs and their lymphatic glands, or where lesions had erupted on the lining membrane of the chest or abdomen.[50] By 1892 there were equally strict laws in Prussia, Bavaria and Saxony requiring removal of a whole carcase when tuberculosis was generalized or the animal emaciated.

The Glasgow trial

On 9 May 1889 Peter Fyfe, a Sanitary Inspector, entered the abattoir in Moore Street, Glasgow, and seized two carcases. One, belonging to a wholesale butcher Hugh Couper, was of a bullock, and the other

---

[47] *Journal of Comparative Pathology and Therapeutics* 2, 1889, 369-86.

[48] Nocard 1895, 87-89; Legge and Sessions 1898.

[49] Stanziani 2005.

[50] [McFadyean] 1888c; *British Medical Journal* ii, 1888, 726.

was a cow owned by Charles Moore, a meat salesman. This apparently mundane incident proved to be highly significant in the history of the meat and livestock industries, and helps us to understand the evolution of this particular system of provision in Britain.[51]

The two butchers were asked if they would agree to the destruction (without compensation) of the carcases, both of which showed signs of bovine tuberculosis. They declined and were prosecuted under the Public Health (Scotland) Act of 1867, which prohibited the sale of meat unfit for human consumption. The Glasgow United Fleshers' Society paid Couper and Moore's £2,311 costs in the court case that followed in the hope that a favourable verdict would protect the future interests of all of their members.

The trial lasted four days. Unusually, the proceedings were published verbatim, and run to 414 pages of evidence, generated from 5,430 questions asked of thirty-five witnesses.[52] These were eminent doctors, veterinarians and MOsH, some of whom had travelled long distances from England. Overall this was a unique amount of effort for four sides of diseased beef but, in the words of Behrend, the case was 'epoch-making'.[53] This was because the trial was a step towards deciding two major issues: first, what is a minimum threshold of food quality that is acceptable; and, second, who in the food chain is responsible: the producer, the retailer, or the state?

The case hinged on whether the local authority had the right to seize a whole carcase that showed signs of tuberculosis, or whether the diseased parts should have been cut out and the rest allowed on to the market. Everybody seems to have agreed that the generalised tuberculosis found in emaciated beasts should mean full condemnation but expert opinion was divided in 1889 on the implications of disease localised to one small portion of the animal.[54]

The Glasgow local authority had not previously prosecuted meat dealers in this way but their MOH, Dr James Russell, took an interest

[51] The Glasgow case was also a significant event in the acceptance of the germ theory in veterinary medicine. Worboys 1992.

[52] Anon. 1889a.

[53] Behrend 1893.

[54] The 'entirely opposite opinions' expressed by scientists at the Glasgow trial caused alarm in the medical press. Anon. 1889c.

in the issue of tuberculosis in the food supply. He had earlier expressed his frustration at the lack of powers to deal with diseased, live animals and he had also spoken out in print on the contamination of milk.[55] No doubt at his instigation, the city's Public Health Committee met on 8 April 1889 and appointed a sub-committee on the inspection of dead meat.[56] On 26 April Chief Constable Boyd changed his orders to the police inspectors, instructing them to 'pass nothing [they] could see a speck of disease upon'.[57] Much hung on what was visible because, as evidence given in the course of this trial proved, there were still doctors and veterinarians who could not grasp the concept of microscopic infectivity and there were still others, not always the same individuals, who were unable even to accept the germ theory of disease.

Care and attention is still required even in modern-day meat inspection because the (occasional) discovery of dry caseous masses in the bovine lung, udder, pleura or lymph nodes is an indication of generalized tuberculosis, which may have reached the muscles due to a breakdown of resistance. Routine inspection of reactor carcases in the UK involves visual inspection, palpation and incision of lymph nodes (retropharyngeal, parotoid, submandibular/submaxillary, bronchial and mediastinal, hepatic, mesenteric and supramammary), as well as the lungs, pleura, liver and udder.[58] Nowadays about seventy per cent of an American meat inspector's time is devoted to necropsy, especially examining lymph nodes for the discoloration or morphological change associated with tuberculosis. In Australia twenty-five lymph nodes must be sliced and checked but there is evidence that even the most conscientious of abattoir inspections miss signs of tuberculosis.[59] In an experiment with one herd, the members of which were all tuberculin test reactors, signs of tuberculosis were found in only nineteen per cent by meat inspection in the abattoir but in fifty-two per cent under the most precise conditions of laboratory autopsy and histology.[60]

---

[55] City of Glasgow, Mitchell Library, MP20.597, 'Report by the MOH regarding animals apparently unfit for human food', 1885; Russell 1889.

[56] Mitchell Library, MP29.168, 'Minutes of Health Committee on the Inspection of Dead Meat, 1889'.

[57] Anon. 1889a, Q194.

[58] Food Standards Agency 2014

[59] Corner 1994; Corner et al. 1990.

[60] Corner et al. 1990.

The universal practice in England in 1889 was to require the removal of the visibly diseased meat only, but in Scotland local authorities were more aggressive. Greenock (since 1874), Paisley (from 1887), Falkirk and Edinburgh had for some time been destroying whole carcases with even the slightest signs of disease.[61] At the trial it became clear that the two Glasgow carcases would have been passed under the city's old rules, but the authority for the shift in policy was said to have come from science: 'no unbiased person fully acquainted with the evidence on both sides can entertain any other opinion than that the only course open to the Sheriff was to declare the two carcases in question unfit for the food of man'.[62]

In his judgement, Sheriff-Principal Berry made several important pronouncements. The first was especially significant, that 'the view that tuberculosis is communicable from one of the lower animals to man must, as the evidence shows, be considered an established scientific fact...'.[63] The judge went on to state that:

> my conclusion from the evidence is that this is not a sufficient protection against the risk of communication of the disease by ingestion. There may be no appearance visible to the naked eye of the action of the tubercular bacillus in a particular part of the animal, and yet it may not improbably be there ... The evidence leads me to the conclusion that it would not be proper to trust to cooking to be of sufficient protection.[64]

Again, this was a bold assertion and one that was not borne out by research. A few years later Woodhead reported that there was little danger to humans from tuberculous meat so long as it was adequately cooked.[65] It seems that the flesh of animals is rarely infected with tuberculosis to the same extent as the internal organs and cavities, and that the danger is therefore mainly in the offal or in the custom of feeding meat juice and raw meat to invalids.[66]

The third aspect of the judgement limited the universal application of the Glasgow case. Although Sherriff Berry commented that the

---

[61] Ibid. QQ.1258, 1911.

[62] [McFadyean] 1889a.

[63] Anon. 1889a, 409.

[64] Ibid. 411.

[65] BPP 1895 (C7703) xxxv.Appendix, Inquiry III. See also Waddington 2006.

[66] Francis 1958; P.P. 1896 (C. 7992) xlvi.QQ.1410, 1694.

present practice 'in various large towns in England' of stripping out tuberculous portions of carcases 'is attended with danger to the public health', he nevertheless felt that:

> I do not think that I require to take up the position that the carcase of every animal shown to have suffered from tuberculosis, however limited in degree or apparently localities, must be condemned ... The disease is shown [in this case] to have been not merely local. It was so far generalized as to extend to the lymphatic glands, and to parts which would have gone out into the market for food.[67]

In other words, the carcases under review were in a category midway between the extremes of having only local signs of disease and of being infectious in every part. McFadyean concluded that the 'decision has much less value as a precedent than it was expected to have'. This was because the trial came to focus on the need to condemn whole carcases of animals with generalized tuberculosis and not on advanced, localised tuberculosis.[68]

Overall, the Sheriff found in favour of the local authority, a judgement that was quickly picked up nationally. Although he claimed not to have read any newspaper accounts, he must have been aware of the publicity that surrounded the case. The *Glasgow Herald* in particular was responsible for stoking up public interest. From 20 April to 17 May it ran a fourteen-part analysis of the issues before the court hearing began, and then a daily report of the trial from 25 May to 21 June. Dugald McKechnie, counsel for Hugh Couper, saw this coverage as prejudicial to his client's interests, and he remarked that 'if I had a jury here, I would have asked your Lordship to call the *Herald* to the bar for publishing on the eve of such an important trial as this'.[69]

Post-trial developments

In retrospect, Sir Thomas Elliott, the Secretary of the BoA, identified the year following the Glasgow case as having been a hinge point. Before that his office had received representations from local authorities and public health societies wanting greater protection for consumers.

---

[67] Anon. 1889a, 412.

[68] [McFadyean] 1889b.

[69] Anon. 1889a, Q. 1,705.

But from then on there was a much greater interest from meat trade associations worried about the seizure of diseased carcases; also from veterinary surgeons arguing that tuberculosis could be prevented from getting into the food chain by establishing a better system of inspection; and from County Councils and agricultural associations, especially in Scotland, urging slaughter with compensation.

Around the country there was also much activity. In Glasgow itself, the local authority sent deputations to Manchester, Liverpool and Edinburgh to gather information on best practice in meat inspection, and they considered increasing the number of their own meat inspectors from two to five, under the management of a 'trained and scientific veterinary surgeon'.[70] The United Fleshers' Society and the Wholesale Butchers' Society immediately demanded representation on the city's Health Committee but the tide was running against them and they were unable to prevent preparation for the relevant clauses in the Bill that in 1890 became the Glasgow Police (Amendment) Act. Nor did they materially influence Section 284 of the Burgh Police Act (1892), which gave local authorities in Scotland powers to replace all private slaughterhouses with public abattoirs. This was gradually adopted over the next thirty years, leaving only the small rural slaughterhouses outside the fully regulated, city-based inspection system.

Following the Glasgow case, there was a tightening of meat control in a number of the other British cities that had inspectors. This was most feasible in what Anne Hardy has called the 'pioneering municipalities', which had a 'modernizing, forward-looking approach to public welfare'.[71] Liverpool, Belfast, Leeds and Newcastle began confiscating whole carcases where there was evidence of tuberculosis, but others remained lenient. Some vets and most farmers and meat traders criticized the 'excess of zeal' shown by a few MOsH.[72] They cited the uncertain science, which made the diagnosis of tuberculous meat difficult, even for experienced inspectors.[73] Most magistrates seem to have concurred because, of the 20,414 tuberculous carcases seized by MOsH between 1892 and 1895, only 2.13 per cent were actually

---

[70] Mitchell Library, MP20.601.

[71] Hardy 2002. See also Koolmees 2000.

[72] Dewar 1895.

[73] [McFadyean] 1891a.

condemned by the courts.[74] In the same spirit the President of the BoA, Henry Chaplin, rejected confirmation of the Glasgow ruling from the centre, claiming that he had no power over meat.[75] He is reported to have said that 'so far as he could learn, there was at the present moment an enormous quantity of meat of this description consumed daily throughout the country without the slightest harm ...' and that 'the question was more for scientists and experts than for the Board of Agriculture. After the experts have settled the question, then it would be for the Board, if necessary, to do their part'.[76] *The Times*, however, was critical of Chaplin's 'light, airy and superficial manner'. To them tuberculous meat seemed like a serious threat and they suggested that what they called the 'butchers' lobby' 'have effectively raised a question of vital importance to the community, and it cannot now be dropped until it is finally decided'.[77]

Such was the level of worry among the farming and meat trade interests about uncoordinated local action on diseased meat that they lobbied parliament immediately after the Glasgow judgement and their supporters, such as Lees Knowles MP, asked questions in the House of Commons and managed to force a short debate in 1890.[78] This was followed by a deputation of MPs to the Presidents of the BoA and the LGB. The influence of the Glasgow case is obvious here because of the several references they made to standards of meat inspection varying between cities. As a result of this meeting, the LGB, along with the Scottish Office, agreed to sponsor research on the effects of diseased meat.[79] This took the form of the first Royal Commission (RC1, 1890-95) on Tuberculosis, which was charged with the task of discovering the facts.[80]

The leader writer of *The Times* mocked the RC1 as 'an absurdity' and 'an admirable machinery for the production of delay'. In his view,

---

[74] *Return of number of carcases seized*, BPP 1893/4 (485) lxxvii.589; BPP 1895 (435) lxxxiv.1159.

[75] *Cowkeeper and Dairyman's Journal* May 1890, 113.

[76] *Meat Trades Journal and Cattle Salesman's Gazette* 1890, 104, 6-7, 9-11; *The Times* 22 March 1890, 11b.

[77] *The Times* 26 April, 1890, 11c.

[78] HC Deb 21 March 1890 vol 342 cc 1547-66.

[79] *The Times* 25 April 1890, 12a-b.

[80] *The Times* 22 March 1890, 11b and March 24 1890, 10c.

the reason that 'this commission dragged along its slow length for four weary years' was because politicians were 'professionally interested in the collective vote of the meat trade'. He argued that the scientific members, if they had been left to themselves, would have completed the enquiry in a 'small number of months'.[81] William Hunting, founding editor of the *Veterinary Record*, was equally scathing. He accused the government of negligence dressed up as 'extreme caution'.[82]

In 1894 the chairman, Lord Basing, died and was replaced by Sir George Buchanan, the recently retired Principal Medical Officer. The Commission was then reconstituted to hear the results of three strands of scientific research. First, McFadyean looked at 'the means of recognising tuberculosis in animals during life'. Second, Martin studied 'the influence upon lower animals of food of tuberculous origin' and was surprised to find transmissibility even when there was no trace of disease in the tissue. Third, Sims Woodhead went into 'the effects of cooking processes upon food from tuberculous animals'.[83]

Buchanan's final report, published in April 1895, commented that the Commissioners regarded the disease as being 'the same disease in man and in the food-animals, no matter though there are differences in the one and the other in their manifestations of the disease'.[84] They also found 'ample evidence' that the consumption of infected meat and milk could produce TB in humans. The tuberculous material in milk 'possesses a virulence which can only be described as extraordinary' and they concluded that this was the greatest risk factor, particularly in milk from urban cowhouses. Boiling would have been sufficient to minimize the hazard, as would the ordinary cooking process of meat, except perhaps in the deepest parts of large joints rolled for spit roasting or cooking in an oven.

Worryingly, McFadyean found that 'extensive tuberculous disease may exist in animals that appear, to his tests, to be in perfectly good health.'[85] This was somewhat misrepresented in the summary report, though, where it was [wrongly as we now know] stated that 'happily,

---

[81] *The Times* 26 July 1895, 9f.
[82] [Hunting] 1894.
[83] For more on the research, see Waddington 2001, 2006.
[84] BPP 1895 (C. 7703) xxxv.624.
[85] BPP 1895 (C. 7703) xxxv.627.

it can, in most cases, be detected with certainty in the udders of milch cows'.[86]

The RC1 also missed an opportunity in its report to set the intervention agenda in stating, somewhat disingenuously, that administrative procedures were 'beyond our province'.[87] The Commission also collectively undermined Martin's important comment that the careful slaughter and dressing of meat 'should be done under supervision' by suggesting that 'the difficulties of such supervision are so great that many years must elapse before any measure of an effectual kind can be carried into practice'.[88] Some years previously McFadyean had similarly found that healthy meat could be taken from tuberculous animals under aseptic conditions but that normal methods of dressing led to contamination from equipment and surfaces.[89]

The RC1's report was not released immediately, presumably because of the General Election that was looming in 1895. William Hunting, the editor of the *Veterinary Record* acidly commented that one reason for inaction, the stated problems of diagnosis, had now been removed with the advent of tuberculin (in 1890), but there had been no change of heart in Westminster or Whitehall. In his view 'everyone is sick of the prolonged exhibition of "how not to do it"'.[90] He later accused the government of being 'afraid to issue it [the report] lest they should be compelled to legislate on a difficult question. The Local Government Board seem to be as timid as the Board of Agriculture about tuberculosis'.[91]

The pan-European consensus about the seizure of diseased meat so painstakingly built in the 1880s began to crumble in the 1890s. Some of the earlier government decrees were repealed, for instance in Hesse Nassau because they 'have repeatedly given rise to erroneous action'.[92] Both Nocard in France and McFadyean in Britain had consistently opposed the seizure of whole carcases and it was their point of view that eventually prevailed at the International Congress of Hygiene and

---

[86] Ibid. 634.

[87] Ibid. 635.

[88] Ibid. 629.

[89] Pritchard 1988.

[90] [Hunting] 1894.

[91] *Veterinary Record* 7, 1894/5, 562.

[92] BPP 1898 (C8831) xlix.767.

Demography in London in 1891 and the Sixth International Veterinary Congress in Berne in 1895.[93] McFadyean went further and was one of the few commentators to publish 'a protest against exaggeration' in the tuberculosis-from-food debate.[94] He was convinced that there was little danger of catching the disease from eating infected meat.[95] For these views he was vilified by some of his colleagues for being 'a special pleader for a cowardly government' and as having appeared 'to minimize the importance of tuberculosis to agriculturalists and to consumers ...'.[96]

Lees Knowles was one of a number of MPs who took a continuing interest in cattle tuberculosis. It had been partly due to his pressure in the House in March 1890 that the RC1 had been established and in March 1896 he moved that another enquiry, of extended scope, should be appointed to consider the administrative procedures that had been largely excluded from its predecessor's report.[97] The LGB assented and commissioners for the RC2 (1896-98) were selected in July of that year. Sir Herbert Maxwell, a Conservative MP, was appointed chairman.

The 1898 Report of the RC2 was an interesting summary of the then current views on bTB (Table 7.3). The Commissioners recommended the systematic inspection of cows by local authorities, powers for MOsH to suspend the milk supply of a farm where it was infected, and the slaughter of obviously diseased animals with compensation only at their scrap value.[98] But they agreed with the agricultural interests that 'any proposal for stamping out tuberculosis by means of slaughter on the lines adopted with marked success in the case of cattle plague, foot-and-mouth disease, and pleuro-pneumonia, is quite impracticable'.[99]

On the one hand the Commissioners played down the risk from infected meat but, on the other, they were in favour of improved, standardised procedures for the seizure of parts of carcases or

---

[93] [McFadyean] 1895d; Anon. 1895b.

[94] [McFadyean] 1899b. He had made similar comments a decade before ([McFadyean] 1888d) and at the 1889 Glasgow trial. Anon. 1889a, QQ.2,823-4.

[95] McFadyean 1899c.

[96] McFadyean 1899d.

[97] HC Deb 21 March 1890 vol 342 cc 1547-55; 3 March 1896 vol 38 c126.

[98] *Royal Commission to Inquire into Administrative Procedures for Controlling Danger to Man Through Use as Food of Meat and Milk of Tuberculous Animals*, BPP 1898 (C8824) xlix.351.

[99] Ibid. 352.

Table 7.3 The principal findings and recommendations of RC2

- Agreed with RC1 that TB communicable from animals to humans.
- Did not recommend scheduling of TB in Contagious Diseases (Animals) Act
- Risk from meat exaggerated; much greater risk from milk
- Local authorities should have powers to erect public slaughterhouses and close private ones, and to require that meat slaughtered outside their district should be brought to a place of inspection.
- Rural slaughtering should be inspected and regulated by county councils.
- Meat inspection should be more general and systematic and inspectors should be qualified by training and examination.
- LGB should be empowered to prescribe the degrees of infection which cause a carcase to be seized in whole or in part.
- Notification should be compulsory for every udder disease of cows.
- Milk should be analysed and tested and milk vendors provide information on sources if required.
- Local Authorities should be required to regulate cowsheds and ensure that they are kept in proper sanitary condition.
- BoA should be funded to produce tuberculin commercially.
- No longer any doubt about tuberculin as a reliable test for cattle disease.
- The BoA should provide free tuberculin tests, with isolation of diseased animals.

Source: BPP 1898 (C. 8824) xlix.356-60

whole carcases (Table 7.4). This was because 'the widest discrepancy prevails in opinion and practice. Chaos is the only word to express the absence of system in the inspection and seizure of tuberculous meat ...'.[100] By a majority of one, the RC2 sparked a major controversy by recommending against compensation being paid to butchers for the seizure of tuberculous carcases.[101]

Table 7.4 RC2's guidelines for the seizure of tuberculous meat

Seizure of whole carcase only when:
- There was miliary tuberculosis of both lungs;
- There were lesions in the pleura and peritoneum;
- Tubercular lesions were visible in the muscular system, lymphatic system, or between muscles;
- Tubercular lesions were found in any part of an emaciated carcase.

Seizure of infected material when lesions confined to:
- Lungs and thoracic lymphatic glands
- Liver
- Pharyngeal lymphatic glands
- Any combination of above but collectively small in extent

Source: BPP 1898 (C. 8824) xlix.358

Crucially, the Commissioners found against the seizure of whole carcases and settled instead for cutting out meat with localized disease,

---

[100] Ibid. 344.

[101] Hunting 1899a.

thus ignoring the possibility of mycobacteria being present in the blood and lymphatic systems. Follow-up circulars from the LGB in 1899, 1901 and 1904, clarifying the issue of seizure, were based on this RC2 recommendation rather than the Glasgow case.[102] These stressed that 'measures more stringent than those advocated by the Royal Commission are not called for' and the LGB recommended that butchers who notify the local authority of diseased meat should not be prosecuted.[103] The latter point had been raised in a Select Committee on the 1904 Bill that we will discuss later.

The RC2 Commissioners thought it essential in future for all meat inspectors to be qualified by passing an appropriate examination. Their guidance to local authorities on the seizure of meat was now much clearer than anything that had been available before but it did not have the force of law and continued for many years to be interpreted very differently from area to area, to the extent that by the early 1920s there had developed a 'concentration of traders of inferior grades of meat in certain districts, where the standards of condemnation were less stringent'.[104] The recommendations on generalized tuberculosis were followed for a time, but by the 1920s:

> many of the best inspectors had long given up following that advice, as savouring of panic legislation ... It was gradually becoming the opinion of many that there was no justification for the wholesale condemnation which took place in some districts of carcases in localized bovine tuberculosis. Many inspectors reached the stage of using their own judgement entirely.[105]

Vested interests and policy-making about diseased meat

A withering attack on government was launched in 1895 by the *Veterinary Record*, which argued for a distinction to be made between 'benevolent neutrality and an active opposition' to change. In their view the BoA

> were not content to do nothing - they solidly opposed any movement, when the experiments with tuberculin showed this agent to be a reliable aid to diagnosis, the old objection, of veterinary inability to recognise

---

[102] *Veterinary Record* 17, 1904/5, 172.
[103] *The Times* 8 September 1904, 5e.
[104] Leighton 1927, 230.
[105] Ibid.

a large proportion of the infected animals, had to be abandoned and another excuse for inaction invented. This excuse still blocks the way, and every attempt to promote legislation is met with the statement that, 'the enormous cost of any effective scheme of suppression renders its adoption quite impracticable'.[106]

Moved to action by the stringent attitude of some local authorities following the Glasgow case, the meat trade embarked on a long campaign to protect their business interests. On the establishment of the RC2 in 1896, a delegation of the National Federation of Meat Traders lobbied the Presidents of the BoA and the Board of Trade and they also gave evidence before the Commissioners. Here they expressed their bitter resentment at what they regarded as an arbitrary threat to their livelihoods. Most rejected insurance as a solution. They preferred instead either shifting the responsibility to the farmer by demanding a warranty of freedom from disease for the fat animals supplied, or, alternatively, asking for compensation from the local rates or the central government.[107]

In 1899 there was another deputation to the BoA and LGB by representatives of eighty-three branches of the National Federation of Meat Traders, thirty agricultural societies and twenty-one MPs. This time the government was able to fall back on the anti-compensation decision of the RC2, and Chaplin, on behalf of the LGB, commented that the 'science was not at present sufficiently advanced upon the subject to justify them in making an experiment involving an expenditure of thousands of pounds'. He suggested insurance as the lobbyists' best option.[108]

The mental model of risk aversion implicit in insurance schemes is an indicator of the attitudes typical of modernity.[109] Life insurance was identified by Foucault as emblematic of the 'practices of the self' that emerged in the nineteenth century, but farmers were more reluctant to buy livestock insurance than they were fire insurance or crop insurance.[110] This was no doubt at least partly due to the collapse

---

[106] Anon. 1895a, 213.

[107] BPP 1898 (C. 8824, C. 8831) xlix.QQ.349-50, 441-7, 585; Perren 1978.

[108] Anon. 1899.

[109] Ewald 1991.

[110] Dean 1999.

of several cattle insurance companies in the 1840s and 1850s as a result of the insufficiency of their premium pots at times of crisis.[111] Informal associations of mutual assistance were an alternative and some tenant farmers were helped in extremis by paternalistic landlords. The notion never disappeared though that somehow the general taxpayer should compensate farmers, particularly for rapid fire epidemics such as rinderpest that seemed likes acts of God.

1899 was a significant threshold. It was the year that the BoA added bTB to the schedule of the Dairies, Cowsheds and Milkshops Order, implying a public interest in this particular cattle disease, and that was also the year when butchers were becoming increasingly aggressive in their views about disease. The Edinburgh Master Butchers' Association took the warranty option, for instance, putting the onus on the farmer or livestock trader for the supply of disease-free animals. Their colleagues in Cardiff did likewise in 1903.[112] Unsurprisingly, arguments over warranties led to ill-feeling between farmers and butchers, with occasional boycotts of markets by one side or the other.[113]

The year after the RC2's report, in 1899, the President of the BoA, Walter Long, made a widely reported speech to farmers in Newcastle. In effect he enunciated five principles that guided government action, or perhaps one should say *inaction*:

1. The data were still too indefinite and imprecise to justify asking parliament for public money for a slaughter policy or to subject livestock keepers to the inevitable financial loss.

2. There was no proof that a slaughter policy would eliminate bovine tuberculosis.

3. The Tuberculin Test could be fraudulently manipulated by the farmer.

4. Experts could not agree on the details of administering tuberculin.

5. Other forms of diagnosis, such as the veterinary inspection of udders, were not reliable.

In short, he suggested that

---

[111] Spinage 2003; Stead 2004; Matthews 2005; Matthews 2010.
[112] *Veterinary Record* 11, 1898, 391; 11, 1899, 391; and 16, 1903/4, 218-19.
[113] Wilson 1896/7.

> at present too little was known, too much doubted, for Parliament to be justified in imposing upon the country heavy expenditure on wholesale restrictions which would be strongly resisted in many quarters, and which might not do anything effectual for the extinction of the disease.[114]

The Secretary of the BoA, Thomas Elliott's, view was similar to Walter Long's: 'even if the adoption of stamping out were necessary, it would not be possible, and that if it were possible, it is not necessary'.[115] Such stonewalling must have been frustrating for a scientific veterinarian such as Sir George Brown - a member of the RC2 - but he was pragmatic about what could be achieved by government. At the 1901 tuberculosis congress, for instance, he commented in his capacity as Chair of the Veterinary Section that:

> I do not think there is any good in saying that certain regulations ought to be made, unless at the same time you can point out to us how ... I think ... the majority of meat inspectors throughout the country have never even read the report which contains [the RC2's] recommendations, and therefore cannot be accused of wilfully neglecting them.[116]

There were difficulties in establishing an efficient system for notifying the authorities of confirmed cases of bTB. At this time the BoA were opposed to compulsory tuberculin testing, and because of the cost they also refused to subsidise tuberculin for farmers.[117] In this they were supported by powerful vets such as John McFadyean, who argued that, although tuberculin was an adequate diagnostic tool, the cost of compensation would be too high: 'we cannot conceive of any sane person seriously advocating the compulsory employment of the tuberculin test on the entire cattle population of Great Britain ...'.[118]

Numerous attempts were made by MPs to introduce compulsion for local authorities to pay compensation for seized meat. In 1901 a private members' Bill was introduced, unsuccessfully, to the House of Commons to amend the law relating to the compensation paid for slaughtered animals, and four other, similar bills were tabled between

---

[114] This quotation is from a speech by Walter Long when he had been President of the Board of Agriculture. Delépine 1902, 239.

[115] BPP 1898 (C. 8831) xlix.Q.174.

[116] Brown 1901, 83.

[117] HC Deb 8 August 1898 vol 64 cc 544; 12 August 1898 vol 64 cc 904-05.

[118] McFadyean 1895c, 147.

1903 and 1906. They all had cross-party support and several MPs co-sponsored two, three or four of these Bills. The 1904 Bill, with support from the Central and Affiliated Chambers of Agriculture (CCA) and the meat trade, was the only one to reach a Second Reading but it also fell eventually because of opposition from MPs who wanted compensation to come from central rather than from local funds.[119] Their objection was on the lines of asking why should the slaughtering districts, usually in or near towns, meet the cost of disease originating in the breeding areas? The Lawson Committee reported on the 1904 Bill but their comment was that the loss to butchers was not great because most disease was concentrated in older stock of lower value and their recommendation was that mutual insurance should pay for half of any loss, with the other half coming from government.

Since the 1870s compensation for animal disease had generally meant a call upon Imperial funds: for instance for outbreaks of cattle plague, pleuro-pneumonia, foot-and-mouth, and swine fever. But in 1907 the Glanders or Farcy Order set a precedent of requiring compensation from the local rates. The government was starting to shift the centre of gravity of responsibility in anticipation of what was to come, an attack on tuberculosis in the national herd.

The question of compensation, either for diseased cattle or meat, became a chronic problem for successive governments over the next quarter of a century. Questions in the House began in 1899 and fending them off became a regular feature of the President of the LGB's performance at the despatch box.

The year 1908 was a flash point because the National Federation of Meat Traders' Associations adopted the Edinburgh model of demanding that suppliers should give a warranty of the health of their cattle.[120] This led to the formation of the *ad hoc* Tuberculosis (Animals) Committee, which stayed active until 1920. Chaired by figures such as Lord Middleton and the Earl of Northbrook, and supported by the eminent veterinarian John McFadyean, the Committee represented farmers' and landowners' societies from all over the country. Its first task in 1908 was to hear the butchers' case for protection from loss incurred when they bought healthy-looking animals, only later to have

---

[119] BPP 1912-13 (Cd 6654) xlviii.68; HC Deb 15 April 1904 vol 133 cc 327-47.
[120] Brooking 1977; Cox et al. 1991.

their meat condemned when tuberculosis was identified by the meat inspector. The Committee deplored the lack of cooperation between the farmers and butchers and proposed that they should hold a joint conference in London to air the grievances on both sides.[121] They, along with the CCA, were ultimately successful in negotiating a climb-down by the butchers but it was the success of their campaigning that made farmers feel empowered to think that they might be able to wield some political power if only they could organize on a national scale. As a direct result of this ferocious dispute about bTB in carcases, various regional groups of farmers joined together later that same year to set up the NFU.

The usual point that is made here is that the farmers and graziers realised that the CCA, despite its success in the 1908 negotiation, would always be dominated by landowner interests and that the voice of tenant farmers therefore needed to be heard separately. There is truth in that but what is usually missed is that this ongoing debate about diseased meat was not just about landlords versus tenants, or horn versus corn, nor even meat traders versus farmers. The furore over diseased carcases from 1889 to 1908 was much more about the relationships and relative power between the various actors in the rapidly evolving food system of Britain's highly urbanised and industrialised society at the turn of the twentieth century. The two major themes here were about quality and trust. Quality was largely vested in the materiality of the foodstuff under consideration. In this case, meat, there was not so much of a concern about adulteration as had dominated thinking about food systems for the previous 150 years. Milk was watered and bread alumed but with meat the issue was its perishability and its widespread contamination with disease. The deterioration of flesh with time could be dealt with through technological means such as refrigeration but disease could only be reduced by trusting the goodwill of all parties not to pass on tubered meat to the next person down the line. Frankly this was not really a public health concern for the stakeholders in the meat chain; it was more about whether they could trust each other and who should take the responsibility for any meat condemned in the market or slaughterhouse.

---

[121] *The Times* 9 October 1908, 9f and 7 January 1909, 8b.

The historical literature has yet adequately to address the issue of the conventions of trust that emerged in the food systems of the late nineteenth and early twentieth centuries. The present author has made a modest start on this in his work on milk.[122] He has shown that the legal concept of warranty was a major development of this period, evolving gradually through case law. As economic networks become more complex and no longer involve face-to-face contact, what Luhmann calls 'system trust' has to be forged through institutional and other mechanisms, formal and informal.[123] The Sale of Goods Act (1893) was one such step, introducing the idea that, in order to be mechantable, goods had to be of an acceptable quality.

Meat after 1908

Despite much lobbying and political manoeuvring, very little was achieved before 1914 in solving the problem of tuberculous meat. It took the disruption of the Great War to facilitate change, when the freedom of the meat trade was curtailed. During the period of hostilities butchers were allocated cattle rather than buying them on an open market and, as a result, they found it impossible to avoid diseased carcases. In recognition of this potential loss they were compensated out of central funds. A Meat Trade Advisory Committee was appointed in May 1919, under the chairmanship of E.H. Blake of the Ministry of Food, 'to consider and report to the meat trade advisory committee of the Ministry of food what steps should be taken to continue the system of insurance of livestock ought to provide for measures whereby compensation will be paid for meat condemned on account of tuberculosis or other diseases'.[124] Of the twelve members, five were from the National Federation of Retail Meat Traders, two were wholesalers, and one from the Cooperative Congress. The rest were civil servants from the Ministries of Food and Agriculture. As far as one can tell, this group met only four times and, given its composition, the conclusions were predictably concerned with the interests of the meat trade rather than the farmer or the consumer. The committee wanted compensation

---

[122] Atkins 2010a.

[123] Luhmann 1979.

[124] TNA: MAF 60/340.

for butchers who had diseased carcases seized and they criticised meat inspection system, alleging that

> the salaries paid are usually quite inadequate to induce the right stamp of men to take up the work. Meat is being inspected in many places by men who are perhaps of the right type for inspecting drains and dealing with sanitary matters, owing to previous connection with the building trade, but to have no real knowledge of the meat trade ...[125]

In 1920 the emergency wartime arrangements ceased and so did the compensation.[126] This caused disquiet in the trade and in June of that year a combined deputation of the wholesale and retail interests visited the MH.[127] Because the government was under pressure in the press and in parliament due a number of meat-related issues, such as decontrol, retail prices, and problems related to imports, an enquiry was set up in the form of a DC on Meat Inspection chaired by Sir Horace Monro.[128] The report of this Committee was completed in July 1921 and the Minister, Sir Alfred Mond, agreed to implement most of the recommendations the following March. The results were enshrined in Memo 62/Foods (1922), the Public Health (Meat) Regulations (1924), and the Rural District Councils (Slaughterhouses) Order (1924). This Memo gave detailed instructions on meat inspection and the most thorough definition yet of the meat that should be condemned.[129] The whole carcase was to be seized only when the animal was emaciated or there were signs of generalized tuberculosis. No compensation was to be paid to the butcher. The Regulations laid down conditions for killing animals and required any disease found by the slaughtermen to be reported to the local authority.[130]

One difficulty was in inspecting and controlling the abundance of small private slaughterhouses; there were 20,000 in 1927.[131] The municipalization of abattoirs, possible since the Public Health Act (1875), was one way of the local state gaining full control and imposing standards, but such slaughter facilities existed in only fifty towns in England and

---

[125] Ibid.
[126] TNA: MAF 60/340.
[127] Jackson 1956, 104.
[128] TNA: MH 56/65-67.
[129] De Vine 1927.
[130] Allen 1925.
[131] McAllan 1925; Collinge 1920.

Wales by 1899 and 100 in 1930.[132] Since 1849 the Scots had been aiming to emulate the German tradition of a public monopoly of slaughtering in cities, a process accelerated by the Burgh Police (Scotland) Act (1892). By 1910 sixty per cent of burghs had public slaughterhouses and in 1930 eighty per cent of home killed cattle in Scotland passed through these abattoirs.[133] Astonishingly this did not become common in England and Wales until after 1966, partly because of the political strength of the farming and meat industries.[134] Shirley Murphy, MOH to the LCC, for instance, had suggested the abolition of private slaughterhouses in 1899 but this brought complaints from the London Butchers' Trade Society, who argued that meat was not the main means by which tuberculosis was spread.[135] In 1912 the National Federation of Meat Traders threatened to sue any local authority that tried to close down a private slaughter house.[136]

For Savage, 1924 was a turning point: 'Previous to the passing of these Regulations it may be said that, apart from a few progressive districts, meat inspection in rural areas was non-existent'.[137] He would have preferred all premises to have been licensed but at least the slaughterhouses were now subject to bye-laws regarding structure and cleansing. He pointed out that in Somerset, where he was MOH, only five out of seventeen rural sanitary inspectors had a special meat inspector's certificate, yet they were the ones responsible for the regulations. Much more meat was condemned in the areas where the inspector had a certificate. 'It is obvious that unless an inspector possesses the necessary knowledge and experience, meat inspection is going to be a farce'. The time devoted to inspection also varied a lot: '… in many rural areas it is a fairly easy matter to deal with unsound meat and dispose of it without any inspection having taken place'.[138]

The Public Health (Meat) Regulations (1924) imposed new quality standards and provided a foundation for a new conventional relationship

---

[132] HC Deb 22 May 1930 vol 239 cc 590-91.

[133] Dunlop Young 1929; Koolmees et al. 1999; Leighton and Douglas 1910; Leighton 1927; HC Deb 21 February 1930 vol 239 c531.

[134] Koolmees et al. 1999.

[135] London Butchers' Trade Society 1899.

[136] *Medical Officer* 8, 1912, 1-2.

[137] Savage 1926a.

[138] Ibid 719.

between the various parties that lasted for forty years. The civil society of food producers, mainly in the form of a vast 'countryside alliance' of clubs, societies and campaigning groups, had been able to mobilise its social capital of contacts and fellow travellers, that inevitably drew in many rural MPs and various elements in Whitehall, to support the cause of the livestock farmer against having to give warranty of disease-free condition for fat animals being sold into a market or slaughterhouse. This had left the meat trade somewhat disadvantaged but they in their turn had fought and won a battle in Parliament to water down disease inspection regimes and to provide for financial compensation when meat had to be condemned.

In September 1937, Memo 62a/Foods provided an update on meat inspection but in truth the situation remained largely unchanged from 1922 to 1963.[139] A major difference, though, was that wartime conditions meant a reduction of slaughter houses from 12,000 to about 550. Although inspection was therefore easier, the costs were a burden to the smaller number of local authorities where these slaughter houses were located.[140]

In the 1950s, even though many tuberculous cows were being slaughtered under the nationwide eradication programme, it was rare to condemn whole carcases. The economic loss would have been too great and 68 per cent of the meat of diseased cows was passed as fit for human consumption.[141] The principle remains, a recent example being the careful butchery and excision of specified bovine offals that in the 1990s was considered sufficient to minimize the danger of BSE to the public,[142] although in practice cross-infection from contaminated abattoir equipment and surfaces has always been a risk factor.[143] According to the EC Regulations,

> All meat from animals in which post-mortem inspection has revealed localised tuberculosis in a number of organs or a number of areas of the carcase are to be declared unfit for human consumption. However, when a tuberculous lesion has been found in the lymph nodes of only

---

[139] TNA: MAF 35/313.

[140] Chief Medical Officer, *On the state of the public health ... 1939-45.*

[141] Francis 1972b.

[142] Smith 1988. The RC2 settled for cutting out diseased meat, but in doing so they ignored the possibility of mycobacteria being present in the blood and lymphatic systems.

[143] McFadyean 1890b; Pritchard 1988.

one organ or part of the carcase, only the affected organ or part of the carcase and the associated lymph nodes need to be declared unfit for human consumption.[144]

Since the Second World War the issue of tuberculosis in meat has disappeared as a matter of public concern. The 1955 Food and Drugs Act gave new powers of inspection to local authorities, but in 1958, when the definitive book on bovine tuberculosis was published, the basis of meat inspection was still essentially that of the Memo 62/Foods (1922). The 1963 Meat Inspection Regulations were an improvement, introducing the trace-back of tuberculous cattle to their point of origin and from 1974 tuberculous carcases have had to be notified – the responsible authority is now the Animal and Plant Health Agency (APHA) – and held until a Veterinary Inspector is called.[145] The regulatory framework is now that of the European Commission.

Conclusion

By way of a first conclusion, this chapter has essentially been about negotiated food quality in the context of relationships between actors constructed through the law courts and regulatory frameworks legislated in Parliament. Such conventions are by no means unusual but an interesting feature here has been the role of science. Between approximately 1885 and 1895 the theoretical consensus amongst vets and MOsH was in favour of the seizure of whole carcases that had even localized tuberculosis, although the practical application of this knowledge varied considerably. After that there was a shift to a much milder view of the risks associated with diseased meat, but the relationships between all of the interested parties, based before 1885 on a combination of ignorance and what amounted to a conspiracy of silence, had been destabilised to such an extent that there was no going back. After 1895 there were thirty years of guerrilla warfare between farmers and meat traders, and between traders and meat inspectors, before eventually the report of a DC in the early 1920s provided the basis for a series of compromises.

In retrospect the meat inspection experience in England and Wales

---

[144] Regulation EC 854/2004, Annex I, Section IV, Chapter IX.
[145] Pritchard 1988.

was significantly different from that on the Continent and for that matter also the evolving practice in Scotland. In the Netherlands, for instance, a national Meat Inspection Act was in effect from 1922 but not in the UK until 1966. The following also had systems of inspection: Belgium (1891), Luxembourg (1892), Germany (1903), Sweden and Norway (1895), France (1905), Spain (1905), Austria-Hungary (1908), Switzerland (1909) and Denmark (1911). According to Peter Koolmees, it was the countries with the strongest traditions of centralization that were most pro-active and able to drive through this kind of sanitary reform.[146] Food politics in Britain were different and their complex contingencies at least partly explain the painfully slow emergence of bTB eradication policy in that country.

A second conclusion from this chapter is about the spread of tuberculosis. We can say that bTB is at its weakest in an opened carcase or dressed meat. Its possibility space is narrowed because dangerous lesions are visible and can be removed. But there are also microscopic lesions that are invisible to the naked eye and these can spread infection if the meat is not thoroughly cooked. *M. bovis*'s great opportunity though came with the dishonesty of some farmers and butchers whose creation of a slink trade in diseased meat was a shameful episode that was extensive in time and space.

---

[146] Koolmees 1999.

CHAPTER 8.

TUBERCULOUS MILK BEFORE THE AGE OF PASTEURIZATION

Introduction

British agriculture was changing in the second half of the nineteenth century. Under pressure from imports of cheap grain from around the world, the nerve of arable farmers was tested from the 1870s, and the same icy chill of competition affected butter and cheese producers as factories in North America, Australia and New Zealand began exporting on a large scale.[1] Some English farmers were bankrupted by these unanticipated market shifts but their entrepreneurial cousins realised that flexibility of outlook was essential, along with the ability to adjust to new market conditions. In the specialist dairy and mixed farming regions, particularly those with ready access to a railway, this meant shifting into liquid milk, for which - coincidentally - there was a rapidly growing demand.

Throughout the twentieth century milk was the most valuable single commodity of British agriculture, with dairy farmers prospering further from the beef of their redundant cows and other minor enterprises such as feeding skim-milk to pigs and the breeding and suckling of calves.[2] Its peak came in 1938/9 with 28.4 per cent of gross farm revenue.[3] The rural restructuring in the late nineteenth and early twentieth centuries required for this achievement created new islands of dynamic change, particularly in the city regions and in corridors of the countryside within carting distance of railway stations. There was also a new sensibility in rural areas of a willingness to engage daily and directly with the urban sphere in a way that yielded a more integrated space-economy and a scaling up of cognitive connexions.

Milk producers signed contracts that by the end of the nineteenth

---

[1] Collins 2000.
[2] Taylor 1976, 1987.
[3] Mitchell 1988.

century demanded a lot of them in terms of quantity and quality. Consigning the morning's meal of milk was no longer good enough. It had to have a certain fat and solids-non-fat content and farmers had to breed and feed their cows to produce above a specified daily minimum quantity. This entrainment of nature was then supplemented by the imposition of commercially-inspired terms and conditions, enforced if necessary by contract law and developments in the common law. Farmers' awareness of these factors on a daily basis amounted for many of them to a new way of thinking and a lock-in to a regime of routine and urgency that would have been unknown to the previous generation.

The political ramifications of these changes were profound. One might think that the creation of legions of milk producers might encourage common cause. But under a regime of mixed agriculture it was difficult to mobilise farmers with multiple enterprises and therefore diverse interests. Profits may have been low – sometimes ruinously so during the recession from the 1870s to 1890s – but at least they had the possibility of spreading their risks across a diversified portfolio.[4] As dairying became more specialised, in the early twentieth century, however, milk-producing dairy farmers gradually became more of a force to be reckoned with, not only through sheer numbers but also because their political power was increasingly concentrated in certain key regions, such as the hinterland of the industrial northern and midland cities, and those parts of South West England having good rail links to London. Issues that seem to have resonated with them were (a) their relations with urban-based wholesalers; (b) debates with cattle dealers and butchers about responsibility for disease in carcases; (c) the cost and reliability of rail transport; and (d) tariffs on imported dairy products.[5]

By 1900 there were rural parliamentary constituencies in the producing areas where milk was an issue that candidates had to take account of and in turn the political parties needed a milk policy that would appeal to these rural voters. Then by the 1920s and 1930s there

---

[4] Fletcher 1961.

[5] Attitudes to the possibility of imposing tariff or quota restrictions on competitively priced imported foodstuffs were conflicted because many livestock farmers were more than pleased to feed their animals on cheap imported grains.

was an oversupply because so many farmers had gone into milk and new policies had to be adopted on a macro-economic scale to deal with this eventuality. In addition, the NFU, which rose to prominence in the very decade, the 1920s, of turmoil in the milk industry, needed awareness of the issues. For them, cattle diseases such as bTB were only a part of an overall picture that was principally about market restructuring.

The situation was further complicated by differentiation amongst milk producers. The important division for our purposes was between (a) those former cheese and butter makers in the deepest countryside who were fortunate enough to have a railway station or a milk processing [pasteurizing] plant close to hand, and (b) the so-called producer-retailers, who were generally small farmers close to a town or city. There were regions dominated by each of these groups, in turn having slightly different needs and approaches to their commodity. The producer-retailers, for instance, between the World Wars were among the principal opponents of pasteurization because they could not afford the necessary heat treatment equipment and were unwilling to cooperate with the middlemen offering them processing services at a price.

Manchesters of the mind[6]

Although tuberculous meat was the first object of policy debate in the 1880s, largely because of the visibility of the effects of disease, it was soon joined, in the 1890s, by milk as a result of the laboratory investigations made possible by the novel science of bacteriology. In the twentieth century this new avenue became the main means of understanding bTB and it was thoroughly and enthusiastically explored at two levels. First there was the micro-scale of the mycobacterium itself, through use of the microscope and of growth media in a petri dish. The second was the mapping of bacteriological results at the regional scale, providing an illustrative service to concerned local authorities. Manchester was in the lead on both levels for at least fifteen to twenty years from the mid-1890s, setting standards that were followed elsewhere.

---

[6] With apologies to Seamus Heaney, *Englands of the mind* (1976).

Story #1: Applied bacteriology and the public health

The story began in 1890 with the appointment of Sheridan Delépine to a chair in pathology and morbid anatomy at Owens College, Manchester. The job description was teaching on Diplomas in Public Health and Veterinary State Medicine but Delépine was energetic and entrepreneurial. In 1896 he used the practical experience he had gained to set up a laboratory capable of bacteriological consultancy work. Within twelve months five local authorities had signed up and by 1900 the laboratory was analysing 4,652 samples a year at five shillings each.[7] The steady income generated enabled new laboratories to be opened in 1902 and 1905. By the time of Delépine's death in 1921 his team were acting for 115 sanitary authorities: six counties, eleven county boroughs, eighteen municipal corporations, sixty-seven urban district councils and thirteen rural district councils.[8] This was industrial scale bacteriology and it was one reason why Britain became a world leader in the detection of pathogenic organisms in milk and other foodstuffs. In 1901 Delépine was made director of what was now called the Public Health Laboratory and in 1904 his intellectual journey was completed with a switch in the title of his chair to Professor of Bacteriology and Public Health.

Delépine began his bacteriological work on milk using experimental laboratory animals. He first tried inoculations with milk samples in 1892.[9] He used guinea pigs because when injected subcutaneously in the thigh they developed lesions quickly if *M. bovis* was present in the milk and the spread of these in the body was a function of the initial infective load of the sample.[10] Anti-vivisectionists focused their anger on these 'cruel' experiments but by the turn of the century the approach was seen as so effective that it was being tried in other public health laboratories.[11] There were wide variations in practice, however. Some gassed and dissected their guinea pigs at four weeks, others at six weeks.[12] The latter is likely to have given more positives but practically

---

[7] Davies 1899.

[8] Fiddes 1937; Stirland 1984.

[9] Delépine 1893, 1909.

[10] But, as Dixey 1937 later pointed out, there was no guarantee that the minute quantity used to inoculate the guinea-pig contained any tubercle bacilli that might have been in the milk.

[11] Loat 1938a.

[12] Pullinger 1934; Sutherland 1938.

speaking the longer period was inconvenient for the development of an efficient and cost-effective control regime. There was also attrition because the guinea pigs died from other infections and it was common therefore to inoculate two for every sample of milk.[13]

An alternative, histological method employed in Liverpool (from 1899), Sheffield (1902-11) and some other laboratories was the use of a microscope to detect tubercle bacilli on specially prepared slides of milk.[14] This rarely gave satisfactory results because the mycobacteria were not numerous enough to be seen on every slide unless the cow had advanced udder tuberculosis.[15] The county analyst of Somerset recognised that such microscopy was fast and cheap but argued that it was three times less likely to detect mycobacteria in a sample than the use of laboratory animals.[16] Centrifuging a sample before analysis sometimes helped and other methods were used to separate and precipitate the mycobacteria to enhance their visibility, for instance by Ziehl-Neelsen staining.[17] These early microscopic investigations were heavily criticised at the time and it was not until the 1920s that the cell groups characteristic of bTB could be properly identified at low magnification.[18] Later, in 1937, again in Manchester, Mary Cowan Maitland developed a microscopic technique, based on stained films of milk, which she claimed was as accurate as any other method, and inexpensive.[19]

A third approach at the beginning of the twentieth century, but again one that took time, was to grow *M. bovis* on media such as a meat broth with gelatine added to make it into a jelly, or on agar, which is a meat broth jellified by the addition of seaweed extract. The latter was particularly suitable because it did not melt and so could cultivate bacteria capable of growing at the temperature of living tissue in mammals (37-42°C). This method was used for distinguishing *M. bovis* from *M. tuberculosis* according to their particular characteristics of growth in the petri dish, and most frequently it was combined with the first approach.

---

[13] Gaiger and Davies 1931.
[14] Lloyd 1927; Jordan 1933; Wright 1929; Smith 1988.
[15] Delépine 1898.
[16] Wood 1930.
[17] Jensen 1909; Bishop and Neumann 1970.
[18] Delépine 1909; Hutchens 1914; Francis 1947.
[19] Maitland 1937; Ruddock-West 1937.

In the early twentieth century all three bacteriological methods had their critics. There were differences in sampling methodology adopted between cities, for instance, that placed question marks against their published data, in the early years at least, and therefore against the comparability of the series of different cities.

Using his guinea pig method, Delépine went further than just tabulating bTB in retail and station samples. He also kept a database of milk on a farm-by-farm basis geo-referenced with the aid of his colleagues, Manchester MOH James Niven, and CVO James Brittlebank. This provided detail in the countryside around the city (Figure 8.1) illustrating the clustering of bTB in Cheshire and the large proportion of farms in the city's hinterland that had had at least one of its milk samples shown to be tuberculous in the period 1896-1908.[20] Of the 1,385 farms

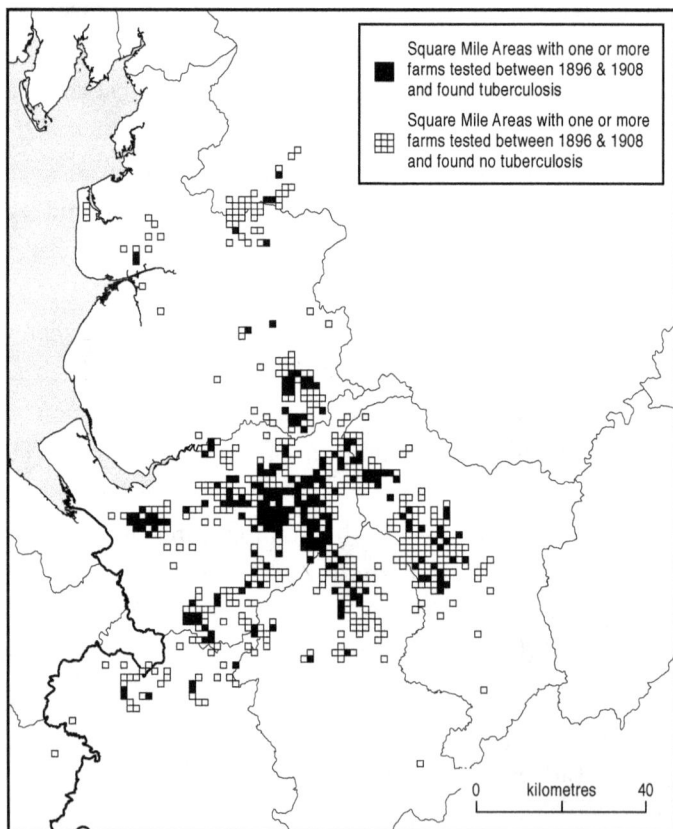

Fig 8.1 Tuberculosis in the areas supplying Manchester's milk, 1896-1908
(Source: Delépine 1909)

---

[20] Delépine 1909; Jones 2004.

tested in that period, 294 sent tuberculous milk, representing 7,669 cows out of 27,032. 276 of these farms were inspected by veterinarians and 68.4 per cent had cows with visibly tuberculous udders.

Bacteriology was applied increasingly to public health matters in the 1890s and the first decade of the twentieth century. In 1905 the LGB checked all of the MOH Annual Reports that were lodged with them and they found data on bTB in milk from Liverpool, Manchester, the City of London, Blackpool and Ilford.[21] Other cities were concerned but most did not have their own laboratories and so for a fee they sent their samples to wherever there was spare capacity. Table 8.1 is a compilation of laboratory results for the period 1896 to 1950 for over seventy cities and counties in Britain. As can immediately be seen, there was a lot of variation from place to place and also through time.

Table 8.1 Tuberculosis in milk samples

City/county	Dates	Samples	TB (%)	City/county	Dates	Samples	TB (%)
Aberdeen	1904-5, 1920-32	1,867	6.4	Lancashire	1924-7, 1929	2,511	9.4
Bangor	1932	103	2.7	Leeds	1904-6, 1913, 1920-30	1,499	4.6
Barnsley	1928-33	135	9.6	Leicester	1929	120	7.5
Bedfordshire	1929	16	6.3	Lindsey	1929	46	8.7
Belfast	1925, 27	352	3.4	Liverpool	1896-1950	43,909	5.5
Birkenhead	1929	81	4.9	London	1908-37	53,195	8.1
Birmingham	1907-45	38,271	8.2	London, City	1924, 1929	74	9.5
Blackburn	1896-1907, 1915, 1920-30	2,069	2.8	Macclesfield	1924-6	39	0.0
Bootle	1925	28	7.1	Manchester	1896-1937	19,747	11.4
Bournemouth	1925, 29	70	0.0	Middlesbrough	1925, 29	155	3.9
Bradford	1923-33	2,115	3.2	Middlesex	1929	277	7.6
Brighton	1915, 1928-37	737	9.2	Middleton	1926	29	10.3
Bristol	1896-1905, 1920-30, 34	562	5.1	Monmouth	1927	213	1.4
Burnley	1929	155	1.3	Newcastle	1913-37	6,819	4.4
Burton on Trent	1904-7	314	14.6	Northamptonshire	1929	39	0.0
Cambridge	1899, 1929	47	21.3	Northumberland	1927, 29	300	5.0
Cambridgeshire	1927, 29	130	2.3	Nottinghamshire	1929, 31	2,083	5.6
Cardiff	1920-30	682	4.6	Oldham	1932-33	14	0.0
Cheshire	1932-33	542	18.6	Plymouth	1924	11	18.2
Chester	1929	14	0.0	Portsmouth	1924-5	100	0.0
Coventry	1909-10	53	15.1	Reading	1920-30	282	11.0
Croydon	1900-21, 25	646	7.0	Reigate	1923-5	272	2.6

[21] TNA: MH/80/3.

Cumberland	1934-41	10,000	1.8	Rotherham	1930-33	145	13.1
Derby	1907, 09, 23-5, 29	247	8.5	Salford	1896-1906, 1913-16, 1920-33	4,808	8.3
Derbyshire	1915-26, 1932	141	7.9	Sheffield	1902-37	21,982	8.0
Dewsbury	1928-33	60	1.7	Somerset	1926-29, 34	1,104	2.3
Doncaster	1932-33	41	4.9	Southport	1902-20	724	8.2
Dorset	1926-7, 1929	336	4.5	Staffordshire	1929	1,238	6.0
Dundee	1922-29, 33	2,838	6.5	Stockton	1929	37	8.1
Eastbourne	1929	37	0.0	Stoke	1929	182	7.7
Edinburgh	1904, 1906-7, 1911-15, 1918-37	4,843	9.6	East Suffolk	1927-33	643	3.7
England and Wales	1929	14,235	6.3	West Suffolk	1929	6	0.0
Essex	1929-31	1,454	9.2	Surrey	1929	1176	3.4
Exeter	1929	16	0.0	Wakefield	1924-33	135	9.7
Glasgow	1908-13, 1921-5, 1928-37	8,031	4.9	North Wales	1933	109	2.7
Hebrides	1934	252	0.0	Warwickshire	1927	85	3.5
Holborn	1929	24	4.2	Watford	1929	158	0.0
Huddersfield	1923-33	955	5.0	West Hartlepool	1925-6	25	8.0
Hull	1924-30	467	6.4	Wiltshire	1929	223	10.3
Kensington	1929	26	0.0	York	1912-31	535	6.7
Kent	1929	96	4.2	Yorkshire, East	1929	156	5.1
Kesteven	1929	24	0.0	Yorkshire, West	1923-33	6,951	5.8

Sources: MOH Annual Reports; Fowler 1908; TNA: MH 56/88; National Milk Conference Committee 1926; People's League of Health 1932a; Fishburn 1932; Pullinger 1934; Savage 1929a; Hopkins Committee 1934.

The cities with the longest comparative series are Birmingham, Liverpool, London, Manchester, Newcastle, Salford and Sheffield, from roughly 1900 to the Second World War. For them we have a collective number of samples amounting to at least 500 a year and the astonishing result of tabulating them and calculating the proportion that were infected with bTB is that throughout these decades the series stays within the range seven to eight per cent on a three year moving mean, with a slight rising trend in the 1920s and 30s. This may sound counter-intuitive given the widespread concern about the disease at the time and one is forced to conclude that measures to control tuberculosis in cattle were failing. We are referring here to raw milk sampled by the authorities in transit to the consumer and no account is taken of the fact that some of this milk was later pasteurized.

The city of Liverpool differentiated between the milk it drew from urban cowsheds and that which came from rural sources. Of the eleven quinquennia in Table 8.2, all but three show a greater risk from the country cows, probably because the town cowkeepers were closely monitored by the city's inspectors. Liverpool, along with Salford and Manchester, also compiled complex databases of their supplies from outside their city limits. Table 8.3 hints at problematic counties where dairy herds were heavily infected.

Table 8.2 Liverpool samples, 1896-1950

	City			Country			All		
	Samples	TB	%	Samples	TB	%	Samples	TB	%
1896-1900	652	20	3.07	641	35	5.46	1,293	55	4.25
1901-1905	1,111	10	0.90	1,763	122	6.92	2,314	132	5.70
1906-1910	1,207	20	1.66	1,514	71	4.69	2,721	91	3.34
1911-1915	1,522	115	7.56	2,233	164	7.34	3,755	279	7.43
1916-1920	773	47	6.08	2,359	138	5.85	3,132	185	5.91
1921-1925	1,298	106	8.17	2,721	262	9.63	4,019	368	9.16
1926-1930	1,404	58	4.13	2,729	154	5.64	4,133	212	5.13
1931-1935	2,350	113	4.81	3,805	199	5.23	6,155	312	5.07
1936-1940	1,840	138	7.50	2,967	238	8.02	4,807	376	7.82
1941-1945	3,265	121	3.71	2,656	155	5.84	5,921	276	4.66
1946-1950	4,717	118	2.50	942	17	1.80	5,659	135	2.39
Total	14,874	866	5.82	24,330	1555	6.39	43,909	2,421	5.51

Source: MOH Annual Reports.

Table 8.3 The source of tuberculous milk received in three Lancashire cities

Source of supply	Liverpool, 1901-14, 1935-48		Salford, 1920-27		Manchester, 1901-47	
	Samples	% TB	Samples	% TB	Samples	% TB
Cheshire	5,030	9.01	1,193	11.2	12,188	12.45
Denbighshire	705	9.22	-	-	2	0.00
Derbyshire	-	-	-	-	3,371	9.14
Flintshire	373	9.12	-	-	-	-
Lancashire	1,122	8.47	829	4.2	2,377	9.13
Staffordshire	40	20.00	-	-	2,907	9.15
Shropshire	881	6.02	-	-	129	11.63
Yorkshire	24	0.0	-	-	308	6.80
Other	71	1.41	297	7.6	112	6.25

Manchester samples, 1901-38, 43-44, 46-47
Sources: MOH Annual Reports

Gradually the application of public health science to milk spread around the world, and in 1937 Marcel Gervois collected the results of 38,718 milk samples analysed in many countries.[22] From this it seems that the British were by far the most enthusiastic dairy bacteriologists but then we could say that they needed to be because they had one of the biggest problems. He found that the global average to that date was 6.9 per cent of milk samples infected with bTB, with Great Britain and

---

[22] Gervois 1937.

Ireland also at 6.9 per cent, and both the USA and Germany on 8.5 per cent. Gervois found analyses of 75,134 samples in Great Britain and Ireland but our collation (Table 8.3) for the same countries over a slightly longer time period manages 264,108 samples, with 7.12 per cent of them containing bTB.

One reason why bTB was so difficult to control was that milk supplies were often bulked when they sent from the country to the city. This sometimes entailed the mixing of milks in the churns that were used as containers on the early morning milk trains. But from the 1920s onwards large tankers were used, on road and on rail. The first road tanker was introduced in America in 1914 though in Britain the Scammell six-wheel 2,500 gallon road tanker was not deployed until 1926. This could carry the milk of up to 1,000 cows, and by August of that year the United Dairies were running regular deliveries the 177 km from Frome to London.[23] By 1927 the Great Western Railway and the London Midland and Scottish had each bought six rail tankers, the former used on journeys from Wooton Bassett to London and the latter from Calveley. The space savings were such that the length of train needed for milk specials was reduced by seventy per cent. The wagons weighed eleven tons and were glass-lined and cork-insulated. This allowed the milk to be cooled to 3°C.[24] By 1933 40 percent of London's milk was being transported in tankers.[25]

There were disadvantages with such large batches. Pullinger showed this in 1934 when he took sixty-three samples from rail tankers at seven depots. He found that every one of the tankers contained live *M. bovis*.[26] The point here is that if only one cow was diseased and excreting mycobacteria then the whole batch was contaminated because tuberculous milk can be diluted 10,000-1,000,000 times and still be infective.[27] Infected cows may intermittently excrete up to five million bacilli per millilitre and one cow can therefore contaminate the milk of 100 other cows. Some commentators thought that the dilution of

---

[23] *Modern Transport* 28 August 1926; Forrester 1927; Roadhouse and Henderson 1941; Davis 1950.

[24] Anon. 1927.

[25] London County Council 1933.

[26] Pullinger 1934.

[27] Forrester 1927; Francis 1947; Kaplan et al. 1962; Kleeberg 1984.

mixing would reduce the risk of disease but the opposite was true.[28] The Department of Health for Scotland found that sixteen per cent of ordinary mixed milk contained *M. bovis*, 37.5 per cent of samples from bulk tankers, and 51.9 per cent in tankers containing over 300 gallons.[29] This was backed up by sampling in England from 1940 to 1952. While 17.5 per cent of ordinary tanker milk contained mycobacteria, the proportion for ordinary milk was 3.4 per cent; Accredited milk 3.7 per cent; TT herd milk 0.5 per cent; holder pasteurized milk 0.16 per cent; HTST pasteurized milk 0.04 per cent; and pasteurized TT milk 0.0 per cent.

This first story has been about the emergence of expertise in knowing the extent of bTB infection in milk. On reflection it is easy to be carried away by the new science of bacteriology and by its 'invention' of the data series that were the raw material of public health activists. Here we have an insight into how milk sampling, laboratory techniques, guinea pigs, and MOH annual reports together formed an assemblage that demanded action and eventually linked forward into arguments for heat treatment technologies and other administrative measures to minimize risk. Looking back this story seems to be mundane but in reality the positioning of health arguments required the deployment of many different strains of argument and the building of networks of allies, from petri dishes and microscopes to paper reports. We know that the outcome was not certain because so many local authorities refused or failed to act, right into the 1950s. Overall we might say that, while bacteriological performances were key to the fight against bTB, it is also true that milk was such an important throughput of all public health laboratories that they were the testing ground of modern bacteriological expertise. Without the disease the history of this particular science would have been very different.

Story #2: the Manchester Milk Clauses

We have already discussed the pre-1914 policy furore associated with tuberculous carcases and meat. Once it was realised, from the 1890s,

---

[28] Gofton 1931.

[29] Department of Health for Scotland 1933.

that milk was also heavily implicated in the spread of bTB, three strands of response began to develop.

The first was the idea that the conditions of milk production were crucial. The certified milk movement in America was already well established by the turn of the century, although its emphasis was upon 'clean' milk rather than offering any guarantee of freedom from *M. bovis*.[30] More relevant for us was the initiative in Denmark of the Copenhagen Milk Supply Company, established in 1879. The 6,000 cows on its forty supplying farms were visited fortnightly by the seven vets in the company's employ and there were also health checks for the milkers and the company's own 400 employees.[31] There were a few attempts in Britain to emulate this model, for instance the Manchester Pure Milk Company (1898-1902), guaranteeing a tuberculosis-free product, but none survived for long because the premium retail price restricted the market. The idea lived on in the clean milk movement that acted as a counterweight to the introduction of pasteurization. It was also supplemented after the First World War by the notion of graded milk, with one grade being described as Tuberculin Tested. Again this played to a very small audience of those able to afford the premium charges.[32]

The second and third ideas were divided by the Atlantic Ocean. In the USA and Canada a tough policy of test and slaughter began in the early twentieth century and this process was completed by the Second World at great expense and with considerable investment of administrative effort. In Europe the approach to bTB control was much milder and slower, with decades of voluntary schemes and encouragement of private initiatives. It was not until after the Second World War that test and slaughter was universally adopted and the problem still remains to be solved in several countries, most notably in the UK and the RoI.

Voluntary slaughter was introduced in Pennsylvania in 1896 and from 1906 in the District of Columbia, where area testing was introduced in 1909. In 1917 the House of Representatives discussed eradication by an 'Attested herds' scheme, and by 1919 this had been

---

[30] Atkins 2010a.

[31] McGregor 1890; Legge 1896; Anon. 1900; Swithinbank and Newman 1903; Jensen 1909.

[32] Atkins 2010a.

introduced in nine states, one incentive being the needs of the large meat-packing industry with its international profile and disease-free image. The slaughter programme was completed for the whole country in 1940 and according to Olmstead and Rhode, 'there are few instances where the police power of the United States government was so ruthlessly exercised in peacetime'.[33] Yet it was only the state of New York that had ever had an infection problem (twenty-six per cent at one point) comparable to that of the UK.[34] It is important to note that the American programme was not without its critics. In the 1920s the American Farmers' Union and the American Medical Liberty League opposed the federal policy of test and slaughter, and in 1931 there were farmer riots in what came to be known as the Iowa Cow War.[35]

The European trend was not at first for slaughter. A Danish Act of 1893 introduced state-sponsored tuberculin testing and another in 1898 prohibited the sale of obviously tuberculous stock and the sale of milk and meat from tuberculous animals. Bernhard Bang (1848-1932) in Denmark and Robert von Ostertag (1864-1940) in Germany wanted to build on this by the gradual lowering of levels of disease incidence.

In Bang's early regime the TT was used to identify diseased animals and these were isolated from others on the farm.[36] However, from 1899 he modified his advice.[37] He no longer advocated testing the main herd and instead concentrated on producing healthy calves as the nucleus of a new and separate herd.[38] Disease-free offspring were separated from their mothers at birth, the animal equivalent of the segregation of human consumptives in sanatoria.[39] Farmers were encouraged to maintain dual herds until eventually all of the infected animals were phased out.[40] Restrictions on breeding from infected animals were part of this policy but an obvious weakness was that farmers were allowed to

---

[33] For fuller accounts see Myers 1940; Myers and Steele 1969; Myers 1977; Olmstead and Rhode 2004a.
[34] Ritchie 1945.
[35] Olmstead and Rhode 2007.
[36] Bibby 1911.
[37] TNA: CAB 58/186.
[38] McFadyean 1927.
[39] Harvey and Hill 1936.
[40] Bang 1908.

sell tuberculous animals wherever and whenever they chose.[41] Byres had to be disinfected and there was careful management of infected manure. Fields grazed by infected cattle were quarantined for at least one month and newly purchased stock were monitored and tested to prevent the importation of disease. Disease was monitored by the tuberculin testing of the animals and the bacteriological testing of their milk.

Bang received some support from workers such as McFadyean and Savage, and there were experiments that reported positive results in Britain and America.[42] But there was little general enthusiasm.[43] On the one hand the cost of establishing and managing a farm within a farm would have been prohibitive for small dairymen and, on the other hand, the intensive nature of lowland British milk production was such that new animals were constantly being bought in as replacements and relatively few farmers bred their own replacement stock.[44] The scope for re-infection was therefore considerable.

As a result of his long experience, Delépine in Manchester developed views about eradication in concert with Niven and Brittlebank. Their close collaboration and similar outlooks produced detailed insights not available in any other British city apart from possibly Littlejohn's Edinburgh. In 1898 Delépine recommended his 'island method', in which small disease-free areas would gradually be built upon until eventually the country was divided into districts for the gradual administrative advance of eradication.[45] The encouragement of tuberculosis-free areas would act as an educational shop window for farmers in areas where little headway was being made against bTB. On reflection Delépine's stress upon the separation of diseased animals was not dissimilar to that of Bang.

But even in the original home of Bang's method, Denmark, use of his procedure diminished.[46] Building up a tuberculosis-free herd from selected cows is simple in theory but in practice very difficult for most farmers who had only one set of farm buildings. Ultimately isolation

---

[41] Moore 1913; Ernst 1914.
[42] Mackintosh et al. 1915; Parker 1917; Adeane and Gaskell 1928.
[43] McFadyean 1895a; Bibby 1911; Buckley 1924; Savage 1929a.
[44] Stockman 1925; Wilson 1942.
[45] Delépine 1902; Brittlebank 1908; Bibby 1911.
[46] Petersen 1938.

methodologies proved to be an expensive failure in all European countries. The Danes finally joined the test and slaughter trend in 1932 and by 1952 they had achieved complete eradication of the disease.

In Germany Ostertag by contrast relied on veterinary inspection as a means of identifying animals for slaughter based on the theory that clinical cases were the main source of infection.[47] He tried to prevent the infection of calves by feeding them on pasteurized milk. Ostertag's approach was widely used in Germany in the 1930s but proved to be ineffective and was eventually abandoned.[48] An eradication programme began there in 1952 at a point when about sixty per cent of cattle and ninety per cent of herds were affected by bTB.[49]

There were many variations of policy in Europe in the first half of the twentieth century, none of them as coherent and effective as in the USA and Canada. Britain's position up to the 1930s was particularly weak, with decades of inaction at the centre. Only in progressive local authorities did anything useful happen. If we go back to Article 15 of the Dairies, Cowsheds and Milkshops Order of 1885, we see that it stated that 'if at any time disease exists among the cattle in a dairy or cowshed, the milk of a diseased cow therein shall not be mixed with other milk; and shall not be sold or used for human food'. But, as we saw in Chapter 4, the definition of 'disease' used at this time was that of the 1878 Contagious Diseases (Animals) Act, which did not include tuberculosis. Considering that the milk of one cow could be consumed by many people, and that only a small dose of bacilli was sufficient to cause an infection, there was little to prevent bTB becoming a serious and widespread hazard.

In the 1880s the risk was increasingly well known though not universally accepted. This slippage was demonstrated by the Public Health (Prevention of Diseases) Bill. In its original form in 1888 it contained a clause that would have allowed Medical Officers to demand a list of a dairyman's customers, with a view to tracing the path of an epidemic, but this was removed from what finally passed as the Infectious Diseases Prevention Act (1890). Sanitary authorities were given powers to stop milk supplies if there was a risk of infection

---

[47] Moore 1913.
[48] Wagener 1949.
[49] Myers and Steele 1969.

being passed on but the procedures were very cumbersome. The MOH had to obtain a magistrate's Order to inspect a dairy or cows and had to be accompanied by a veterinarian. Another Order then had to be made forbidding the local sale of the milk, with a penalty for default. In practice there was nothing to prevent the dairy farmer or dairyman from switching the milk to an area other than the one mentioned in the prohibition order, or indeed from selling the infected cow to another, unsuspecting dairy farmer. As a result, few prosecutions were ever attempted and the measure was later described as 'quite worthless'.[50]

The law in Britain therefore remained weaker than the precedent set by the French milk legislation passed in 1888.[51] Having said that, the Dairies, Cowsheds and Milkshops Order of 1879 did prohibit the sale of milk from animals certified by a vet to be diseased and the Diseases of Animals Act (1894) in theory also enabled the BoA to enforce compulsory notification of the clinical signs of disease in cattle. Yet in neither case did 'disease' encompass bTB and, anyway, both of these measures were also deemed to be dead letters according to a survey conducted by the *British Medical Journal* in 1903.[52]

In the absence of any bold and focused central government initiative, Glasgow was the first city in Britain, in 1890, to take powers for its own medical and sanitary officers to inspect any cowshed supplying the city, including those located outside its administrative boundaries, and to prohibit the sale of milk thought to be 'dangerous or injurious to health'.[53] Edinburgh followed in 1891, requiring that milk dealers provide lists of their customers to help with tracing infection if and when disease broke out.[54] The Public Health (Scotland) Act of 1897 then gave local authorities the power to insist upon the removal of a tuberculous cow within twenty-four hours, but this provision was flawed because there was no guidance on how the animal should be disposed of and there was no compulsion on any new owner to notify the authorities if it was taken to another area to resume milking.[55]

---

[50] Dodd 1905, 11.

[51] McFadyean 1888c.

[52] Anon. 1903, 1488-92.

[53] Glasgow Police (Amendment) Act, 54&55 Vict chapter ccxxi; BPP 1898 (C. 8831) xlix.Q.155; Pennington 1982, 89-91.

[54] McFadyean 1891b.

[55] Mitchell 1914.

Meanwhile, the LCC was trying to upgrade its own legislation, with disappointing results. Clauses in both their 1892 and 1902 General Powers Bills, which would have enabled the slaughter of tuberculous animals, were struck out in the House of Lords and were not successfully revived until 1904. Further progress was in small increments. In 1907 it became possible for LCC officials to take country samples at railway stations and thereby to prevent tuberculous milk being sent to London. Further powers were sought in 1908 but the relevant clauses were withdrawn when the government gave an assurance, falsely as we will see below, that they were about to enact legislation that would standardize and generalize the control of the country's milk supplies.[56]

The problem for the LCC was that they were consistently and vehemently opposed in the House by MPs representing farmers' interests on the grounds that there were already too many local provisions, and that what was really needed was a general Act. There was also pressure from campaigning interest groups such as the Tuberculosis (Animals) Committee.[57]

Manchester was also active in seeking to protect its citizens from bTB. The formation of its Sanitary Committee in 1890 introduced a different view of public health from that of its predecessor, the Nuisances Committee, which had been principally responsible for the inspection of housing.[58] A new, epidemiological sensibility is evident in their minutes at this time and various initiatives followed, such as the tracing of infected milk to country suppliers. This involved the Corporation in establishing links with the relevant rural authorities, who were then asked for their assistance. In 1895 the MOH, James Niven, went further and made a number of suggested improvements, including the slaughter of tuberculous cows, with compensation for the farmers, as mentioned in the RC1. The previous year, when newly appointed, he had also leafleted consumers in Manchester advising them to boil their milk to minimise the danger of contracting a number of diseases, including bTB.[59]

From 1896 to 1898 detailed examinations of cattle supplying the

---

[56] HC Deb 5 March 1908 vol 185 cc 966-87.
[57] *The Times* 4 February, 1909, 6c.
[58] Redford and Russell 1940.
[59] Niven 1923.

city were made by the corporation's Chief Veterinary Inspector, and of their milk by Delépine, in his new laboratory. In practice though it was difficult to track down tuberculous milk because dairy companies mixed their supplies at rural depots before consignment.[60]

In September 1898 Manchester's Sanitary Committee resolved to seek powers along the lines of the Glasgow Police (Amendment) Act, with additional powers of compulsory slaughter of animals found to be suffering with bTB. Other cities were considering similar measures but the opposition was focused on Manchester. The city's annual Ratepayers meeting was consulted about this tightening of controls, including a prohibition of the sale of contaminated milk, and the officers present were surprised that these were 'considerably watered down' by a show of hands. In retrospect the explanation was straightforward; the slaughter provision would have been a charge on all ratepayers, and it was therefore removed from the Corporation's Bill. This dislike of local taxes was coupled with 'persistent opposition from the organised traders in foodstuffs'.[61] Nevertheless an important remnant of the milk provisions in the Bill survived and became known as the 'Manchester Milk Clauses'. These were soon seen as a rallying point for other authorities seeking their own local acts. With the passing of the Manchester Corporation (General Powers) Act in 1899, the authorities were now enabled to:

- prosecute anyone knowingly selling milk from cows with udder tuberculosis;
- demand the isolation of infected beasts;
- demand the notification of any cow exhibiting signs of tuberculosis of the udder;
- inspect cows and take samples from herds which supplied milk to the city;
- summons any dairyman thought to be putting the citizens of Manchester at risk of bTB and, if required, make an order terminating that supply.[62]

In 1899 the LGB issued a Dairies, Cowsheds and Milkshops Order at last adding tuberculosis to the list of diseases which could be dealt

---

[60] Niven 1908; Delépine 1909.
[61] Redford and Russell 1940, 74.
[62] Niven 1902, 1908.

with by Local Authorities. In theory this enabled the sale of milk from animals with udder disease to be stopped. The Order was adoptive, however, and was simply ignored by those councils which felt unable to afford a veterinarian to make the necessary checks.[63] By 1905 675 sets of regulations had been made (Table 8.4).[64] A LGB circular, issued in 1899, encouraged veterinary inspections and by 1907 a further 768 sets of regulations had been made, leaving 346 local authorities yet to make arrangements.

Table 8.4 A summary of regulations mentioned in 1905 annual reports of MOsH.

	Regulations under Article 13 of 1885 Order	Regulations based on LGB Circular of 1899	No regulations	Less than 10 cowsheds	Total
County Boroughs	39	30	4	0	73
Other Boroughs	86	127	40	8	261
Urban Districts	330	345	131	50	856
Rural Districts	220	266	171	34	691
Total	675	768	346	92	1,881

Sources: TNA: MH/80/3; BPP 1907 (152).

The 'milk clauses' (Table 8.5) were included in the *Model Bills and Clauses of the Houses of Parliament*.[65] But they did not go unchallenged. In the House of Commons in February 1899 Arthur Jeffreys MP sought, on behalf of his agricultural constituents, to remove all milk clauses in corporation Bills.[66] Various meetings were held in April that year, including one between government officials, representatives of the big cities, and the farming side under the auspices of the CCA.[67] Collectively they agreed to concentrate in future private Bills on eliminating udder tuberculosis rather than the wider definition of disease which has been proposed in some in the past. From then on there was less variation of wording between the new milk clause Acts. Also the CCA managed to win several concessions. In 1900 a right of appeal by dairymen to the BoA was added to the standard wording, as in 1901 was the right of dairymen to compensation when their milk supply had to be stopped.

---

[63] Malcolm 1901.

[64] In 1907 the number making tuberculosis regulations had increased to 906.

[65] Anon. 1907.

[66] HC Deb 21 February 1899 vol 67 cc 16-17.

[67] Lloyd 1902; Matthews 1915.

1903 was a key date. After that, clauses were denied to smaller authorities, especially if they did not have a full-time MOH and staff to enforce them. All clauses were now vetted by the Commons' Police and Sanitary Committee, and the LGB was asked for its opinion on all of them. From 1911 the truce was shattered when the CCA finally decided that government prevarication was no longer acceptable. They asked the BoA to implement the 1909 Tuberculosis Order and opposed all further private Acts.

Table 8.5 Local Acts with Milk Clauses

Boroughs unless stated otherwise
1899 Blackpool, Bootle, Darwen, Derby, Salford, Stockport, Warrington
1899 and 1901 Leeds
1899 and 1904 Manchester
1900 Bradford, Coventry, Croydon, Farnworth UDC, Halifax, Hastings, Ilfracombe, Lancaster, Liverpool, Oldham, Preston, Rochdale, Scarborough, Sheffield, Southport, Taunton, West Bromwich
1901 Barrow-in-Furness, Blackburn, Bolton, Brighton, Burton-on-Trent, Chesterfield, Harrogate, Lowestoft, Mansfield, Rhyl UDC, Ripon, Rugby UDC, Shipley UDC, Smethwick, Stratton and Bude UDC, Wallasey
1901 and 1909 Bury
1902 Cleethorpes UDC, Dartford UDC, Huddersfield, Knaresborough UDC, Leamington, Swansea, West Ham, Whitstable UDC, Wigan, York
1903 Beckenham UDC, Birmingham, Ebbw Vale, Erith, Gateshead, Hyde, Kingston-upon-Hull, Leigh, Middlesbrough, Nantwich UDC, New Hunstanton UDC, South Shields, Sutton Coldfield, Willesden UDC, Wood Green UDC
1904 Acton UDC, Birkdale UDC, Bridlington, Carlisle, Doncaster, Ilford UDC, Kettering UDC, Leyton UDC, Lytham UDC, Radcliffe UDC, Rotherham, Selby UDC, Skipton UDC, Stretford UDC, Swindon, Wolverhampton
1905 Bristol, Ealing, Morley, Otley UDC, Rhondda UDC
1906 Newport
1907 Brighouse, Devonport, King's Norton & Northfield UDC, London County Council
1908 Burnley, Finchley UDC, Leicester, Merthyr Tydfil, Padiham UDC, Widnes
1909 Cardiff, Mountain Ash UDC

Source: HC Deb 2 March 1914 vol 59 cc 71-73.

In the final analysis, the Manchester Clauses and similar enactments had educational value but it seems unlikely that they ever made much impact on the incidence of tuberculosis on the farm. In 1929 Joseph Brittlebank, Manchester's chief vet, reflected on his career enforcing the clauses:

> In my honest opinion, in the light of nearly 30 years' experience of controlling the milk supply of one of our largest cities ... much of the money which has been spent and much which is being spent at the present moment, may be unproductive expenditure.[68]

---

[68] Brittlebank 1929, 518-19.

This was because producers, when confronted by a well organized sanitary effort in one city, simply sent their milk to another where there were no regulations. [69] He also suggested that

> ... the milk clauses may have been a positive hindrance to general progressive measures in that the mere existence of such restricted powers as the clauses provided tended to lull the health service generally into a false sense of security.[70]

Anyway, all of the milk clauses were repealed in 1926, ending the power of the cities to visit cowsheds in rural areas.

John Burns and preparations for central legislation in the UK

The presence of *M. bovis* in milk became increasingly well known in the first decade of the twentieth century and this fuelled a debate about the need for action that went beyond the local remit of the milk clauses. There were calls for a legislative response at the centre. In 1904, for instance, the Royal Institute of Public Health formed a committee chaired by W.R. Smith and with eighteen members, including many of the top names in the dairy and veterinary worlds. They held ten meetings and in December 1906 their findings were presented to Sir Edward Strachey by a delegation.[71] Their estimate of the prevalence of udder tuberculosis was two per cent but ten to twenty per cent for other forms of bTB, including cows with sub-clinical disease. In order to help cope with this hazard they made a detailed list of suggestions for alterations to the Dairies, Cowsheds and Milkshops Orders, making them compulsory in rural districts, and for improvements generally to the milk supply.[72] Strachey's response was defensive on behalf of farmers:

> I assume that you do not wish for unreasonable precautions or to harass a great industry which is not in a very prosperous condition ... I think you will scarcely be anxious to make it more difficult for farmers

---

[69] Savage 1912, 1929a.

[70] Brittlebank 1925, 173.

[71] It is not clear in what capacity Strachey was acting. He seems to have spoken in the Commons for the President of the LGB, Earl Carrington, and was also chair of the Parliamentary Committee of the CCA.

[72] See also Anon. 1928.

to earn a living with what seems at present to be almost their best standby.[73]

It was John Burns, President of the LGB from 1905 to 1914, who was responsible for any legislation that might come forward. He was the first working man to reach cabinet rank, and an isolated socialist in a Liberal administration. Yet contemporary observers and historians have been hard on him. He has been called vain and incompetent, and even reactionary, and he was certainly unable to galvanize his civil servants into any significant action.[74] Christopher Addison commented that his term of office was notable 'only for a self satisfied waste of precious opportunities'.[75] Ensor observed that the culture of the LGB was forged out of the old Poor Law Board's tradition of 'cramping Local Authorities and preventing things from being done'.[76] When Burns was appointed, his officials, such as Sir Samuel Provis, who had been with the Board since 1872, were successful in recruiting him to their deeply conservative philosophy and it has been said that change was not possible until Provis retired in 1910 and Burns himself was reshuffled in 1914.[77]

We must remember three further points here. First, this was the time of radical Liberal governments, which had policy priorities other than food safety. Second, the structure of the LGB was overloaded to breaking point with recurrent routine administration, not to mention policy matters such as housing and the unemployment that worried Burns so much. But, in the words of Christine Bellamy, 'the culture and organization of the LGB – both at headquarters and in the field – was adapted much more successfully to a role of the state as the guarantor and arbiter of private interests and individual rights, than to the development of collectively consumed services'.[78] Third, in Burns' defence we can see from a reading of the files of the LGB and the MH that the milk issue received fuller attention at the highest level, of Permanent Secretary and Minister, during this than in most eras,

---

[73] TNA: MH 80/3.

[74] Kent 1950.

[75] Addison 1924, vol. I, 39.

[76] Ensor 1936, 517. See also Bellamy 1988.

[77] MacLeod 1968.

[78] Bellamy 1988, 155.

even in the 1920s and 1930s, a high point of political interest in milk. A fair conclusion therefore seems to be that policy implementation was attempted but stalled by the power of the farming lobby, coupled with a system of governance that was not geared to challenging vested interests in the name of public health.

In 1905 a summary was produced in the LGB of the Annual Reports of local MOsH. A long section in this on the Rural District Council, County Council and urban reports indicates conclusively that the Dairies, Cowsheds and Milkshops Orders were not applied in many rural areas and small towns. The reason for this indolence was that milk producing areas were rarely big consumers of their own product, and they therefore did not wish 'to spend money to protect a milk supply for the benefit of their urban neighbours'.[79]

A short exchange on 'the milk supply' in the House of Lords in 1907 made it clear that powerful legions were drawn up demanding government action on milk. Opening the debate, Lord Kenyon asked for a government response to a recent deputation to the BoA from representatives of the CCA, the leading dairy associations, forty-six affiliated societies and sixteen other outside bodies. All were calling for centralized legislation rather than clauses in local Acts. Answering, Lord Allendale promised a consultation between the BoA and the LGB, the latter representing the public health interest, with a view to the preparation of a Bill.

The promised meetings took place over the summer recess. The key sessions were in the form of an inter-departmental conference between the LGB and the BoA. This was thought likely to yield quicker results than a more formal Inter-Departmental Committee (IDC). The concerns of the deputations of the previous December and February were addressed, along with how to react to the milk clauses in the pending Public Health Bill and LCC (General Powers) Bill. These meetings were significant because they represented the first rumblings of the turf war that was later to break out between the two ministries. The LGB staff, for instance, were keen to lead any policy-making from a position of strength:

---

[79] TNA: MH/80/3.

> The interests of the two departments are necessarily somewhat antagonistic, and to leave to a committee upon which they are equally represented to recommend legislation would probably lead to no useful result.[80]

The weakness of John Burns as President of the LGB was demonstrated hereafter. He repeated several times from 1907 to 1914 that he would legislate on milk but somehow the opposing powers always seemed to be too strong for him and he backed down. As a result of a promise he made in 1908, the milk clauses that had been included in the LCC (General Powers) Bill were withdrawn so as not to complicate the future Milk Bill. The same fate befell J.W. Wilson's private member's Public Health Amendment Bill (1907) in which he attempted to incorporate milk control into a nationwide legal framework.

Farmers' and landowners' campaigning organizations, such as the well-established CCA and the Tuberculosis (Animals) Committee, supported the notion of general legislation on standards of milk production, and wanted compensation for slaughter to be from 'Imperial' funds rather than the pockets of local ratepayers, but on the other hand they opposed any local Bill which gave inspectors the right of what the CCA Secretary, A.H.H. Matthews, called 'invasion'. This was the legal ability of municipal authorities to inspect the premises of any farmer sending milk to their citizens. Farmers were in difficulties if they sent to more than one city because the standards of facilities required varied but this was mitigated to some degree by their collective action at the local level.[81]

In March 1908 the LGB's Permanent Secretary demanded a progress report on the proposed legislation and an indication of how much action could be taken with and without legislation because 'the President is about to receive some deputations about milk and is anxious to know this'.[82] When the deputations came, some of the exchanges were tense. Sir George Barham, for instance, founder of Express Dairies, somewhat tetchily reminded Burns that

> For a number of years we have been in a state of ferment owing to different Bills being introduced into Parliament by different authorities,

---

[80] Ibid.

[81] BPP 1912-13 (Cd. 6654) xlviii.67.

[82] Ibid.

which although defeated, are re-introduced the following year at the expense of the ratepayers. Many of us have given more time to public affairs in connection with these Bills than to our respective businesses. What we want now is one Bill.[83]

In reply, Burns was equivocal. He did not give any hope of getting rid of local milk clauses and was not optimistic about money from the Exchequer to fund a programme of slaughter with compensation, although he seemed to dismiss the significance of the latter issue because he did not think many cows would be found with clinical signs of tuberculosis. His only concessions were that airspace in cowsheds should not be an issue and that County Councils should be responsible rather than local authorities.

In early 1908 Burns was said within the Board to be 'very desirous of having a Milk Bill prepared. He is much pressed by the Board of Agriculture and Fisheries on the subject'.[84] The Bill eventually appeared in draft form on 8 April. The main provisions with regard to bovine tuberculosis were as follows:[85]

1. Registration required but can be removed if MOH reports unsatisfactory conditions. Licensing in districts over 10,000 population.

2. Model Milk Clauses 2-4 into force everywhere. Any udder disease to be notified to a MOH. Tuberculous cows to be isolated, branded, and sale of their milk prohibited.

3. County Councils and Boroughs over 10,000 population to be required to appoint vets. LGB to make regulations about their employment.

4. LGB to make Dairies, Cowsheds and Milkshops Orders.

5. Section 4 of the 1890 Act into force everywhere except London, where already in force under its own 1891 Act. Applications make inspection in other areas now have to be made to the MOH and Clerk of District, rather than to a JP.

6. Every Borough and Sanitary Authority over 10,000 population should have the powers of Milk Clauses 5-12.

---

[83] Ibid.

[84] Ibid.

[85] Ibid.

7. Authority for cows to be Counties, County Boroughs and Boroughs over 10,000. Authority for the Dairies, Cowsheds and Milkshops Orders to be the Sanitary Authority.

A key calculation in the process of Bill-making was the likely cost of compensation. It was thought likely that about two per cent of cows had udder tuberculosis, and if compensation was to be given at the London rate throughout the country then £500,000 would be required to deal with these animals, plus a further £1 million for the 200,000 cattle that had the disease but had no udder symptoms and were not 'wasters' or 'piners'.[86]

It was not until 1909, after years of discussion, that it seemed possible that a Milk and Dairies Bill would at last receive the royal assent. In February the King's Speech promised legislation and this time the LGB sponsored a measure that would in effect have made the Manchester Clauses generally applicable. There would have been a prohibition on the supply and sale of milk likely to cause disease, including bTB. But, despite a number of inter-departmental conferences, the LGB and the BoA found common ground difficult to achieve. The former consistently took the line of the local authorities in wanting stringent regulations, and the latter were wedded to the 'agricultural' cause of minimal change. An example was the tuberculin test, which might have been a starting point for a slaughter campaign but Sir Thomas Elliott of the BoA showed his hand in the following unguarded statement:

> It [the tuberculin test] finds out too much. Very few cows would pass such a test. Indeed, it is considered a pedantic test. [The BoA] consider that the number of animals who would react to such a test would be numerous.[87]

The BoA worried 'that there would be little short of a revolution among farmers, if we segregated their cows and gave them no compensation' and they objected to branding, which might have been a means tracing diseased cattle.

After much deliberation, the Milk and Dairies Bill reached its eleventh and final draft on 25 May 1909, and the following day the sixth draft of BoA's Tuberculosis Order was formalized and an official circular

---

[86] Ibid.
[87] TNA: MH 80/3.

sent out to local authorities.[88] The publication of the Bill stimulated debate and encouraged many representations. These are preserved in the National Archives and range from handwritten notes from concerned citizens to the official views of public health bodies, local authorities, trade associations, and even resolutions passed at public meetings.[89] The arguments raised (Table 8.6) were not new but the anger and anxiety of all concerned were palpable. There was energetic lobbying from the milk trade and farming interests. Mass meetings were held by the Dairy Trade Protection Society, and retail dairymen's associations in cities such as London, Leeds and Manchester.[90] The new Permanent Secretary of the LGB, Sir Horace Monro, understatedly summed up the situation as 'somewhat contentious'.[91]

Table 8.6 A summary of arguments surrounding the Milk and Dairies Bill, 1909

- Which authority should be responsible? Many wanted the County Councils but these were not health authorities and did not have the experienced staff found in Local Authorities
- Farmers continued to object to inspections ('invasions') by city authorities.
- The milk trade lobby sought to prevent the LGB having power to make Orders in Council rather by direct legislation after debate in Parliament. Alternatively they wished the BoA to see and approve any Orders.
- The trade did not want the abolition of the warranty that they usually demanded from their suppliers that milk was free from disease. This was a matter of who bore responsibility.
- Where compensation for slaughter should come from. Those wanting it to be a government responsibility included 12 agricultural/dairy societies, 9 RDCs, 15 CCs, 2 UDCs, 2 TCs, the NFU, and the CLA.

Source: TNA: MH/80/4

But the Bill fell in August. The Treasury had refused any central funds and the cost, estimated at £60,000 in the first year, would therefore have had to come entirely out of the local rates, a situation that was politically impossible. As a consequence of the Bill's failure, the LGB was forced to withdraw its parallel Tuberculosis Order. This would have given all local authorities powers of inspection and slaughter, as specified in Section 19 of the Diseases of Animals Act (1894).[92]

In the next parliamentary Session the LGB restarted discussions

---

[88] TNA: MH 80/3; *The Times* 25 May 1909, 10d; 1 June 1909, 7d.
[89] TNA: MH 80/4.
[90] *Cowkeepers' and Dairyman's Journal* July 1909, 365-66.
[91] TNA: MH 80/4.
[92] HC Deb 16 June 1909 vol 6 c1086.

of the Bill but the new draft had not been finalized by the opening of parliament in February 1910 and other priorities soon intervened. George Courthope MP introduced his own version, as a Ten Minute Rule Bill, but, like all such private members' initiatives, it had little chance of success.[93] It was heavily weighted to the agricultural agenda, in keeping with his chairmanship of the CCA. Courthope's Bill had support from groups as varied as the Conservative Party, the LCC, and the dairy trade press. Courthope was typical of a loose group sometimes called the 'agricultural MPs'. The names that cropped up regularly in parliamentary debates and delegations to ministers opposing progressive measures on bTB included Courthope, Charles Bathurst, Sir Edward Strachey.

Once more, in January 1911, the LGB geared itself up for a possible Bill. They knew that compensation was a major focus of dissent and set about thinking of ways to persuade the Treasury that this was desirable. It was estimated that one per cent of dairy cows had clinical tuberculosis of the udder, of which half were so advanced that they should be prevented from infecting the milk supply. If farmers were paid £2 each for at slaughter if the disease was proven and £12 if they were clear, then the total bill would have been about £120,000.[94] All of these estimates were on the low side, so as not to sully the prospectus.

The draft Bill was ready by March 1911. It included two major compromises: that the responsible authority should be the County Council rather than the local authority, and that 'invasion' by big city inspectors should cease. All of the local milk clauses were to be abolished and the warranty defence removed. Courthope was consulted and approved the changes but he was unable to vouch for all of his agricultural member colleagues. In the event, the Bill went to revise number five in July before being put on ice with a view to reintroduction in the following Session. But it was not until May 1912 that the matter was revived again. By then Burns was again said to be 'anxious' to make progress.[95]

Drafts of the 1912 Bill seem to have benefited from the various compromises struck since 1909. In particular, County Councils were to have control of implementing the Dairies, Cowsheds and Milkshops

---

[93] BPP 1910 (123) iii.503.

[94] TNA: MH 80/4.

[95] TNA: MH 80/4.

Orders and 'invasion' was to be replaced by the approach taken in Section 87 of the Burgh Police (Scotland) Act (1903), where one MOH was responsible for telling another of any problems. This would not have been possible in the 1909 Bill because County Councils had not yet been required to have a Medical Officer. In addition, the milk clauses in local Acts were to be abolished. The main difference, though, was that when Burns wrote to the Treasury in July, he received a favourable response in October that they would pay half of the compensation required for a slaughter programme, although only for a limited period of five years. After four further revisions, the Bill was finally ready in December 1912.

It was not until 1913 that the LGB felt it was making progress with the Bill. By then Burns was hopeful and thought the matter would be 'substantially uncontested' because 'the long interval of time [since 1909] has enabled the various interests that were previously almost irreconcilable to come together and to adjust some of their differences'.[96]

Meanwhile, there were more deputations.[97] One in particular stands out, involving eighty-seven delegates from twenty-three dairymen's associations, introduced to Burns and supported by fifteen MPs.[98] They objected to the loss of warranty, by which milk traders had been able to shift the responsibility for milk adulteration and disease on to the producer, and they also disliked the provision for a dairyman to be struck off the register upon conviction of a second offence under the Act. Nevertheless their attitude was less hostile than it had been in 1909 and Burns commented on this: 'I do not know the reason why your demeanour towards the Milk Bill has changed but I welcome the change'.[99] But he also issued a clumsy threat about the future.

> In the House of Commons there is practically a consensus of opinion in favour of it; there is only one objection and that is a gentleman who, if we had a Bill to bring in Arcadia and Utopia combined, would oppose it ... I would advise you not to add to the difficulties of passing this Bill because I can assure you that if this Bill does not pass the next

---

[96] HC Deb 5 June 1912 vol 39 c197.

[97] TNA: MH 80/5.

[98] TNA: MH 80/4.

[99] Ibid. 8.

> one will be a more drastic one. You had better deal with me whilst
> you have me in the gate, and I am prepared to deal with you in similar
> circumstances.[100]

Not for the first time, Burns was proven to be incorrect; once more the Bill had to be dropped in the face of concerted opposition.[101] This in itself was uncomfortable, for instance when the BMA protested at 'the continued shelving of such important measures'.[102]

On the whole MPs mouthed the opinions of outside bodies, for instance the so-called farmers' members who vigorously opposed any measure which would have affected the interests of their constituents. They also reflected the full range of popular views and prejudices about the effect of meat and milk upon public health. However, occasionally fresh ideas came forward that cannot be traced elsewhere. For instance, Charles Bathurst MP, a notorious opponent of any legislation on bovine tuberculosis, in 1911 proposed the establishment of a national register of sound cattle that presumably would have been examined by a vet and tested with tuberculin.[103] This positive idea was decades ahead of its time.

The government's continuing inability to get pure milk legislation on to the statute book was put down by the press to there being 'no votes in milk'.[104] The issues in parliament at this moment blocking progress were said to be Irish home rule and the disestablishment of the church in Wales.[105] The Astor Committee on TB reported at this time and did not buy such excuses. In their view, the duty of the government was plain:

> the best way to eradicate tuberculosis from the cattle of this country
> is entirely to eradicate tuberculosis from the cattle of the country ...
> the ultimate eradication of animal tuberculosis is not impossible of
> achievement, but is likely to be a slow process, and must depend upon
> co-ordinated and continuous effort ... [106]

In 1913 once again the BoA was outflanked and embarrassed by the LGB which launched a Tuberculosis Order into the void left by their

---

[100] Ibid. 11.
[101] HC Deb 16 July 1913 vol 55 c2012.
[102] Wellcome Contemporary Medical Archives Centre: SA/BMA/F105.
[103] HC Deb 20 July 1911 vol 28 c1277.
[104] *Daily Express* 6 February, 1913, 4.
[105] *Daily Express* 8 January 1913, 4.
[106] BPP 1912-13 (Cd. 6641) xlviii.38.

indecision. It was made on 13 February and came into effect on 1 May. The all important compensation-for-slaughter package was seventy-five per cent of the animal's value to the farmer if it was tuberculous but only twenty-five per cent if the diseased was advanced.[107] Half of this sum, net of the value of salvage, was to come from the centre and half from the local rates, an arrangement to last for five years.

Conclusion

It is easy to see why Smythe claimed in the 1920s that 'milk, under present conditions, is a dangerous food'.[108] This can be seen as the long-running failure of politicians to find a legislative and regulatory framework that suited all parties, from farmers and dairy industrialists through to consumers. As the latter part of this chapter has shown, it is easy to be drawn into the minutiae of the policy decision-making and consultation process, which is interesting in situations like this where there is a balance of forces for and against a measure and therefore the story has a certain energy. But ultimately such an approach is only one explanatory cut through the complexity of bTB history. A further problematization was provided early in the chapter by three further perspectives. First, we saw that the development of bacteriology needs to be taken into account. This was the scientific means of knowing the extent of the infection of the milk supply and thus making *M. bovis* present and visible. This was fundamental to alerting both the milk consumer and the public health profession to the need for action. There were limits, however, as demonstrated by Delépine's laboratory. There were only so many samples that could be processed and therefore the veil was only partially lifted, and the use of animal testing meant that results were produced very slowly. At the national level there were also shortages of trained experts available for testing. Our second insight was one of contingency. It was Manchester and a small number of other progressive authorities with both the political will and the resources who were prepared to pioneer this scientific means of protecting their citizens. The variability in time and space was therefore profound and lasted for a further half century until the 1950s; the solution finally

---

[107] TNA: T161/1177.
[108] Smythe 1927.

was not one of all local authorities at last following best practice but rather the dairy companies installing sufficient capacity to pasteurize all milk. Our interest in politicians and administrators was finally made redundant by a technical resolution. In this case it was necessary to mix policies with materials and technologies in order to develop the picture fully.

The third point is one of scale. The framework of many aspects of governance in nineteenth Britain was permissive, with legislation frequently allowing local authorities to adopt or ignore measures according to local needs and preferences. Although both legislation and regulation shifted increasingly towards nationwide norms, the underlying notion of local preference continued, as we will see in subsequent chapters. The standardized macro-spaces of modernity never wholly triumphed in the bTB sphere and as recently as 2012 cattle were being tested on a spatial template of parishes.

Although it was known from the 1890s that the infection of milk with bTB was a hazard, it took decades for the extent of the risk to be known. As we have seen, Manchester was a progressive authority and the city was fortunate in the quality of the individuals responsible for its milk. The city was a leader but other local authorities lacked the resources and leadership to match Manchester's initiatives, with the result that the risk map was a patchwork mainly of unknowns and partially knowns right through into the middle of the twentieth century. In the 1950s pasteurization swept away risks that in some areas were never acknowledged, let alone quantified. This chapter has discussed the specifics of milk and in Chapters 9-11 we will move on to discuss the more general politics of bTB split into the periods 1914-29, 1930-37, and 1937-71. The logic for this periodization will become apparent as we proceed.

CHAPTER 9.

INDETERMINACY IN POLICY MAKING: 1914-1929

Introduction

Jessop sees the state as a 'site, generator and product of strategies.' In his view 'any theory of the state must produce an informed analysis of the strategic calculations and practices of the actors involved and of the interaction between agents and the state structures. However the relationship is always dynamic and dialectical.'[1] The present book attempts to add a further layer of understanding to recent reconstructions of the complex nature of bTB policy-making in Britain. There is a risk, however, that the impression might be given of a reductive view of state action. It is therefore important to make two cautionary points.

First, the slow advance in bTB policy before 1950 did not mean a lack of progress in veterinary public health across the board. Several initiatives *were* undertaken by government and by commerce. Graded milk, for instance, was introduced in 1917 and relaunched in 1923, although it did not have much impact for a decade after that. There was also the idea of Attested herds, which was altogether more significant, starting shortly before the Second World War. Finally, and most important, pasteurization was introduced gradually by dairy companies in the inter-war period. This method of heat treatment was primarily designed to increase the shelf life of retail milk, but in its technically more efficient guises it had the beneficial side effect of killing the mycobacteria that potentially could have been passed on by infectious cows.

Second, the local state was heavily involved in making and implementing policy with regard to bTB. This point has already been made about the milk clauses and there will be further comments later about the geographically uneven responses of local authorities, with large cities such as Manchester, Liverpool, and Glasgow in the lead.

Chapters 9-11 will develop this theme of the problems of central

---

[1] Jessop 1990.

state policy-making, from both the legislative (Westminster), regulatory and administrative (Whitehall) perspectives. The present chapter begins in 1914, which was an important threshold because of the rather different imperatives of wartime conditions and because of the ministerial reshuffle that took place immediately beforehand. It then looks at the chaos and inertia of the 1920s when government seemed incapable of anything worthwhile with regard to bTB. Chapter 10 then deals with the strategic shifts of the 1930s, which were radical for some aspects of the dairy industry but less so for disease control. Chapter 11 commences with the Agriculture Act (1937), which laid the foundation for the era of area eradication, and it finishes in 1970 when bTB in cattle appeared, falsely as it turned out, to have been defeated.

Policy-making after Burns

At the end of Chapter 8 we left the despised John Burns, embarrassed and outflanked once again with regard to milk legislation. Following his departure in February 1914, the Bill-drafting recommenced but, this time, 'to the delight of radicals everywhere', Herbert Samuel succeeded him at the LGB, which 'had been moribund for eight years'.[2] The new Bill was said to be a 'compromise'.[3] There was a new urgency because no local milk clauses had been allowed since 1909, so there were many local authorities keen to have a central Act in order to protect their citizens.

Samuel's style was different from that of Burns. He invited likely opponents of the Bill, such as the CCA, to the Board for talks. Others he met at the House of Commons. This way he learned about their underlying fears, such as the possible expense of having to modify cowsheds, and their wish for the BoA to participate more in the administration and so dilute the public health zeal of the LGB. An example of this misplaced enthusiasm, in their view, was the Bill's threat to deregister, and therefore effectively put out of business, any milk producer convicted of two offences. They also worried about

[2] TNA: MH 80/5; Rowland 1971, 297.
[3] HC Deb 12 May 1914 vol 62 cc 945-48; 9 June 1914 vol 63 cc 239-45; 14 July 1914 vol 64 c1725.

competition from imported milk and the proposed end of the warranty defence in adulteration cases.[4]

With the political will it was surprising how quickly action could be taken. Samuel had been President of the LGB for only two months when he made the following statements in advance of the passing of the Milk and Dairy Act:

> The measures which have so far been taken to deal with the milk supply are totally inadequate to safeguard the public health. Our laws date back to a time before the importance of bacterial contamination was fully realised. We do, indeed, take the utmost pains to guarantee the purity of our water supply, and yet we allow our milk supply to go almost unprotected ... I find every interest anxious for legislation.[5]

In his short time in office he received fifteen deputations on this subject alone. The LGB was therefore not short of advice and encouragement. The problem was that:

> Unless a measure of this sort [the Milk and Dairy Bill] is generally acceptable in all quarters of the House, it is unlikely to pass. The experience of the last five years has shown how easy it is to stop the progress of this Bill.[6]

Samuel observed wryly that 'the subject of milk, which ought to be a peaceful topic, and the very name of which summons up ideas of all that is meek and mild, has, in fact, been a matter of heated and almost burning controversy'.[7] His Bill was a reduction in length by one third of its predecessor, losing many of the most controversial clauses.

Once the Tuberculosis Orders were sidelined by the War the agricultural industry returned to its former practices. The trade in diseased animals continued unabated, often under the noses of the inspectors hired by the more conscientious urban authorities. Even those cities with Milk Clauses found it difficult to exercise control. Between 1920 and 1922, for instance, the City of Bradford's vets noted that 86 per cent of the cows that they had found to be tubercular were immediately

---

[4] TNA: MH 80/5.

[5] HC Deb 22 April 1914 vol 61 cc 1058-59.

[6] Ibid. c1066.

[7] HC Deb 12 May 1914 vol 62 cc 945-48; 9 June 1914 vol 63 cc 283-91; *The Dairyman, The Cowkeeper and Dairyman's Journal* June 1914, 425-6, 428-33.

sold on to dealers, who then recycled them in their neighbourhood or beyond.[8]

Wasserstein comments that the Milk and Dairies Act was Samuel's only significant piece of legislation at the LGB.[9] Ironically, it became law in September 1914 but never came into operation because it was almost immediately repealed by the Milk and Dairies Consolidation Act (1915), which in turn was suspended until after the war by the Milk and Dairies Acts Postponement Act (1915). This was because of representations from the dairy trade that the war effort made the Acts impossible to implement and also because there was a shortage of inspectors to carry out their various tasks.[10] The *Dairyman* noted that 'the postponement of the M&D Bill until after the war synchronises with the advent of Mr Walter Long, an old friend of the agriculturalist, as President of the LGB'.[11] Long had in the past been President of the BoA (1895-1900) and was well known for his opposition to radical state interventions in livestock farming. He took advantage of his brief stay (May 1915 to December 1916) at the LGB to reshape legislation to the advantage of the farming interests. His Milk and Dairies (Consolidation) Act was simply a means of bringing together in one piece of legislation all of the relevant clauses from other Acts which had relevance to the dairy food chain. Parts of it were permissive. A local authority could control milk at the point of sale, forbid the sale of milk from cows with tuberculous udders, and prohibit the sale of milk from open churns. In addition, notified consumptives could be excluded from dairy employment. This used the principle established in the Public Health Amendment Act (1907) which had empowered inspectors to forbid a notifiable infectious person from distributing milk before the end of a six week period of quarantine.[12]

A regressive provision of the 1915 Act was the curtailment of the powers in the local city 'milk clauses', to inspect cowsheds in areas outside their direct jurisdiction. To achieve the same object more red

---

[8] HC Deb 5 March 1923 vol 161 c196.

[9] Wasserstein 1992.

[10] *Dairyman, The Cowkeeper and Dairyman's Journal* September 1914, 6; January 1915, 158; May, 325; June, 373, 385-90; July, 421.

[11] The Act was again postponed in 1917.

[12] Smith 1988.

tape was now required and inevitable delays occurred because the country MOH had to be contacted over every case of infected milk and requested to make enquiries. Meanwhile the cowkeeper was informed and he had plenty of time to offload his suspect animals.

The Astor Committees and milk in the immediate postwar period

The decade 1910-20 had potential for change. There had been progressive legislation and milk had become an issue for the popular press. Even the war represented an opportunity because of the resetting of agricultural priorities and restructuring of hitherto stable food systems.

It was with the uncertainties of war in mind that a DC was established to investigate the 'Production and Distribution of Milk'. This sat from 1917 to 1919 under the chairmanship of Waldorf Astor. Although the committee had a broad remit, it is of interest to us because throughout his career Astor was involved in the politics of tuberculosis and of milk.[13] The committee accepted the findings of the RC3 which had reported in 1911 that human abdominal disease was largely the result of drinking infected milk, and commented that both of the two commonly mentioned solutions - the disposal of reactors or their separation from the rest of the herd - would be financially disadvantageous for farmers if they had to bear the cost themselves. Since most dairy farmers of the day operated on a small scale, their financial resilience was limited and, because precautionary measures were out of the question for many of them, they stood in the front line of any cattle disease hazard. Astor took the opportunity to highlight a third solution, the Accredited Herd Scheme that had been pioneered recently in America. This would have involved the provision of free tuberculin for regular testing by full-time state vets and the issuing of certificates to herds that were deemed to be free of the disease. In order to optimise such a scheme, the committee also recommended that the manufacture of tuberculin should be a monopoly of the government laboratory at Weybridge, and that the tuberculin dose should be standardized.

Astor also used his committee as a vehicle for advocating his and Wilfred Buckley's agenda on graded milk, which again would have meant

---

[13] Atkins 2010a.

state control of quality, this time with regard to standards of hygiene.[14] But the committee's findings were quickly undermined by a political crisis associated with milk prices in the winter of 1918/19 and by an avalanche of criticism of the state participation it advocated in both the wholesale and retail milk trades.

Completely unconnected with these tribulations at the Ministry of Food, in 1919 the second Lloyd George coalition government created a MH out of the old LGB. The inaugural Minister, Christopher Addison, had for some years taken an interest in milk and had been a member of the first Astor Committee, on tuberculosis, in 1912-13. No doubt drawing upon this memory, Addison appointed Astor as chair of an informal ministerial advisory committee, this time on a draft Milk and Dairies Order in anticipation of a reactivation of the 1915 Act.[15] Its deliberations were progressive and influenced policy-making over the next few years. To give a brief flavour, Astor recommended that bTB in milk should be taken seriously and that the 1915 Act should be amended to enable local authorities to hire specialist veterinary staff to inspect cattle and to administer the tuberculin test. He also wanted legal backing for certified milk, the licensing of all milk sellers, and power for the state to classify grades of milk according to health and quality criteria, and to define pasteurization.

The Milk and Dairies Consolidation Act (1915), which had been postponed by the war, did not come into immediate effect after the end of hostilities because the war was not deemed to be over until the peace treaty was signed in 1919. Following Astor's advice, in 1920 Addison then prepared an Amendment Bill to modify the Act in three substantial ways. He sought to provide for: the licensing of milk producers and dealers; the grading of milk; and the appointment of whole-time veterinary officers to check livestock for tuberculosis.

The dairy press immediately attacked the new Bill as the idea of 'cranks at the Ministry' and there was the usual chorus of objections from trade associations.[16] But the deal breaker was the Bill's empowerment of local authorities to municipalize milk distribution in their areas. In

---

[14] Atkins 2010a.

[15] TNA: MH 56/92.

[16] *Dairyman, The Cowkeeper and Dairyman's Journal* July 1920, 395, 398, 402; August, 439, 444.

response to this, an editorial in the *Milk Industry* called the Bill 'a step, and a long one, upon the downward path to a socialistic bureaucracy' and there was certainly widespread concern that milk policy was moving in the direction of nationalization.[17]

Most stakeholders on the producer and retailer side preferred to give the 1915 Act a chance without amendment, no doubt because it was already a dilution of the more radical 1914 legislation. They need not have worried because the Bill fell anyway before the summer recess of 1920. Addison blamed 'considerable interested opposition to one clause', meaning the one dealing with municipalization.[18] Among the ranks of the dissenters were the CCA, whose Dairy Products Committee and Council rejected the need for further legislation until the 1915 Act and the 1914 Tuberculosis Order had come into operation and could be judged either a success or a failure.[19] Another factor was a delay due to 'difficulties with the BoA until it was too late to attempt to proceed with it at all'.[20]

Eventually a Milk and Dairies (Amendment) Act was passed in 1922 but it was a small and insignificant piece of legislation. To have some legislation was necessary, if only as a delaying tactic, because the 1915 Act would otherwise have come into force automatically on 1 September 1922. The Minister of Health stated clearly in the Second Reading debate in the House of Commons that the government could not afford to implement the more comprehensive 1915 Act because it would have required large staffs of Inspectors and incurred administration costs of about £1 million per annum.[21] The further postponement until September 1925 was supported by the MAF, the CCA, the NFU, and the Association of Grade A Milk Producers.[22] The only significant steps forward were:

[17] *Milk Industry* 1, 1, July 1920, 7.

[18] HC Deb 11 August 1920 vol 133 c400.

[19] Jeffcock 1937.

[20] MH 56/81.

[21] The Earl of Onslow stated that an IDC had concluded that it would cost £700,000 per annum to implement the 1915 Act, and a further £150,000 to pay for compensation under the Tuberculosis Order. HL Deb 26 June 1922 vol 50 c1172.

[22] HC Deb 19 July vol 156 cc2199-2200. The support of the CCA was conditional on the inclusion of a clause insisting on the parliamentary tabling and scrutiny of

- the power to refuse registration and to de-register dairies;
- formalization of graded milk;
- banning of colouring additives;
- it became an offence knowingly to sell tuberculous milk;
- regulation of imported milk;
- County Councils now able to make bye-laws concerning cowsheds, dairies and milkshops.[23]

This whimper of a measure was greeted with derision by some MPs and indifference by others. Sir Francis Acland, who rose to speak in the accompanying debate at 9.45 p.m. regretted 'that there are so few Members present ... There must be many hon. Members who at present are more practically interested in other fluids than milk'. But the fiercest speech in the debate was delivered by Addison, who had resigned as Minister of Health only the previous year and whose idea this measure had originally been. He called it a 'little Bill ... an exiguous affair'. The government was said to be afraid to take on too many additional civil servants 'because the *Daily Mail* or some other paper would have headlines about swarms of inspectors'.[24] Allowing for some parliamentary licence and maybe some bitterness at the manner of his departure from the front bench, Addison nevertheless caught the mood of many MPs.

That so little was achieved in the early history of the MH is hardly surprising. From its foundation in June 1919, there were no less than seven Ministers of Health in five years. A lack of managerial continuity tended to militate against progressive measures, coupled to which the troubled last years of the Lloyd George coalition saw a retrenchment against some of the ministry's expensive schemes.

More dairy politics

At this point, in the early 1920s, cracks began to open in the previously united opposition to dairy legislation. The abandonment of wartime control led to chaotic conditions and over-supply and in 1920 the NFU

all Ministerial Orders. Lord Strachie was the force behind this amendment. Jeffcock 1937, 59.

[23] Robinson 1923, 30-31; Smith 1923, 129-30.

[24] Ibid. cc2223, 2226.

and the National Federation of Dairymen's Associations (NFDA), the latter acting for the larger dairy companies such as United Dairies, clashed over producer prices. So heated did the atmosphere become that there were farmer milk strikes and shortages in the London market.[25] In the spring of 1922 a rapid fall in prices led to even greater tension but through the good offices of the Minister of Agriculture, Sir Arthur Griffith Boscawen, there were negotiations and these differences were sunk in an experiment in collective bargaining known as the Permanent Joint Milk Advisory Committee (PJMC).[26] This new relationship between the two sides was noisy and at times bitter, and the Committee was unable to impose its agreed prices on the whole industry, but the very existence of the PJMC demonstrated that the major players in the market were willing to compromise for *their* own mutual benefit. The smaller retail dairymen were left to fend for themselves. Their views were articulated in trade journals such as the *Dairyman* and it was clear that they resented their exclusion and feared the likely increased competition from the large companies.

Together the parties to the PJMC made recommendations to the government about the 1922 Bill, including the idea that all milk should be designated and that large cities should be allowed to enforce regulations that might include compulsory bottling and pasteurization.[27] The latter in particular infuriated the *Dairyman* whose constituency of small traders was the most likely to suffer as a result. The NFU and NFDA were accused of having misrepresented the views of the trade in their meeting with the CMO.[28] Matters came to a head with an editorial in the *Dairyman* entitled 'Federation openly declares war on small distributors', which referred to an article in the *Milk Industry* which predicted the rationalization of the trade towards larger sized firms.[29] Nor was agreement about prices guaranteed in the PJMC, for

---

[25] *Dairyman, The Cowkeeper and Dairyman's Journal* May 1922, 385.

[26] Forrester 1927; Cox et al. 1990.

[27] *Observer* 8 January 1922, 16.

[28] There was also a bare knuckle fight between *The Dairyman* and *The Milk Industry* over the NFDA's attempt to make the latter a compulsory element of Federation members' subscriptions. *The Milk Industry* 2, 8, February 1922, 48. Roper (1925) claimed that *The Dairyman* had 'no authority among the leading and progressive firms in the trade'.

[29] *Dairyman, The Cowkeeper and Dairyman's Journal* January 1926, 271-72.

instance in the late 1920s and early 1930s acrimony again broke out as the agricultural depression bit and milk supplies exceeded demand.[30]

When the 1922 Bill was published in the House of Lords, ordinary dairymen held their largest ever protest meetings, angered by the annual contracts which the NFU was now negotiating at a national level.[31] Bad feeling was exacerbated by disagreements over pasteurization. The NFU advocated the 'holder' method of pasteurization, which required expensive equipment but produced safer milk, and this begged questions among smaller distributors who could not afford such an investment.

The NFU also argued for the prohibition of misleading designations but felt that grading was best applied to milk as delivered to the consumer rather than as produced in the cowshed. This latter view was transparently self-interested but the NFU argued for a standard that would take account of visible dirt because this would help to educate producers - their members. A pamphlet of theirs published in 1922 showed that they were fully aware of the latest methods of milk production and distribution in the United States, even if they chose to ignore the aspects that would have been expensive for British dairy farmers.[32]

This vigorous reaction from the NFU followed their reconstruction in 1918 with a view to exercising more effective pressure. By 1923, membership was over 100,000 and the NFU had arrived as a heavyweight lobby group in Whitehall; no Minister of Agriculture could ignore a voice this loud.[33] One might have expected them to espouse Tory values but even Conservative politicians found it difficult to deal with such an irritant. They were 'a bitter disappointment' to Stanley Baldwin and Neville Chamberlain, for their 'selfish, unconstructive, greedy and ungrateful' attitude and their 'dishonesty, ignorance, and stupidity'.[34] The NFU was accused of relying upon the emotion generated by mass meetings, as reported in the press, to exercise pressure, and of resorting

---

[30] Cohen 1936.

[31] *Dairyman, The Cowkeeper and Dairyman's Journal* January 1922, 197; February, 241.

[32] Langford 1922.

[33] According to Self and Storing (1962) the peak of membership was about 210,000 in 1953, representing approximately seventy-five to eighty per cent of full-time farmers.

[34] Cooper 1989, 68, 97.

to criticism of proposed legislation rather than suggesting any positive alternative.

The NFU drew strength in the 1920s from the pivotal role of its Milk Committee in the PJMC.[35] The trust of the ever-growing membership to represent dairy farmers' interests and their exercise of negotiating power was a key platform for their grasping of the benefits that fell out of their role in the setting up of the MMB in 1933 and later the close relationship with government from the 1940s onwards. It is not farfetched to say that milk was an essential commodity stepping stone in their rise to becoming one of the most powerful special interest groups in Britain.

The growth of the NFU represented a major challenge to established bastions of rural interests, such as the CCA, and even the newly formed CLA, whose influence was through channels opened by status and privilege. The NFU harnessed the raw power of numbers and they began to fill the vacuum left as they influence of the landowners fell away in British agricultural politics.[36] Martin Smith cannot have been thinking of the dairy industry when he commented that until the late 1930s 'the influence of farmers on agricultural policy was not strong'.[37] Maybe he wanted to contrast the pre-war period with the MAF/NFU deal-making of the 1940s and 1950s, but even so in the 1930s, as we will see in Chapter 10, the NFU were gifted a position of considerable power in British milk politics in that decade.

The Tuberculosis Order (1925)

Many in the public health and veterinary worlds were in favour of an early resumption of the Tuberculosis Order that had been suspended in 1914 and in May 1919 the government gave an undertaking to do so when the Milk and Dairies Act came into operation.[38] But four years later the Minister of Agriculture stated in Parliament that only a minority of Local Authorities were now in favour.[39] The pressure was coming disproportionately from Scotland. In England only four County

---

[35] Barnes 2001.
[36] Ashby 1939.
[37] Smith 1988.
[38] HC Deb 8 May 1919 vol 115 c1152W.
[39] HC Deb 18 June 1923 vol 165 c982.

Councils asked for implementation, whereas in Scotland sixteen out of thirty-three passed resolutions. In England 33 out of 203 Boroughs expressed a view in favour but in Scotland thirteen of the thirty-one burghs.[40]

Such figures make public health measures over zoonotic disease sound discretionary. There were few voices arguing for compulsory slaughter if any sign of bTB were found in the products or the body of an animal. One was Wilfred Buckley, who in 1924 wrote to the MAF arguing that no compensation should be given for the compulsory slaughter of diseased cattle under the Tuberculosis Order because 'a producer is acting immorally in selling milk from a cow that is suffering from the diseases enumerated in the Order'.[41] He argued instead for cattle insurance. In his moral crusade, one might have thought that Buckley was most likely to find common cause with consumers, but instead his closest ally was Ben Davies, a director of the largest dairy corporation, United Dairies. Talking about clean and disease-free production methods, Davies argued that it was farmers who should bear the responsibility:

> Those surely are merely the fundamental decencies of the production of human food, and failure to observe them must be regarded as a culpable and penal offence involving even disqualification as a producer.[42]

Buckley and Davies were at one end of the spectrum of opinion and at the other was Sir Daniel Hall, Chief Scientific Adviser to the MAF, who in 1925 asked his colleagues in a memo 'is it really necessary to attempt to eliminate all tubercle in milk?'[43] It is important not to judge this with the benefit of hindsight because at the time the thinking behind the question was both mainstream and seemingly logical. A few weeks after Hall's memo his implicit caution was amplified at a meeting between the CVO and representatives from the MH and the MRC. They agreed in effect that incremental action was the best course, that vaccination was as yet in its infancy, and that compulsory tuberculin testing should be postponed, because 'the number of reactions would

---

[40] TNA: MAF/35/309.

[41] Ibid.

[42] Davies 1934, 488.

[43] TNA: MAF/35/309.

be far too many and would create an unmanageable situation'.[44] There is more than a hint here that the truth about bTB was so bad that it should not be revealed by the scientific precision of a test. This political instinct for secrecy surfaces from time to time elsewhere in the MAF's archives. One official in 1929, for instance, chose to send out only confidential correspondence to Local Authorities: 'I prefer that means of communicating ... rather than a Circular Letter because the letter becomes public, and might excite the zealots who think that tuberculosis could be eradicated by a stroke of the pen'.[45]

In July 1924 the MAF wrote to the Treasury asking for the re-introduction of the Tuberculosis Order. This was, they said, because of lobbying from a large number of local authorities, bodies such as the Association of Municipal Corporations, who represented most of the towns, and twenty County Councils. The reply was that a decision had already been taken in 1920 that the financial situation was such that they would not be providing any compensation from the Exchequer.[46]

When the Order did finally came into operation in 1925, it was framed to operate 'as cheaply as possible and not as a preventative measure'.[47] Levels of compensation were to be low, and therefore there was little incentive for farmers to cooperate.[48] As a result, the eminent veterinarian John McFadyean correctly predicted that the Tuberculosis Order would have little effect upon prevalence of disease in the national herd.[49] This was later confirmed, as we will see, by the Hopkins Committee in 1934:

> The evidence that we have received all points to the fact that the Tuberculosis Order of 1925 has done nothing to reduce the incidence of disease. Nor has it done much to protect the public from infected milk, as the majority of cows are not reported until towards the end of their lactation, or when in an advanced state of the disease.[50]

The issue of valuation and compensation was central to this debate;

---

[44] TNA: MAF/35/309.

[45] TNA: MAF/35/312.

[46] HC Deb 8 May 1919 vol 115 c1152W.

[47] Savage 1929, 90.

[48] HC Deb 16 February 1926 vol 191 c1804.

[49] Pritchard 1988.

[50] BPP 1933-4 (Cmd. 4591) ix.469.

indeed financial considerations were the main topic in MAF internal memoranda and the science case was hardly mentioned.

The Tuberculosis Order (13 July, 1925) was actually made before the Milk and Dairies Consolidation Act came into effect on 1 September in order that preparations could be made by Local Authorities.[51] The Order was then quickly supplemented by a second, this time seeking to prevent diseased carcases being sold before they were cleared by an MOH or by a meat inspector. Farmers and vets both had a duty to notify cases of animals suffering from TB of the udder, emaciation, or chronic cough with clinical signs of the disease, but in practice this was not usually done until the disease was well advanced and it proved difficult to prevent tuberculous animals being recycled in the slink trade.[52]

The well-known MOH of Somerset, William Savage, was contemptuous of this Tuberculosis Order.[53] He pointed out that it was based upon Ostertag's principle of slaughtering open cases of tuberculosis but not backed by Ostertag's insistence on regular veterinary and bacteriological examinations. In 1926 Savage listed five major flaws in the implementation of the Order:[54]

- Local Authorities were not advertising the provisions of the Order to farmers and were not alerting them to symptoms to watch for.

- Very few cases of udder tuberculosis were being reported.

- Little use was being made of the available laboratory facilities to clear up uncertain cases, even though their use was free.

- Despite the encouragement of the Ministry of Agriculture's 1925 Circular, vets were not examining other animals in herds with known cases of tuberculosis.

- Under Section 13 of the Order, disinfection of premises was left to the police. This had proved to be unsatisfactory.

As Savage pointed out, the Tuberculosis Order, even if it was carried out successfully, did not address in any significant way the issue

---

[51] TNA: MAF 35/312.

[52] Savage 1927a.

[53] Savage 1927b.

[54] Savage 1926b.

of diseased animals infecting milk.[55] The Order only dealt with animals near to death, by which time 'they have been infective for long periods and have done most if not all the harm they are likely to do. The Order only interrupts their careers some short while before they would reach their natural destination, the knacker's yard'. In his view, the Order was 'being administered by the wrong people in the wrong spirit' and was 'looked upon as an administrative measure to be worked as cheaply as possible'.

Despite his blunt and critical language, Savage was not always negative. His various writings show him to have been one of the sharpest and best informed commentators of the day on this subject. His recommendation was that the preventative public health mindset of MOsH would yield better results than veterinary examination. What he had in mind were the powers in the 1915 Act that enabled Local Authorities

> bacteriologically to examine milk for tubercle bacilli and, if they are found, give ample powers for the Medical Officer of Health of the area of production to have the cattle examined and to take other steps to detect and eliminate the animals which yield the tubercle bacilli.[56]

He was thinking of the city authorities because most of their milk came from rural areas outside their jurisdiction. Sampling and laboratory testing was therefore the main weapon in their armoury.

As the MAF themselves pointed out, it was publicity in the farming media and lectures by veterinary staff that boosted the numbers of animals brought forward, as did the increasing number of inspectors employed by local authorities. Another factor in the late 1920s was the falling value of carcases at knackers' yards, which encouraged farmers to seek state compensation.[57]

The MAF later acknowledged that the 1925 Order 'was neither designed nor expected to eradicate tuberculosis completely ... [which] cannot be achieved in any comparatively short space of time, without a great and sudden depletion of the herds of this country and very large expenditure in compensation'. The Tuberculosis Order was designed,

---

[55] Savage 1928.

[56] Savage 1928, 342.

[57] Ministry of Agriculture (1931) *Report of proceedings under the Diseases of Animals Acts* London: HMSO.

rather, to remove those animals of greatest danger to human health and at risk of spreading the disease amongst other animals.[58]

From 1926 to 1936 215,413 cattle were slaughtered under the Tuberculosis Orders in Britain. Of these 67.7 per cent were found on post mortem to have had *advanced* tuberculosis, and only 0.6 per cent had no visible lesions. 18.5 per cent had tuberculous udders, 36.5 per cent were emaciated, and 43.0 per cent had a chronic cough or other clinical signs of the disease. Figure 9.1 shows the number of animals taken each year, diminishing after the Second World War and effectively disappearing in the 1960s. These data are for the Tuberculosis Orders only and therefore relate mainly to animals identified at veterinary inspections, with some voluntarily declared by farmers. They do not include animals tested with tuberculin and slaughtered as part of the Attested Herds Scheme from 1935 and during area eradication in the 1950s (see Chapter 11).

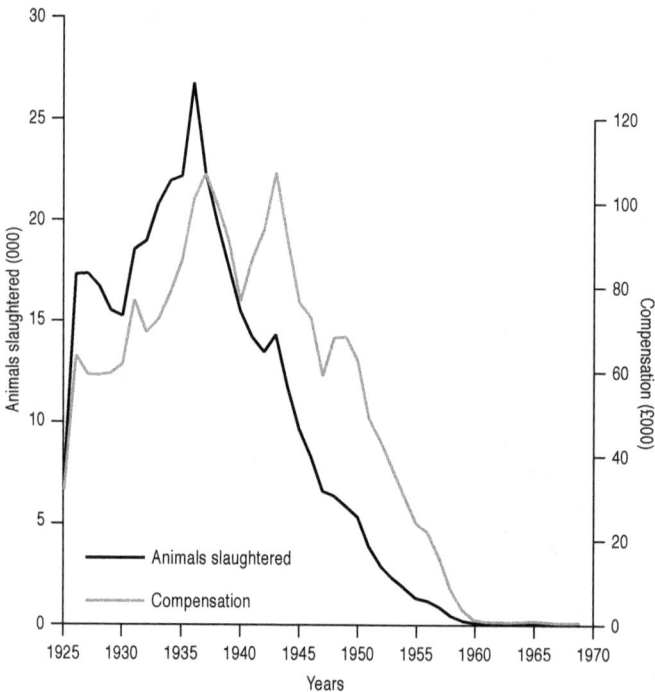

Fig 9.1 Animals slaughtered under the Tuberculosis Orders, 1925-1966
(Sources: MAF, *Report of Proceedings under the Diseases of Animals Acts*; MAF, *Report on the Animal Health Services*; MAF, *Animal Health: Report of the Chief Veterinary Officer*)

---

[58] Ibid 1930.

Figure 9.2 displays the geographical distribution of cattle taken for slaughter 1926-40 under the Tuberculosis Orders 1925 and 1938. The North West of England, and the centre and South West of Scotland were the most consistently and seriously affected. Many of the worst counties were also the chief milk producing areas. Cheshire, for instance, in the mid 1940s still had sixty to eighty per cent of its cows infected, when the estimated average for Britain was thirty to thirty-five per cent.[59]

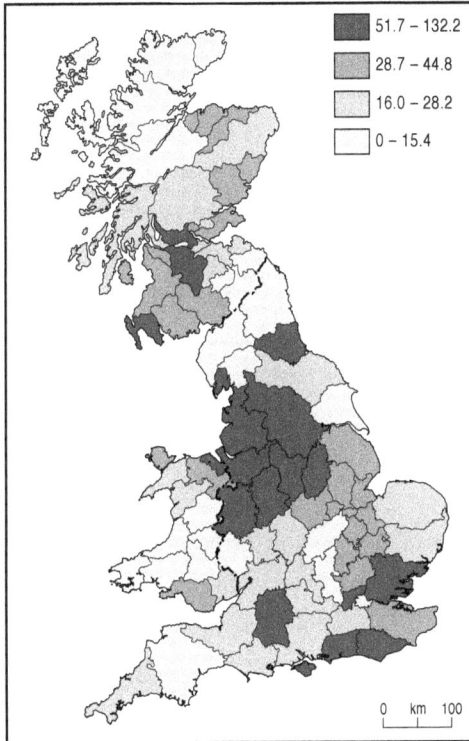

| 51.7 – 132.2 |
| 28.7 – 44.8 |
| 16.0 – 28.2 |
| 0 – 15.4 |

0   km   100

Fig 9.2
Cattle slaughtered under the TB
Orders per 1000 head, 1926-1940
(Source: Francis 1947)

The Milk and Dairies Orders (1922-26)

As we saw in Chapter 5, a Milk (Special Designation) Order was made in 1922 to facilitate the introduction of graded milk of a higher quality, including Certified and Grade A (Tuberculin Tested) milks that were in theory free of bTB.[60] The producing cows had to have a skin test every six months. There was also Grade A and Grade A (Pasteurized), where the cows had to be inspected every three months by a vet and certified free of tuberculosis; and there was also one (Pasteurized) for

---

[59] Francis 1947, 27, 32.
[60] Made under the Milk and Dairies (Amendment) Act (1922).

which there were no special provisions because it was assumed that heat treated milk would by definition be disease-free.

In early March 1923 Joseph Lamb MP, acting on behalf of the NFU, put down a motion in the House of Commons for the annulment of the 1922 Order.[61] His point was that twice yearly veterinary inspections would be a sufficient safeguard against TB in the human food chain without the need for further regulation. In response Neville Chamberlain, then Minister of Health, made the Milk (Special Designations) Order (1923), in which the bacteriological standard of pasteurized milk was slackened to placate the farmers.

Despite these concessions, some MPs were still arguing as late as 1925 and 1926 for the postponement of further dairy legislation.[62] Chamberlain claimed that that it was his judicious use of flattery that won the cooperation of the NFU.[63] But he also admitted that '... I never can keep the details [of the Milk & Dairy (Consolidation) Act] in my own mind. Its not my Bill, but one which was passed I think in 1915, and only now has come into operation'.[64] In his view 'the difficulty has been with the farmers. We don't consider at the M/H that the bill is satisfactory but the B/Agriculture got shot at pretty heavily and we had to compromise'.

On 1 September 1925 the Act finally came into operation. In theory all consumers would now be protected by the prohibition of the sale of diseased milk. Previously, cities with milk clauses in their private acts were safe but the milk could be sent elsewhere. Now the relevant MOH had to be notified if tubercle bacilli were found in milk. The idea was that suspect cattle could be given a veterinary examination and, if necessary, be isolated or eliminated. But there were two major flaws in this plan. First, in the 1920s milk was increasingly being bulked before being transported to the cities and sampling at the receiving end could therefore no longer play a part in this detective work.[65] Second, a period of four to six weeks elapsed before guinea pig results were available, by

---

[61] HC Deb 13 March 1923 vol 161 cc1284-5.

[62] HC Deb 20 July 1925 vol 186 cc1837-38; 2 December 1926 vol 200 cc1357-58.

[63] Cooper 1989, 97.

[64] Letter dated 10 October 1926. Self 2000, 368.

[65] By the end of the decade there were 120 rail tankers in use, mostly of 3000 gallon capacity. MAF 1933.

which time the infected cow might have been moved on, possibly to spread its disease elsewhere.

It was intended that a Milk and Dairies Order would accompany the Act but it was delayed by a rearguard action from the CCA. They expressed concern about the powers to stop the sale of milk from farmers unable or unwilling to improve their cattle sheds to the standard required by inspectors. The issue was one of cost and the tactics used were to raise a scare about the price of milk. In the event they only managed to get a postponement for a few months.[66] The Order came into operation on 1 April, 1927, revoking the Dairies, Cowsheds and Milkshops Orders of 1885, 1886 and 1899 and replacing them with stricter provisions. It insisted on the compulsory registration of cowkeepers, dairymen and purveyors of milk, and their premises; the proper storage of milk; and it took a view about what we might call the infrastructure of milking: cowshed drainage, lighting, ventilation, water supply, the cleansing of vessels and utensils, and conditions under which cooling, bottling, sterilization, and pasteurization could take place. Milkers had to keep their clothing and person clean and notify the MOH of any disease in their family. The opening of churns in transit was forbidden, except for checking or sampling, and all practicable precautions had to be taken to prevent exposure of the milk to heat and contamination by dirt, dust or rain water.[67]

The Order also transferred the responsibility for investigating suspect samples to the County Councils and County Borough Councils, and it widened the definition in the 1922 Act of bTB that would require slaughter. Now any cow in a comatose condition, having a septic disorder of the uterus, or any infection of the udder or teats likely to spread disease had to be killed. Several loopholes were also closed, for instance the tactic employed by some cowkeepers of withdrawing their animals when an inspector gave notice of a visit. The largest remaining loophole was that there was no statutory requirement in England and Wales for the authorities to undertake the routine examination of dairy cattle.[68]

The Milk and Dairies Order, then, had potential for eliminating dirt

---

[66] Jeffcock 1937, 62.

[67] Rhodes 1929.

[68] CMO 1926.

and disease from milk through onsite inspections, but this was theoretical because there were such large gaps in the biosecurity map. In practice there were too few inspectors and there is strong evidence that poor cowshed practice persisted. According to one County MOH, 'it would be difficult to visit a series of farms in any rural district without finding on all of them extensive and serious evasions of its provisions.'[69] A more cost effective system would have been the bacteriological testing of the milk output of farms.[70]

Although certified/graded/designated milk was intended to provide a premium for farmers willing to rid their herds of diseases such as bTB, progress in the 1920s was very slow. A continuing handicap was that the public did not understand the complex system of grades on offer and the retail market for tuberculosis-free milk coming through this route was therefore limited.

The Milk Advisory Committee (1923-30)

It seems that the financial explanation for the absence of radical regulatory changes in the milk industry was not the full story. A coded insight into the cross-cutting interests at stake was given by a Committee appointed after the General Election in 1922 by the new Conservative Minister of Agriculture, Robert Sanders. Reporting very speedily, only three months later, the Linlithgow Committee recommended the appointment of a Milk Advisory Committee (MAC).

This part of Linlithgow was accepted and it was decided that the brief of the new MAC would be 'to advise … on matters concerning the production, handling and distribution of milk and dairy produce, including questions relating to education and research, and any legislation, orders and regulations which may be under consideration'.[71] Revealingly it was seen as 'a sort of mouthpiece of the milk industry', and an early warning system for the potential conflicts that might arise.[72]

In August 1923 an inter-departmental conference was held to determine the composition of this committee, attended by representa-

---

[69] Savage 1931a, 543.
[70] Savage 1932.
[71] TNA: MH/56/75.
[72] Ibid.

tives from the Ministries of Agriculture, Health and Labour, the Board of Trade, and the Scottish Office. The MAF took the lead, packing the meeting with four key staff, including their Permanent Secretary and the Chief Scientific Adviser. By comparison the MH sent only one representative.

The initial make-up was to be a neutral Chairman, two officials each from the Ministries of Health and Agriculture, eight trade representatives, one delegate from the NCMS, and two MOsH. During and immediately after this meeting there was sparring between the Ministries of Health and Agriculture as to who would pay the committee's expenses. Eventually this was settled when the MAF agreed to use its exchequer grant and, as paymasters, they inevitably gained leverage over the business.

Despite the modest brief of this committee, it attracted a disproportionate amount of political attention. First, it proved difficult to find a chairman acceptable to both the MAF and the MH. The MAF's preferred candidate, Lord Kenyon, who was eventually appointed. He had a proven interest in milk, including asking questions about it in the House of Lords.

Second, many representations were made about the composition of the committee, mainly objections to the preponderance of trade voices and the omission of interests such as the trade unions and women's groups.[73] For such lobbying to be worthwhile there must have been expectations that the committee might deliver policy changes after such a long period of stagnation. Discussion between the Ministries eventually led to an expanded committee with a marginal shift in the gender balance.

Third, there were scandals about interests served or not served. In June 1925, for instance, J.H. Maggs offered his resignation because of complaints from some members of the Federation that he had ignored their interests in the Advisory Committee when they clashed with those of United Dairies, of which he was Chairman. This was rejected by the MAF who argued that the members of this committee had not been intended as delegates representing some narrow interest, but rather as well-informed traders who could share their knowledge

---

[73] HC Deb 2 April 1924 vol 171 cc 2154-55; *Dairyman, The Cowkeeper and Dairyman's Journal* May 1924, 470.

with the Minister.[74] This annoyed the Federation who had all along wanted a placeman to represent them and they began an irritable correspondence with the Ministry asking for clarification.[75] They could not have guessed that all along there was a reserve option, revealed in the policy documents. If Maggs had persisted with his resignation, which actually he did not, the MAF intended to re-appoint him anyway as an independent cooptee, who just happened to be the most powerful dairyman in the country.

The Committee's minutes indicate that it met formally on only eleven occasions, all in the period 1924-1926. The death of Lord Kenyon in 1928 left a vacancy that was not filled. At that point the MH's internal memoranda show that they placed little store by the Committee.

The Vice-Chairman, Mr Langford, took over as Acting-Chairman but he was undermined in 1930 when it was discovered that he had used his position in an advertisement for a new company with which he was involved.[76] The Committee seems to have been dissolved at that point.

Topics that had reached the Committee's agenda included technical matters such as whey disposal, the sealing of churns in transit, or the quality of cheese; more general issues like dairy education; and just occasionally controversial discussions such as the advisability of legislation and regulation affecting dairy products. The minutes of the first meeting were dominated by the proposed Tuberculosis Order. Wilfred Buckley from the National Clean Milk Campaign argued against compensation for slaughtered animals and J.H. Maggs did not want the Order at all.

The demise of the MAC left a vacuum that needed to be filled, not least in the face of representations from the Council of Agriculture and various other bodies for a comprehensive Milk Act.[77] Throughout its existence, the Committee had failed in its task of providing unbiased advice because each of the groups represented had voted along the lines of self-interest, even on relatively trivial issues.

---

[74] TNA: MH/56/75.
[75] Ibid.
[76] TNA: MH/56/76.
[77] TNA: MH/56/91 and MH/56/88.

Conclusion

It is difficult to draw conclusions about bTB policy from this period, 1914-29. It makes sense to postpone our thoughts until the end of the next chapter. But as an interim general point we can maybe put the lack of progress down to what is sometimes characterised as Britain's predilection for an incrementalist policy style and decision-making system that avoids controversy and conflict by taking seriously the views of powerful vested interests.[78] This was pragmatic and negotiative but the bureaucratic accommodation involved did not necessarily amount to full consultation, at least in the sense of a balanced appraisal of all of the current views and values.[79] Certainly with regard to our policy area, bTB, the managerial momentum in Whitehall was reactive rather than proactive until the end of the Second World War. Then a short period of uncharacteristically radical thinking and planning from the late 1940s to the mid 1970s was followed by another phase on the back foot, right through until the last decade or so when new ideas have come forward.

How can we explain such a cautious, 'conservative' style? Did it emanate from a 'culture' of the Whitehall or Westminster elites? This seems unlikely; indeed, given the changing ideological frames of successive governments and the extraordinary shifts of fortune brought about by wars and economic collapse, it is stretching credulity to imagine stability in any single style that one might call a conscious anticipatory strategy or even a 'cultural' preference. Nevertheless the taken-for-granted assumptions of each ministry acted as upstream frames that provided a starting point and then a contingent context for policy making.

Inspiration can be drawn here from Law and Wilkinson who are interested in how values and goals are shared and communicated within organizations.[80] In the case of Whitehall ministries, this is less a 'culture' than a set of discursive practices and non-verbal performances mediated through materials. Nor can we read off the MAF's or Defra's

---

[78] Jordan and Richardson 1982.

[79] France by contrast is said to have greater secrecy and less consultation, combined with an autocratic style that lends itself to a paradoxical combination of stasis and occasional bold initiatives. Richardson, Gustafsson and Jordan 1982.

[80] Law 1994; Wilkinson 2011.

(Department of Environment, Food and Rural Affairs) intentionality directly from their publications or even indirectly from their confidential in-house minutes. Their 'modes of ordering' are rather implicit in the stories they tell each other and their colleagues in other ministries. This is partly textual but is also concretized in, say, the bodies of the animals that were their responsibility and also in the bacteria that swerve around their defences.

Perhaps then the 'styles' were institutional? In the case of Britain the Civil Service has traditionally been politically neutral and civil servants continued in post whatever the colour of the political party in power. According to this model, a combination of elitism and meritocracy gave the continuity needed to moderate the wilder fluctuations of policy. And yet even a cursory glimpse at the papers of Whitehall ministries preserved in the National Archives reveals significant differences between the implicit mission statements of the ministries in our policy area - MAF, MH and Treasury - and also between the leadership styles of the powerful individuals managing them, especially the Permanent Secretaries.

Policy-making style amounts to methods of filtering and processing business and for us this yields performative or behavioural insights into the mind-set of the participants. According to Bevir and Rhodes, this is best pursued in the present day through on-the-ground ethnography but the historian also has written evidence in the everyday internal communications and administrative paper trail of officials and their dealings with the rest of Whitehall and the outside world.[81] The Thirty Year Rule means that most of these papers remain confidential for recent decades and beyond the moving time threshold one finds that many files have been weeded in order to economise on shelf space. Nevertheless, we can build up a detailed picture of activities on the formulation of particular policies and their implementation as laws or regulations. If one had the time or funds to hire research assistants, it would theoretically be possible to look across the full range of a ministry's daily business and so recreate the action sphere of each senior civil servant. Even in the narrow range of bTB policy we can learn from the tone of an individual's memos, their personal relationships

---

[81] Bevir and Rhodes 2003.

with their working colleagues, and the routines of hierarchical power. Cynicism, idealism, resignation, aggression, humour, erudition and many other emotions and skills are all on display and together they are an extraordinarily rich source of raw material for the researcher.

One possible mode of processing the archival material is via the conventions theory of Laurent Thévenot and Luc Boltanski.[82] They are leaders of the French 'pragmatic turn' in social theory and their programme is an attempt to reconstruct the notion of human action. They are less motivated by an understanding of intentionality than by the constitutive nature of action. For them it is important to build from below a grasp of the way people come to appreciate their commonality and coordinate their efforts into conventions of action. Thévenot and Boltanski are sceptical of any theory of institutional structure that does not take such regimes of engagement into account, and their approach is encouraging for the micro-focus adopted in the present volume because of their interest in the capability and competences that agents bring to any situation of social negotiation.

Boltanski and Thévenot in their *On Justification* identified a number of 'cités', dimensions of common values or orders of worth. For our purposes the most relevant are what they call the 'civic', 'market' and 'industrial' worlds. Through the performances of their participants we can detect a differentiation of approaches, mindsets, and behaviours. In the civic world the stress is upon unity, collectivity, authorization, representativeness and legality. The market world is driven by value, quality and luxury, and the industrial world by functionality, reliability, efficiency and expertise. We may hypothesise that the differences observable between ministries, and to a lesser extent within ministries, is the result of circuits of value and action differentiation along these lines.

An illustration of this is the 'sectorization' of policy issues, with different styles and modes of accommodation being deployed according to the nature of the problem at hand. Institutionally Whitehall seems to have had some flexibility in this regard, although the friction visible in the system from time to time proves that attempts did not always run smoothly. As we have seen, conflicts did break out within and between

---

[82] Boltanski and Thévenot 2006.

ministries and, given the resourcefulness of the individuals involved, these were conducted in numerous subtle and indirect ways. At times it seems that civil servants felt that they had more in common with the key members of their policy community than they did with colleagues in other ministries. In Boltanski and Thévenot's terms the staff of the MAF thus operated in and shared the mindset of the industrial and market cités, whereas those of the MH were clearly in the civic world. There is no implication here of a 'culture' or of clientalism. Nor was technical or other specialist expertise necessarily a factor. Veterinary expertise was a source of tension in the MAF, and in other ministries it was common right up to the Second World War for both internal and external experts to be marginalised in the policy-making process by the generalist mentality of civil servants. There seems to have been a common feeling in that period that expertise was somehow divorced from the gritty reality of day-to-day administration.[83]

---

[83] Lowe 2011.

CHAPTER 10.

1930 TO 1937: WHITE HEAT IN WHITEHALL

Introduction

In Chapter 9 we saw that the legacy of the First World War was a delay in the implementation of legislation that had so painstakingly been formulated in the LGB under Burns and then Samuel. It was judged that the regulatory framework of the Milk and Dairies Consolidation Act (1915) and the accompanying Tuberculosis Order would be expensive to put into effect and the Act was therefore postponed until 1925. There was some modest progress on the milk-borne disease front in the 1926 Milk and Dairy Order but precious little in terms of cooperation between ministries. The MAC did not achieve much from 1923 to 1930 and resembled a low-level skirmish, with forces on either side advancing or retreating according to the issues that came up. It was to no-one's surprise or regret that it ceased to exist in 1930 and was replaced by an 'informal' IDC on milk.

In this chapter we will illustrate how the new IDC highlighted the differences in conventions between the MAF and the MH, which were then repeated in several policy struggles with regard to milk and disease. The 1930s were a momentous decade for the MAF, with the successful creation of the MMB but the abject failure of its Milk Bills from 1937 to 1939. They found zoonotic diseases particularly challenging and, despite the creation of Attested herds in 1935 and the National Veterinary Service in 1937/8, the level of risk at the end of the decade was no lower than at the outset.

The Inter-Departmental Committee on the Law Relating to Milk (1930-31)

The IDC was appointed in December 1930 but this did not heal the wounds left by the failed MAC. The trenches vacated by the warring delegates of the farmers, distributors and retailers were occupied instead by foot soldiers from the disputatious Ministries of Health and

Agriculture. This Whitehall-only affair did at least have the advantage of confidentiality, with very few headlines appearing in the press of the kind that had been so embarrassing in the 1920s. Rather, it was a form of institutionalised struggle in which the parties employed a variety of tactics to develop their respective causes, and in which the departments concerned seem to have had a strong will to succeed. The flavour of this was less like Jeremy Richardson's 'policy styles' than the 'institution-alised conflict' described by ex-civil servant Clive Ponting.[1]

The IDC had been established 'largely at the insistence of Dr Addison, the new Minister of Agriculture.[2] Addison no doubt saw himself as a potential bridge between the interests of the producer and consumer. He had been Minister of Health from 1919 to 1921 and knew about the ministry's long-established antagonism with the MAF. However, in the event Addison was not an ideal broker of disinterested policy. He had had a chequered career himself, including a switch from the Liberals to the Labour Party and a period out of Parliament after losing his seat in the 1922 General Election. Ultimately his success as Minister of Agriculture (June 1930 to August 1931) lay in the initiation of collective marketing and not in the encouragement of inter-departmental collaboration.

From the outset, officials in the MH had private misgivings, but they did proceed and the Committee was established, with two members each from the Ministries of Agriculture and Health, and one each from the equivalent departments of the Scottish Office.[3]

Like a poultice, the IDC drew out poisonous disputes that had festered for years, but the cleansing process was incomplete. The idea of a Royal Commission on bTB was rejected by the Committee, as were policies such as extending the veterinary inspection of infected cattle, and the encouragement of the heat treatment of milk to kill the bacteria of tuberculosis and brucellosis. The Scottish Office was especially keen on the veterinary policing of the dairy herd, as this had been accomplished effectively north of the border for several years, but in England and Wales the responsible department would have been the

---

[1] Richardson 1993; Ponting 1986.
[2] TNA: MH 56/88.
[3] TNA: MH 56/88.

MH and they had to admit that they were unable to find the £200,000 annually that would have been required to hire the necessary staff.

In the IDC the MAF was 'primarily concerned' about the effects of pasteurization upon producer-retailers, almost all of whom were small farmers.[4] They also objected to the main alternative, municipal pasteurizing stations. Here their problem was that the 'milk would lose its identity' and the personal connection between producer-retailers and their customers would therefore be lost. There would also be delays and additional transport costs.[5] With these small players being forced out of business a greater proportion of the general milk supply would come under the control of the big combines. By a logic that is not entirely clear, the MAF concluded that the loss of producer-retailers would slow down efforts to reduce the incidence of bTB in cattle and discourage attempts to produce milk of a higher hygienic quality.

With regard to consumers' interests, the MAF objected to pasteurization on four principal grounds. First, the effect of pasteurization on milk was as yet only partially understood and using the technology was therefore a 'leap in the dark'. Second, in those cities where the bulk of the milk supply was already pasteurized, there was no conclusive evidence to show that the incidence of tuberculosis was less than in the country as a whole. Third, the processing technology was not always reliable and 'no regulations can insure that it shall be always effective'. Fourth, they dismissed Manchester's proposals for compulsory pasteurization because the continued sale of raw milk would have been allowed if it was Certified or Grade A (TT) and, while those milks would presumably be free from bTB, they might carry other bacteria. Finally the MAF asked that pasteurization legislation be delayed for the completion of the cattle vaccine work at Cambridge by Professor Buxton and Dr Griffith (BCG) and in Northern Ireland (Spahlinger).[6]

In an internal memo in March 1931, Dr Thomas Carnwath, a Senior Medical Officer at the MH, regretted his ministry's inability to make 'a clear pronouncement ... in favour of pasteurization.' Although he was scathing about the producer-retailers who were 'peddling milk

[4] TNA: CAB 58/184.
[5] Ibid.
[6] Ibid. For more on Buxton, see Waddington 2004, 2006.

from door to door in open tins' and accused them of being 'the people who have kept us sitting on the fence all these years', he nevertheless admitted that inaction by the MH meant that 'we are as much or more to blame than they are.'[7]

Collectively the staff of the MH were disappointed but probably not surprised at the inconclusive outcome of the IDC. A.B. Maclachlan (Principal Assistant Secretary) reported to his Permanent Secretary:

> I am afraid this Committee has not proved very useful from our point of view. Its first report dealing with bovine tuberculosis was distinctly disappointing and its third report on adulteration contains majority recommendations for the amendment of the law which we should have to resist ... It is difficult to suggest any forward step in present circumstances.[8]

Possibly the most interesting outcome of the IDC procedure was the emergence of a new tactic on the MAF side. They were determined, if at all possible, to avoid any expensive and disruptive intervention against zoonoses, such as the isolation or slaughter of cows infected with tuberculosis. Throughout the 1920s and early 1930s they consistently emphasised the need to avoid ruining small farmers by excessive inspection and regulation. It was with barely disguised triumph, therefore, that MAF officials attending a conference on bTB, which had been called in January 1932 to provide expert opinions for the IDC to consider, seized upon an idea of Professor Basil Buxton of the University of Cambridge. He was engaged on a series of experiments to see if BCG could be employed as a vaccine to protect cattle against tuberculosis, as it already had been used across Europe to immunise humans. Buxton is reported to have said that 'in the light of the results already obtained, and as the work was nearing completion, it would be indefensible at present to institute any important new administrative measures dealing with the problem'.[9] For some time to come the MAF quoted this opinion as definitive and they counselled against any policy or administrative changes with regard to bovine tuberculosis until

---

[7] TNA: MH 56/81.

[8] TNA: MH 56/88.

[9] TNA: MH 56/90.

Buxton's results were known.[10] The IDC and its reports were therefore effectively dead.

Following Buxton's remarks, the MAF/MH tussle broadened to include other departments. It is worth recounting in some detail one incident involving the MRC because it demonstrates the sharp personal animosity that could be generated within the broader clash of discourses.

A few days after the January conference, Sir Walter Fletcher, Secretary of the MRC, wrote an angry letter to Sir Charles Howell Thomas, Permanent Secretary of the MAF about the minutes that had been prepared.[11] Fletcher effectively accused Howell Thomas of distortion in suggesting that the meeting had accepted Buxton's view that action on TB should wait for his results on BCG. According to Fletcher, 'the meeting did not agree upon anything of the kind and did not even discuss it'. Sir Walter suggested that the views of Buxton's co-worker, Stanley Griffith, that immunisation was not the solution, had been 'suppressed' and Fletcher was especially irritated that the MRC was in effect being used by the MAF to sell a particular policy option to the Cabinet:

> What I am sure you will not defend is that the Ministry, without any consultation with us on this subject, should represent to the Cabinet committee that the Council have been consulted upon it, and that they acquiesce in certain views of which, so far as I can judge, they would probably hold the exact opposite.[12]

Later, in a private letter to Sir Robert Greig of the Scottish Office, Fletcher confided that Howell Thomas's reply to his complaint had been unsatisfactory.[13] 'If I did not feel sure that Thomas had been simply misinformed by ignorant or stupid subordinates, I should think his reply a piece of amazing effrontery'. However, Sir Charles Howell Thomas, far from withdrawing his report or conceding any errors, wrote

[10] His *Lancet* paper (Buxton and Griffith 1931) was published later that year but Buxton published several other papers on BCG and calves up to 1939. Ultimately his work was not a success.
[11] TNA: FD 1/5084.
[12] Ibid.
[13] Ibid.

a stinging riposte. His letter to Sir Walter is full of heavy sarcasm that fizzes on the page.

> If, as it now appears, you then felt so strongly on the subject, what opportunities you missed for enlightening us on your views! How you might have told us that an overwhelming reason for declining a Royal Commission was that the real object of those who asked for the Commission was so obviously sound that we ought to proceed forthwith to recommend immediate initiation of some such scheme as eradication as they had proposed … A mere hint from you at that time on this subject would obviously have affected our conclusions.[14]

In a sympathetic letter, Greig informed Fletcher that Howell Thomas had recently visited the Scottish Office and had asked the Secretary of State, Sir Godfrey Collins, whether 'he had been deceived by the paragraph [in the minutes] quoting the MRC in regard to immunisation'.[15] The unwanted reply had been 'yes', that it had been assumed that the MRC were being quoted as supporting the MAF's policy.[16]

> We both tried to make him understand that you were not accusing him of deliberate falsehood, but of giving the wrong impression through the careless construction of the paragraph by an uninformed subordinate. I told him he was guilty of producing an incorrect impression of the result of a meeting, and that he better confess it and be done with it and it was not a matter to bother about as any subordinate could let one down in such a way … But he would not be placated and left much astonished and disappointed by the attitude of the Secretary of State and telling us that he was determined to carry the matter further … I wish I was in London, as I think I could induce that doubting and unreasonable Thomas to admit his mistake over a bottle of port.[17]

It seems that the controversy was eventually settled, months later, over lunch at Brooks's club. By then the politics of milk had moved on and Fletcher himself was seriously ill. Leaving aside the personalities involved, the vicious infighting revealed in this correspondence suggests that the issues were very important to the MAF. Fletcher admitted that he actually had 'no strong feelings' on bTB, and it seems that for him

---

[14] Ibid.
[15] TNA: FD 1/5084.
[16] Ibid.
[17] Ibid.

the issue was one of the tactics employed by Sir Charles. The latter was clearly anxious that his position was being undermined by a marginal player in this particular Whitehall game. Postponement of action on cattle disease was Howell Thomas's immediate tactic. He won this skirmish but the war with other parts of Whitehall was not over yet.

By the time of the IDC's final report in October 1931, there had been a change in government. The planned system of veterinary examinations was quickly dropped for financial reasons and so was the Bill that had originally been contemplated by Addison. Interestingly, his intention had been to suggest a 'public committee or commission (including MPs) ... to hear all interested parties who might have points to urge and of objections to raise ... (I believe that something like this procedure was adopted in the case of de-rating)'.[18] Such innovation would have involved a certain loss of control and it is not surprising, given the deeply conservative culture of the MAF, that postponement was once more in the air. The recent appointment of a Reorganization Commission for Milk to start work in 1932 was given as a reason for delaying any decisions about legislation.

There are two lessons to be learned from this case study. First, in terms of the everyday performance of governance, the contacts between the parties were extensive but the positions were so entrenched, and at times so close to the core values of the respective departmental views, that compromise was impossible. The MAF, in the end, translated outside 'expert knowledge' to its cause in order to re-establish the force-field of its power relationship with the MH. This prompts the second conclusion, about governmentality. 'The conduct of conduct' is one way of looking at the exercise of power and our case study illustrates that the MAF's tactic of using science to stall further action was embedded within a system of implicit, low-order trust.[19] Their mistake was a clumsy and arrogant solidification of their victory on the doctored minutes that frankly amounted to a breach of trust. Civil servants were usually slicker and more professional than this in getting their own way.

---

[18] TNA: MAF/52/8, TD/2549.

[19] Foucault 1991.

The People's League of Health report (1932)

An important letter to the editor of the *Lancet* was published in December 1930 from Viscount Dawson of Penn, physician to the Royal family, and seven other leading scientists. They called for pasteurization and the revision of milk grades. This was widely cited and by February 1931 the MH was taking the opportunity to admit that the 1915 Act had failed with regard to the reduction of bTB.[20] They were probably hoping that lobbying by the elite of the medical profession would help to push their own agenda forward and further assistance soon came in the form of an influential speech by Lord Moynihan in the House of Lords on 10 February in which he revived the idea of a Royal Commission.[21] The collective feeling in the IDC had been that a Royal Commission was not necessary in view of the vast amount of information, scientific and administrative, already in the public domain. Any limitations to research were due to the 'lack of able workers and not lack of funds'.[22]

Following the *Times* letter, one of the most influential reports published in the decade before the War came in 1932 from the campaigning group, the PLH.[23] It was the fruit of meetings that had started in February 1930. One of the most useful aspects of the report was its survey and compilation of data concerning rates of bTB infection in cattle and humans.

The PLH argued for modifications to the Tuberculosis Order in order to make it more effective.[24] In particular they wanted owners of tuberculous stock to have a duty to notify any clinical symptoms of bTB immediately - incentivized by more generous compensation - to close the loophole that allowed farmers knowingly to keep diseased animals until the end of their economically useful life.[25] The report also called for more full-time local authority veterinary inspectors and more extensive milk sampling programmes. In addition, the League, following

---

[20] TNA: MH 56/81.

[21] HL Deb 10 February 1931 vol *79 cc 891-8*; TNA: MH 56/81; Anon. 1931, 444; People's League of Health [1932b], 2.

[22] Walter Fletcher, MRC, TNA: MH 56/81.

[23] People's League of Health 1932a.

[24] Ibid.

[25] This change was not made until the Tuberculosis Order (1938).

its mentor William Savage, suggested animal isolation centres and compulsory slaughterhouse registers of where animals were sourced.

The League's report was launched in January 1932 at the Mansion House by Savage, Lord Dawson of Penn and Lord Moynihan of Leeds.[26] It had been compiled from the thoughts of a committee of one hundred doctors, veterinary surgeons, laboratory scientists, farmers and milk dealers chaired first by E.B. Turner and later by Savage.[27] They also concluded that more research was needed on cattle vaccination, that all milk should be graded, and that permissive powers should be given to local authorities to enforce the compulsory pasteurization of all milk other than certified and TT grades.

The Hopkins Committee (1932-34)

In February 1932, shortly after the PLH report, the new Minister of Agriculture, Sir John Gilmour, made a unilateral announcement in the House of Commons that there would be an investigation of 'the means of seeing a reduction of disease among dairy herds'.[28] This prompted another flurry of activity in Whitehall. With the IDC barely cold in its shallow grave, officials and politicians realised that a new departure was necessary, not least because the broader medical debate demanded it. In addition, Gilmour showed his sensitivity to the coming crisis in dairying by setting up a Milk Reorganization Commission under the Agriculture Marketing Act (1931) to consider a major restructuring of the milk industry in Britain. In due course this would offer opportunities for a variety of economic and health-related initiatives.

A meeting was held in March 1932, just a month after Gilmour's statement to Parliament, comprised of delegates from the Ministries of Agriculture and Health, the Scottish Office, and the Agricultural and Medical Research Councils. The National Archives have preserved a verbatim transcript of the proceedings of this meeting, which is interesting because it is much blunter in tone than the sanitised minutes

---

[26] Anon. 1932a.

[27] Anon. 1932b.

[28] TNA: MH 56/84.

later circulated.[29] Sir Charles Howell Thomas was in the chair and he declared at the outset that:

> If I felt that any one department was in a position to tell the government exactly how to proceed, we would not be sitting here today. It is because of these different points of view, the different considerations that we have met to consider how we can best face up to this problem, and it seems to me that we can hardly hope to avoid – much as I dislike it – the setting up of another Committee to go into the several questions.

In the discussion that followed, a fundamental incompatibility re-emerged about the need for compulsory veterinary inspections to identify tuberculous cattle. Pasteurization and milk grading also remained controversial. The meeting concluded, against the wishes of the officials of the MH, that the Economic Advisory Council, a Cabinet committee, should appoint a sub-committee to advise on cattle disease.[30] This would in effect be a form of arbitration because disagreement was so great between the MAF and the MH. In private Sir Arthur Robinson[31] explained to his Minister that it was better to go to an overriding authority such as a Cabinet committee because inter-departmental meetings were mostly unfruitful:

> When we confer officially with the Ministry of Agriculture and Fisheries, the interests are conflicting and there are cases on record where, when we came to put into an actual Bill, what had been agreed at such conferences, the Ministry of Agriculture, under pressure from the farmers, went back on the agreement.[32]

As the reply from the Minister, Hilton Young, indicates, his greatest worry was rather the cost of veterinary inspection to his Ministry if a state veterinary service was ever implemented:

> The moment is not favourable for an active effort that needs more money: so we may be content with the reference to the committee, which postpones the effort.[33]

The Cattle Diseases Committee, as it came to be known, was officially appointed by the Prime Minister in November 1932, with Sir

---

[29] TNA: MAF 35/435.
[30] TNA: MH 56/84.
[31] Ibid.
[32] Ibid.
[33] Ibid.

Frederick Gowland Hopkins as Chairman.[34] In retrospect, the format of this 'committee of experts' enquiry was much more likely to yield results than the MAC or the IDC because its participants were less beholden to vested interests. The Ministries tried to get their placemen on to the Committee but it seems that the Economic Advisory Council and the Cabinet Office prevented this.

After receiving written submissions from the interested departments, and taking evidence verbally from selected witnesses, the Committee had its report ready in draft by November 1933, and in final form by April 1934. The MH argued for the compulsory clinical examination of all cattle and they were also very keen on the pasteurization of milk. In contrast, the Department of Agriculture for Scotland wanted a voluntary eradication scheme with free tuberculin testing to identify tuberculous cattle, and the MAF pressed for an Attested Herds Scheme, giving a financial incentive (1d per gallon) to farmers who were willing to rid their herds of tuberculosis.[35] What Hopkins actually recommended is complex and did not meet all of these needs (Table 10.1).

Table 10.1 Main recommendations of the Hopkins Committee

- Universal and routine veterinary inspection, cost falling on Local Authorities;
- Farmer to pay for six-monthly tuberculin testing by local authority and enter into agreement about purchase of new animals, isolation of reactors, and disinfection of buildings. Such agreements to be called 'Supervised Herds';
- Supervised Herds that pass two consecutive tests to qualify for the list of disease-free 'Accepted' herds (later called 'Attested');
- Loans or loan guarantees to assist herd owners with eradication;
- A higher price should be paid for milk from tuberculosis-free herds;
- Tuberculosis-free stock to be kept separate from other cattle at markets and shows;
- Four new grades of milk;
- Compulsory pasteurisation in towns and cities over 100,000 population five years after start of eradication and after two years notice;
- Reject idea that immunisation of cattle is ever likely to prove a solution of the public health problem;

Source: BPP 1933-4 (Cmd. 4591) ix.427.

In its evidence before the Committee, the MH submitted two documents, one on compulsory pasteurization and the other on the public health control of milk. They claimed to be 'the central authority mainly concerned with the public health problem of the milk supply' but admitted that consultation with the MAF was often desirable in

---

[34] TNA: MAF 35/435.

[35] Ibid.

areas affecting their interests.[36] The report and subsequent correspondence indicate that the MH's case was the most compelling for Hopkins. Although the Ministry's officials were annoyed by the report's proposed delay in pasteurization in order to allow producer-retailers and small dealers to make the necessary technical arrangements, they expressed their general satisfaction with the findings, and characterised it as 'a valuable document from the public health aspect'.[37]

In the months between the draft and final reports, there was time for negotiations between the two Ministries. Feeling now that they were in a stronger position than for years, the MH agreed to the MAF's proposed Attested Herds Scheme, provided that it was coupled with a full-time veterinary service paid for by the local authorities. The MH also felt they had a 'clear understanding' that a *quid pro quo* of this compromise would be the implementation of local pasteurization on the expiry of a five-year moratorium. But the Permanent Secretary made it plain to his Minister that he did not take this for granted:

> The G. Hopkins report contained a good deal which the M. of Ag. do not like - notably as to pasteurisation, and it is quite likely that they may try to shelve the matter, on the plea of having their hands full with a Bill ... It seems advisable that Mr Elliot's attention should be drawn to the matter ...[38]

An inter-departmental meeting was held on 12 May, 1934, to discuss the outcome of the Hopkins Committee.[39] It was agreed to proceed with the Attested Herd Scheme but soon afterwards it transpired that 'the MAF are not proposing to take any action on the report until the present Milk Bill is through. I presume that this means that they would like the question of further legislation to be postponed indefinitely'.[40]

In October, 1934, Hilton Young had a private meeting with Walter Elliot and managed to extract an agreement to legislate for pasteurization. Within a month Elliot had changed his mind, however, and proposed another round of meetings between officials. In Sir Arthur Robinson's

---

[36] Ibid.

[37] TNA: MH 79/326.

[38] TNA: MH 56/85.

[39] TNA: MAF 35/313.

[40] TNA: MH 56/85.

view, the Hopkins Report 'raises questions of such difficulty that the govt have not yet been able to make up their mind about it', and he challenged his Minister to 'decide whether you will or will not accept Mr Elliot's device for shelving the report by starting another series of departmental conferences which, from the start are condemned to futility'.[41] Robinson saw an appeal to the Cabinet as 'the only way out'.

The Minister of Health ignored the very clear view of his Permanent Secretary and agreed to one more inter-departmental meeting, in order 'to clear the air'.[42] Foot dragging is a time-honoured Whitehall device where the Civil Service disapproves of instructions and in this case ten weeks elapsed before A.B. Maclachlan of the MH wrote to the MAF conveying the message. When the meeting was eventually convened, in April 1935, there were recriminations. Sir Arthur Robinson for the MH made his irritation clear at the lack of progress on the Hopkins recommendations with regard to pasteurization as a solution to the problem of bovine tuberculosis.

> There is ... a most urgent health problem, and in the view of the department which has to bear the responsibility no solution except through pasteurisation is in sight. The Ministry of Agriculture had always contested this view and finally a Committee had been set up by the Cabinet machinery to form an independent opinion and the Ministry of Health had had no hand in its setting up. This Committee has supported the Ministry's view that a measure of compulsory pasteurisation was required in the interests of public health and that, subject to certain conditions, it should be imposed. Nevertheless the Ministry of Agriculture now proceeded to question the findings of the Committee and further enquiry and further delays were suggested. This attitude was profoundly disquieting to the Ministry of Health and seemed quite out of keeping with the principle of using Cabinet machinery to resolve departmental differences.[43]

The immediate and robust reply was that 'the Committee had convinced nobody, for they had failed to produce satisfactory evidence in support of their conclusions'.[44] However, the MAF did offer a compromise whereby a local authority could apply to the MH for a

---

[41] Ibid.
[42] Ibid.
[43] Ibid.
[44] Ibid.

pasteurization Order, which would be granted so long as it was approved by both Ministries. Sir Arthur Robinson rejected this overture because they 'would repeat the battle each time'.

Further points of difference arose when no agreement was possible about funding for veterinary inspections, and also when the MH announced its intention to seek minimum standards of cleanliness for all milk. This latter was a bold move because they were rowing away from the relatively sedate backwater of enforcing the quality of designated milks into the rougher mainstream of the milk industry, where much of the milk produced was still of a very low standard. The MAF representatives at the meeting rejected this out of hand, claiming that it 'would arouse a storm in the agricultural community'.[45]

In a memo to his Minister, Sir Arthur Robinson described this meeting as having achieved 'complete deadlock'.[46] He was scathing about the MAF, who, on the subject of pasteurisation, he described as

> so terrified of the farmers that they will have recourse to any manoeuvres to dodge this issue … and, when they cannot dodge any further, will fight to the finish against the recommendation. In these circumstances, and with a general election on the horizon, when county seats will be a pretty weighty element, I should judge that we must give this matter up as a bad job … The impression made on my mind is that we cannot do anything more than we are doing, and that we shall have to reconcile ourselves to the situation. Since one element in the situation is that we have, say, two thousand deaths annually from bovine TB, it is not a very happy one for a Minister of Health, but I fear the sons of Zeruiah are too strong for us.[47]

The Minister remained more optimistic than his Permanent Secretary, however. He gave instructions to accept the MAF's compromise of treating each local authority request for pasteurisation on its merits.[48] One or two of the more junior civil servants agreed with this strategy and in private correspondence they pointed to imminent changes among the MAF staff as signs of hope.[49]

---

[45] Ibid.

[46] Ibid.

[47] Ibid.

[48] Ibid.

[49] Atkins 2010b.

> The opposition comes from the more old fashioned part of the Ministry, who accept the view of the National Farmers Union that a policy of compulsory pasteurization would be detrimental to the interests of the producer-retailer. The importance of the producer-retailer is undoubtedly on the wane, and two of the principal advocates of this point of view, Mr Dale and Mr Blackshaw, are likely to retire at the end of this year.[50]

Although in the Cabinet, Young was a minor figure in the National Government of 1931-35, constantly in the shadow of high-profile politicians such as his successful predecessor as Minister of Health, Neville Chamberlain. He seems to have been weak in his relations with other Ministers and unable to forge a strong policy agenda against criticism in parliament and the press.[51] By contrast, Elliot saw through revolutionary policies at the MAF, particularly on marketing.[52]

The Grigg Commission (1932-33)

With world agricultural commodity prices falling rapidly after the financial crises of 1929 and 1931, there was pressure to abandon cherished policies of free trade.[53] The debate was about whether any re-imposition of tariffs should include food products and whether some level of preferential treatment should be given to imports from farmers around the Empire.[54] Such imperial preference was opposed by British dairy farmers for fear of a flood of competitively priced butter and cheese from Canada, Australia and New Zealand. An alternative, at least in the minds of the hard-pressed politicians, was improving British market structures to make them more efficient and profitable. One possibility was the better grading of commodities according to quality and another was improving the articulation of retail distributive systems. But most significant politically was the idea of creating marketing collectives in which risk would be shared mutually. This notion was pioneered in 1931, near the end of the Labour administration, by Addison's Agricultural

---

[50] TNA: MH 56/85.

[51] He has been described as 'dead wood' by one historian of the 1930s. Smart 1999, 91.

[52] Cooper 1989; Taylor 1979.

[53] Brown 2000.

[54] This was controversially negotiated in the 1932 Ottawa accords.

Marketing Act. This was not welcomed at first by the farming world because of perceptions of bureaucratic interference but the NFU were soon persuaded by their branches in the dairy counties to at least see what might be on offer. As Cooper points out, three-quarters of their members were milk producers so the NFU leaders had no choice but to take their views into account.[55] What the dairy farmers had spotted was that the Act was offering them the extraordinary possibility of additional power in their negotiations with distributors such as United Dairies. This relationship, which had been so problematic in the days of the PJMC would eventually be resolved in favour of the farmers; and the farmers had to give very little in return. All that was asked was their voluntary and financially incentivised participation in schemes to reduce bTB in cattle and improve the cleanliness of milk.

In retrospect this was a remarkable turnaround for a group of farmers who had been rendered weak in the 1920s by dairy product imports that had forced them into dependence upon a fluid milk market dominated by the wholesalers.[56] They now plunged into a more lucrative dependence upon a government-inspired but producer-led institution that was a monopsonistic buyer and monopolistic seller of milk. In early 1932 the MAF was involved, with the NFU and others, in the preparation of a milk scheme under the Agricultural Marketing Act that was passed in 1933. In April a Reorganization Commission for Milk was established under the chairmanship of Sir Edward Grigg, former Governor of Kenya.[57] He immediately appointed a committee to consider a standard quality for milk and they discussed the possibility of a bacteriological standard that would be enforced by sampling and by testing at laboratories strategically placed around the country.

Walter Elliot's arrival at the MAF in September 1932 as Minister in the National Government convinced a sceptical NFU that farmers themselves could occupy a position of unprecedented influence.[58] Their main task then was to heal divisions between farmers from different regions and enterprises whose inevitable concern was that a sector of marketing collectives might mean some groups were getting ahead of

---

[55] Cooper 1989.
[56] Barnes 2001.
[57] TNA: MH 56/100.
[58] Self and Storing 1962; Baker 1973.

others in terms of favourable treatment in government policy. Elliot's achievement was to turn the sketchy and at times hostile relations between government and farmers into a relationship that subsequently became close, to the point that for the period during and immediately after the war it has been called a prime example of corporatism.[59] It has even been suggested that 'the MMB was ... arguably, the single most important development in agricultural policy during the interwar years'.[60]

Elliot was a member of the 'YMCA' group of reform-minded Conservatives, who argued for radical solutions to stave off a collapse of the economic status quo.[61] He favoured collective organization in order to restore efficiency. This meant a partnership between government and various core interest groups in a corporatist architecture that provided politicians with clearly identifiable sites of negotiation and investment. In agriculture he did not approve of subsidised prices but rather sought to empower the producers to establish and run their own marketing boards. This was the basis of his Agricultural Marketing Act (1933) that built upon the foundations laid by Addison.

By the time Elliot had mastered his brief in the MAF, the Grigg Commission's work was well under way. Their report was presented in January 1933 and the NFU was given the task of preparing the practical detail, which they did by March. A poll of farmers in September was 96.4 per cent in favour and the Board was formally established on 6 October.[62] This was the England and Wales MMB, and there were three other Boards in Scotland (established 1933-34) and one in Northern Ireland (1955). The NFU had the final say on what came to be known as the Milk Marketing Scheme (MMS). They rejected Grigg's wish for balance with a Central Producers' Board and a Central Dairymen's Board both reporting to a Joint Milk Council.[63] The producers ran the scheme and it was not until 1954 that they were forced to accept the need for a Joint Committee with the distributors and manufacturers.

In essence this new MMS was a producers' monopoly with statutory

---

[59] Cox et al. 1986; Cox et al. 1990.
[60] Cox et al. 1990, 83.
[61] Cooper 1989.
[62] Raison and Ashby 1934.
[63] Hammond 1956, 180.

powers over price, grading, transport, marketing and advertising. It was based on regional pool prices, with the producers in each region getting the same price. The milk was then sold on for manufacture or retail liquid consumption. Although ideas about quality did eventually emerge, the MMS was initially about its lowest common denominator: the most basic milk produced on the vast majority of farms. Much of this came from small herds of cows that were not well nourished, and which were milked in unhygienic conditions.

By no means everyone was happy with these new arrangements, particularly the producer-retailers, many of whom had only small businesses. 46,801 of them were registered with the Board and had to pay a levy, which was the way all dairy farmers shared the burden of having a manufacturing price that was lower than the retail price of milk. The producer-retailers felt that manufacturing had nothing to do with them and they also resented the imposition of a minimum retail price when price competition had previously been their principal advantage.[64]

The other group that did not fit the structure of the MMS were the producers of high quality milk, including two grades that were in theory tuberculosis-free (Certified and Grade A (TT) and two with a reduced risk of tuberculous cattle (Grade A and Grade A (Pasteurized). Their numbers were small, only 1,000 in 1933, but the NFU nevertheless saw them as a distraction from the vast majority of their members, who were unable or unwilling to think about producing designated milks. Such milk was said to be produced by 'gentlemen farmers' and they were treated with a mixture of suspicion and contempt by the majority. It was in this context that various suggestions were made to reduce the complexity of the grading system or to undermine it altogether by introducing a new grade that the majority of farmers could aspire to.

Accredited and Attested Herd Schemes and the Milk Act

American ideas about the eradication of tuberculosis in cattle using Accredited herds were well publicized in Britain but it was often pointed out that conditions were different. The initial percentage of diseased animals was said to be low across the Atlantic along with a low density

---

[64] *The Times* 6 December 1937, 20b.

of cattle, whereas the British rate of infection was one the highest in the world.[65] Also, part of the British livestock economy was wedded to a rapid turnover of cattle, in so-called 'flying' herds, in order to keep milk yields high, particularly in winter.[66] This was maintained, and still is, by frequent sales between farms and through cattle markets in country towns, which were foci of cross infection. But overall cost was the main factor. In the words of the CVO, Sir Stewart Stockman:

> It is obviously not within the scope of practical politics, in this country, at least, to adopt a policy of testing all cattle, or even all milch cows, slaughtering the reactors, and paying compensation to the owners.[67]

This cost issue was repeated so often that it became a mantra of the MAF, for instance in 1929 when the Minister, Christopher Addison, commented privately that

> the occurrence of tuberculosis in herds was so widespread that any attempt at eradication by slaughter and compensation would be quite out of the question and we are a long way off being able to eliminate tuberculosis from herds.[68]

This was because the CVO, Sir Ralph Jackson, in the same year had estimated that over one million cows were tuberculous, and that the cost of slaughter and compensation would be £30 million.[69] It is hardly surprising that the MAF baulked at this. Hopkins neatly summarised the dilemma:

> The total eradication of bovine tuberculosis is generally agreed to be the only complete solution of the problem of tuberculous milk ... But any such scheme must take account of conditions peculiar to Great Britain. In the first place, the incidence of tuberculosis among our cattle is so high that the wholesale slaughter of infected animals ... is out of the question. Not only would its immediate cost be prohibitive, but it would also seriously contract the supply of milk.[70]

With regard to improving milk purity, the MAF's big idea in the 1930s was Accredited herds and Accredited milk. The terminology was

---

[65] Wilson 1942; Rich 1944.

[66] Crossley 1959.

[67] Stockman 1925a, 36.

[68] TNA: FD/1/4335.

[69] Ibid.

[70] BPP 1933-4 (Cmd. 4591) ix.478-9.

borrowed from North America, but in Whitehall there seems to have been some confusion as to its precise meaning and its purpose.[71] In 1931, Jackson, reported that he had carefully studied the Accredited herd schemes of Canada and the USA, but it was clear his interest was really in the tuberculin testing and slaughter part of accreditation rather than in milk hygiene in the broader sense. He had a detailed animal health plan for Britain but there was resistance to his ideas within the MAF because of their radical nature.[72] Jackson's successor as CVO in 1932, John Kelland, seems to have ignored these politics and provided continuity of concept.[73]

The usage of the term Accredited was picked up by the Grigg Commission in 1933 but with a meaning that was more to the liking of the MAF.[74] Their idea was for the official certification of Accredited producers who would have to meet certain conditions for producing quality milk, such as satisfactory buildings, hygienic conditions of production and handling of milk, and surprise sampling that confirmed that the milk was within certain bacteriological limits. In addition, famers would be expected to facilitate the regular veterinary inspections of their cattle and the slaughter of those showing clinical signs of bTB. Grigg recommended county-based whole-time veterinary services but made no mention of tuberculin testing.

Grigg's plan for accreditation was accepted by the government and the legal basis for Accredited milk was introduced in October 1933 under Section 33 of the MMS. Accredited milk then replaced Grade A in the Milk (Special Designations) Order, 1936, and, with the incentive of a bonus payment per gallon from the new Milk Marketing Boards (MMB), a rapid take-up was expected. Three certificates were to be required for admission to the roll of Accredited Producers: the first confirming that the herd had been clinically examined twice a year; the second indicating that the methods of production had been officially approved; and a third to the effect that two consecutive milk samples

---

[71] TNA: MH 56/92.

[72] TNA: MH/56/90.

[73] TNA: MAF/35/435.

[74] Grigg Commission 1933.

had been examined at intervals of not less than fourteen days, within the two months prior to the date of registration.[75]

In November 1933 the MAF convened a small group on 'the milk and milk products situation' under the chairmanship of Sir Horace Wilson. Although this was mainly about milk prices and help for cheese and butter producers, they did consider other matters, including bTB. They agreed with Grigg that a whole-time veterinary service was needed and that the cost should be borne by the MMBs, and like St Augustine, they sought this ultimate state of grace but 'not yet'. Instead they favoured launching 'an efficient campaign for cleaning up herds' and a publicity campaign to advertise milk.

Acting on the Wilson Committee's advice, in February 1934 the Minister, Elliot, introduced a White Paper on milk policy in the House of Commons. He pointed to the predicted twenty per cent surplus in the current winter contract period, due to end in March, and a forty per cent surplus in the summer. To deal with this and other issues, he first announced that £1.5 to £1.75 million would be spent each year for two years by the government to subsidize the manufacture of the surplus milk into butter and cheese. Second, £750,000 was to be spent over four years on encouraging 'a pure milk supply' and after that the Boards would take on the responsibility themselves.[76] No details were given of how pure milk was to be achieved, however. Finally, there was to be up to £1 million per annum over two years for a milk publicity fund, with equal amounts coming from the government and the MMBs.[77] Payment was conditional on a satisfactory plan to include the provision of milk in schools at a subsidised rate.

Elliott moved speedily from his White Paper to a Bill, which was submitted in draft to the Cabinet's Home Affairs Committee in March. By June it had already been presented to parliament and reached its committee stage.[78] It then received the Royal Assent and became the Milk Act (1934) at the end of July.

Soon after this it emerged that the MAF had decided against spending on veterinary services in favour of bonuses to farmers to be

---

[75] TNA: MH 56/101.
[76] TNA: MH 79/327.
[77] Anon. 1934.
[78] TNA: MH 56/106.

paid through the MMS if they joined a scheme for bTB-free herds.[79] This was to be a roll of 'Attested' herds and the MAF hoped that the farmers would pressurise local authorities into providing the veterinary services to make this possible. The term Attested had been coined to distinguish this policy from the Accredited Herds Scheme.

We saw above that the MH agreed to Attested herds in order to make progress with pasteurization but they were privately outraged by the idea. They estimated that attestation would touch only 1,000 herds and leave the other ninety-nine per cent of the milk supply unaffected. The reason was that no special designation was established for what might have been called Attested milk, and producers received only a bonus of 1d per gallon for sale into the MMS pool (Table 10.2). As a result, only a tiny minority of producers of TT milk thought it worth their while to seek Attested status, preferring instead the premium they gained from retailing their milk as Certified or Grade A (TT) milk. In addition they avoided the MMB levy since designated milk at this stage had not yet been admitted to the MMS.

Table 10.2 Incentives to join the Attested Herds Schemes in England and Wales

---

Milk bonuses
1935-40 Bonus of 1d per gallon to owners of attested herds for attested milk, payable through the Milk Marketing Scheme operated by the Milk Marketing Boards.
1939-44 Entry to scheme limited to Certified or Tuberculin Tested herds.
1940-50 Bonus at 1d for 3 years only. No bonus for new entrants 1944-50.
1950-66 New entrants 2d per gallon for 4 years, then 1d for next 2 years.

Capitation bonuses, alternative to above mainly for breeding and feeding herds
1938-50 £1 per head for 3 years. No bonus for new entrants 1944-50.
1950-66 New entrants £2 per head for 4 years, then £1 for 2 years.

Additional premium on TT milk from attested herds
1938-43 2¼d per gallon for accredited attested herds, 1d for unlicensed attested herds.
1943-50 4d per gallon, 1d for milk from attested herd not T.T. or accredited.
1950-57 2d per gallon for T.T. milk
1958-59 3d per gallon for T.T. milk
1959-64 4d per gallon for T.T. milk

When they were both launched in 1935 there were now two separate and parallel schemes. Voluntary attestation was officially introduced on 1 February 1935 under Section 9 of the Milk Act, 1934.[80] The Accredited Herd Scheme came soon after on 1 May 1935. Attested herds were

---

[79] TNA: MH 79/327.
[80] Ritchie 1959, 3.

subject to strict rules preventing contact with the cattle of neighbouring farms, the movement of animals on and off the property, and attendance at agricultural shows.[81] Cattle from Attested herds were supervised at markets and kept in compounds separate from the other animals, and any animal brought in from an infected herd had to spend sixty days in isolation and then pass a tuberculin test before it could join an attested herd. Retests were at annual intervals. The scheme was altogether more stringent than the conditions required for the TT milk producer who only had to remove reactors at the six monthly test.[82] However, it was the farmer's own vet who, provided they were 'approved' by the licensing authority, carried out the tuberculin tests and this situation of inevitably divided loyalties continued until the National Veterinary Service was fully functional from 1938 onwards.

The Attested Herds Scheme was very slow to become established. In October 1937, after two years, there were still only 500 Attested herds in England producing a paltry 0.6 million gallons between them.[83] So the scheme had to be modified in 1938 under the provisions of Section 20 of the Agriculture Act (1937). This extended the financial underpinning of the scheme and brought the various anti-tuberculosis measures under the control of the MAF. But the surge in applications that came in 1938 was mainly due to additional financial incentives. Those herds that were both Accredited and Attested were entitled to 2¼d per gallon for milk that was sold as TT. In addition the concept of Supervised Herds was introduced in the Agriculture Act. If a herd was tested and found to have no more than ten per cent reactors, once these animals were removed the farmer could now apply for free testing on up to three occasions.[84]

In May 1939 there were 4,039 Attested herds in England and Wales and 1275 in Scotland, with a collective output of 2.6 million gallons. The scheme was closed on the outbreak of war except for TT herds.[85] When it reopened in 1944, only the TT quality milk premium was paid, at 4d per gallon, with no payment to beef or rearing herds. By 1950

---

[81] Boundary fences had to be solidly constructed and maintained. Fishwick 1947.

[82] TNA: MH 79/367.

[83] Ibid.

[84] *The Times* 7 June 1937, 20a.

[85] TNA: MAF 35/785.

twenty per cent of all cattle were in Attested herds (Table 10.3). The engagement in England was considerably less than in Scotland or Wales, although it was by then beginning to catch up after a very slow start. Most progress was made in counties that we might regard as the low hanging fruit: Zetland (100 per cent of cattle), Scilly Isles (100 per cent), Bute (90.4 per cent), and Ayr (90.0 per cent). But the dairy counties where bTB was mainly concentrated were far behind. Farmers there knew their guilty secret might be costly for them in a transition to attestation.[86]

Table 10.3 Attested Herds Scheme, 1950

	Attested herds	Attested cattle	Attested cattle as a percentage of total cattle population
England	20,568	944,840	14.1
Wales	14,204	291,270	29.6
Scotland	12,527	619,070	39.5
Britain	47,299	1,855,180	20.0

Source: MAF.

At a meeting of the Royal Society in 1945, H.T. Matthews estimated that only 8 per cent of milk in England then came from attested and tuberculin tested herds (Table 10.4) and 'he did not think that any great reduction in bovine tuberculosis was to be expected over a period of years'. [87]

Table 10.4 Tuberculosis-free milks (million gallons)

	TT and Attested	TT only	Accredited and Attested	Attested only
1943	92.5	16.7	10.4	22.0
1945	122.6	48.9	7.8	23.7
1947	181.8	80.9	7.1	32.0
1949	304.6	105.4	7.9	50.1

Source: Anon. 1945b.

The Cutforth Commission (1935-36)

From the moment of their establishment in 1933/34 there was immediate friction between the MMBs and the larger distributors. There was, for instance, no agreement on prices, which then had to be set by three independent 'appointed persons'. In September 1935 the Central

---

[86] Wynne 1953, 8.

[87] Anon. 1945b, 340.

Milk Distributive Committee made a formal complaint against the Board for its high wholesale prices and they argued that decisions had been made that had disadvantaged dealers and depot owners.[88] Indeed such was the rancour surrounding the MMS that, only eighteen months after it had been set up, a Commission was appointed in 1935 under the chairmanship of Sir Arthur Cutforth to undertake a fundamental review. This took much longer than the politicians expected and it was therefore necessary to pass two interim measures - the Milk (Extension of Temporary Provisions) Act (1936) and the Milk (Amendment) Act (1937) - to keep the 1934 Act in play.

Reporting at last in November 1936, Cutforth found that the new MMS had encouraged farmers to sell more liquid milk, which had then flooded the market, much of the surplus going for manufacturing.[89] He recommended far-reaching changes to the MMS, including the establishment of a National Milk Commission. Cutforth showed little interest in milk quality or disease but, in his minority report as a Commissioner, Sir John Orr suggested that the new Commission should be required within two years to produce a report on the public health implications of its policies.

Giddings in his analysis of Cutforth notes the disquiet that the Commission engendered.[90] The NFU objected to what they saw as the undermining of the MMB by a reduction in its price-setting powers. They issued an 'unqualified condemnation' of its report and in this they were supported by the Conservative Parliamentary Agriculture Committee. Cutforth therefore faced formidable hurdles if any attempt were to be made to implement the Commission's proposals.

The Poole Corporation Bill 1936

In the 1920s and 30s there was a series of severe outbreaks of milk-related disease. In 1929 there was an outbreak of septic sore throat in Brighton that affected 1,000 families and caused sixty-five deaths. But politically more momentous was the 1936 outbreak of typhoid fever in Poole, Bournemouth and Christchurch that involved 700 cases and

---

[88] Committee of Investigation for England [1936].

[89] Cutforth Commission 1936.

[90] Giddings 1974, 173-89.

fifty-one deaths. The significance lay in the local council's subsequent decision to promote a Bill to enforce the compulsory pasteurization of any milk to be consumed locally. This they did in the absence of any government action on the health risks associated with drinking milk. This initiative immediately came to the attention of the MH, which in February 1937 called a meeting with their colleagues in the MAF.[91] Here they heard that the NFU was planning to organize opposition in the House of Lords that would cause the Poole Bill to fall but it was nevertheless agreed that it was embarrassing to the government that a private Bill was making the running on such an important issue. Tactically they also worried that drawing up battle lines in parliament might antagonise the farming community and ruin the prospect of general legislation on pasteurization in the future.

In April 1937 the Cabinet authorised a statement to head off the Poole and Glasgow Bills. This was on 27th by Lord Halifax, in his capacity as Leader of the House of Lords, to the effect that: 'The government intend to bring forward long-term legislation dealing with milk policy in the near future'.[92] He was saying that no local measure was necessary since the government was just about to introduce its own general policy. Upon these reassurances the Poole clause was withdrawn but the government spent the next two years dealing with the painful and embarrassing consequences of their rushed statement.[93]

Shortly after, in June 1937, the MMB produced a 'Memorandum on compulsory pasteurization of milk circulated for the consideration of members of the Milk and Dairy Produce Committee' of the NFU.[94] This suggested that pasteurization had been a matter of contention under the ancien regime of milk marketing when the distributors had the upper hand. But the MMB was now in effect a farmers' collective, so the risk of such domination had disappeared. It recognised the opposition of small producer-retailers but commented that they could always act cooperatively to purchase the necessary equipment and be given a number of years' grace to adjust.

By July 1937 the MAF delivered a document to the Cabinet Committee

[91] TNA: MH 79/352; MAF 52/130.
[92] TNA: CAB 23/88. Cabinet 16(37)5.
[93] Anon. 1937a.
[94] TNA: JV 5/316.

on Agricultural Policy promisingly entitled 'Proposals for long-term milk policy'.[95] This recognised that 'It is held in responsible quarters that the introduction of some measure of compulsory pasteurization should no longer be deferred'. Although about half of the milk supply was already pasteurized there were obstacles to further progress such as worries about the efficiency of pasteurization technologies and, because of the capital outlay, about concentration in the hands of large firms. The Cabinet Committee met on 7 July and endorsed these outline proposals, which by then had been discussed by the MH, the MAF and the Scottish Departments.[96] Local authorities were to be allowed to apply to the MH for an Order making compulsory the pasteurization of retail milk in their particular areas. But the process was not to be straightforward. The MAF had to be consulted on whether the local authority would be able to administer it efficiently; and the Order would only come into effect after a two year delay, enabling all stakeholders to make the necessary adjustments. Right from the outset the NFU's Subcommittee on Pasteurization made their opposition clear, on behalf, they said, of the producer-retailers.[97]

Although pasteurization was contentious, the main element of the new policy was about arrangements for milk supply. This meant extending the Milk Acts of 1934 and 1936 and thinking about pricing structures, including bonuses for Accredited herds. In order to drive through the improvements in milk distribution asked for by Cutforth, the proposed Milk Commission was to provide services of conciliation and arbitration between the major players in the industry. In recognition for their cooperation in this complex political process, the MH wanted something, ideally in both the policy statement and the Bill, on the need for more mother and child welfare milk, and improved arrangements for disease-free milk.[98]

Tuberculous udders and veterinary inspection

Diseased udders usually meant diseased milk and local authorities were therefore inspired to take administrative action and it seems, from Table

[95] TNA: MH 79/352.
[96] TNA: MH 79/367.
[97] TNA: JV 5/316.
[98] TNA: MH 79/352.

4.4, that their inspectors were more likely to find udder tuberculosis than the country vets who knew the farmers. Inspection was easiest among beasts tethered in urban settings but some local authorities also employed inspectors to tour the country areas supplying milk. The results were varied at first but gradually farmers came to realise that diseased animals threatened their livelihoods and, as we have already noted, offloaded them to the 'slink' trade in 'wasters' and 'mincers', the hidden circuit in the livestock economy found in several regions.[99] These animals were slaughtered outside the municipal jurisdiction and their meat was either turned into sausages or sold in the poorer parts of towns where there was less inspection.[100] The vets employed by the City of Manchester found that twenty-four per cent of the cows they judged on inspection to be tuberculous (1901-9) could not be traced later because they had been sold.[101] This informal resistance from farmers drove the problem underground. According to Worboys, 'for sound economic reasons there was effectively no diseased livestock' at this period.[102]

It seems to have been the large city authorities, such as the corporations of Manchester and Liverpool, who were first persuaded of the need to employ veterinary consultants, and later full-time veterinary inspectors, to discover the extent of disease amongst the herds supplying milk to their citizens. Manchester first sent out instructions to farmers concerning TB in 1898, and in 1899 they appointed a veterinarian to enforce their Milk Clauses.[103] By 1907 seventy Local Authorities had made arrangements in addition to the County Councils which had been required to do so by the Diseases of Animals Act (1894).[104]

It was not until Part IV of the Milk and Dairies Order (1926), made under Section 8 of the Milk and Dairies (Consolidation) Act (1915) that the need for inspection was recognised but even then there was no insistence upon a particular frequency. The problem was that in the absence of 'regular inspection of cattle, famers are tempted not to report cases falling within the scope of the TB Order, and the milk

---

[99] Niven 1923, 130.
[100] BPP 1888 (C. 5461) xxxii.290; Behrend 1893.
[101] Savage 1912.
[102] Worboys 1991, 312.
[103] TNA MH/80/3.
[104] Ibid.

supply might be grossly contaminated before the affected animal was discovered'.[105]

Tuberculosis of the udder, a relatively rare complication of the disease and difficult to detect until it was well developed, was found in up to three per cent of animals. Estimates varied. McFadyean thought 2.0 per cent udder tuberculosis likely, Stockman 2.0 per cent, and Dewar 1.2 per cent, but Savage considered all of these to be too high. The MAF found that 1.0-1.5 per cent of herds in which tuberculosis had been found actually yielded infected milk, whereas Hopkins guessed at 0.5 per cent.[106] The figure for cows supplying Sheffield was 0.27 per cent clinical udder disease during the period 1903-26 and in England as a whole in 1926/7 it was 0.12 per cent for the 136,380 animals inspected. Modern researchers, however, think that these historical estimates were too low.[107] In India modern veterinary inspection methods reveal rates of six to seven per cent of udder tuberculosis in the milking herd there.

Table 10.5 Percentage of cattle tuberculosis reported by various parties in Lanarkshire, 1928

	Farmers	Local vets	Inspectors
Udder tuberculosis	25	14	61
Emaciation	60	24	16
Chronic cough	50	27	22

Source: Savage 1929a.

As we saw above, in 1931 the IDC recommended veterinary examinations and Addison, as Minister of Agriculture, was keen to press ahead but the MH backed out at the last minute when challenged by the Treasury to foot the bill.[108] They subsequently made enquiries to see if farmers would be willing to bear the cost but the NFU was resolutely opposed.[109]

In 1933 the Ministries of Health and Agriculture met again to discuss the possibility of a state veterinary service. This was partly because the matter was under consideration by the Grigg Commission and partly because of their proxy battle in the Hopkins committee over

---

[105] TNA: FD/1/5084.

[106] Ministry of Health 1931; BPP 1933-4 (Cmd. 4591) ix.451.

[107] O'Reilly and Daborn 1995.

[108] TNA: MH/56/88.

[109] TNA: MH 56/81.

the policy territory of milk. The MH was persuaded to agree but they fought a rearguard action by insisting that the vets should undertake work currently done by Sanitary Inspectors under the Milk and Dairies Order.[110] This would have made them full-time and justified the expense being borne by local authorities rather than the Ministry. They also reasoned that part of the £750,000 promised by the government for improving the quality of the milk supply under what was to be the Milk Act (1934) should be used to assist the local authorities in arranging for veterinary inspections.[111] As we saw above, in the event the Minister of Agriculture, Elliot, changed his mind.[112] He no longer wanted to spend the £750,000 on aiding veterinary services and decided instead to spend through the Milk Marketing Scheme on production bonuses for Attested herds.

Conclusion

Chapters 9 and 10 have covered the period 1914 to 1937, a period of febrile dairy politics in a context of momentous national and international change. In Chapter 9 we concluded that the conventional styles of the MAF and the MH were very different and that it was this, rather than any departmental 'culture', that promoted different visions of bTB policy and friction in day to day implementation. To this we can now add some more detail about the four ministries involved in bTB policy.

The Treasury is by far the best known, although it was in reactive mode rather than making a direct input in policy about livestock disease. Throughout our period it had a well-grooved cost-minimizing strategy and was frequently criticized for holding back promising policies. What Heclo and Wildavsky call 'Treasury norms' were based on this informed scepticism but also upon performances. Even today their officials cannot be convinced unless a department 'pushes and stands up to questioning' and there is a ritual of negotiation in which the Treasury bargains the applicant down.[113] With regard to bTB, no view was ever taken on policy

[110] TNA: MH/56/84.
[111] Ibid.
[112] TNA: MH 79/327.
[113] Heclo and Wildavsky 1981, 45.

as such but, as Chapters 9-11 show, the Treasury several times blocked what they saw as unnecessary expenditure.

Responsibility for livestock disease and for food production lay principally in our period with the BoA (1889-1903), the BoAF (1903-19) and the MAF/MAFF (1919-2001). The old BoA/BoAF was staffed by specialist examination and by promotion from the junior ranks of those with specialist knowledge of the unrelated and frankly miscellaneous functions gathered under the Board's wing: animal disease, fisheries, forests, Ordnance Survey, Kew Gardens, and others. The new MAF taking over from 1919 operated differently, selecting from the general civil service examinations. Given the diversity of their tasks their senior staff remained few in number, however, with only 25 administrative class officials in 1927 and no specialized principal assistant secretaries until 1928.[114] Dale suggested that both the BoAF and the MAF in its early years were of low status in Whitehall. The MAF was also particularly unpopular with farmers in the period following the rescinding of the promises it made about guaranteed prices immediately after the First World War. Dale suggested that government saw the MAF's main duty to farmers in terms of protecting them from disease in their crops and livestock. Their attempted post-war realignment towards price support would have turned it into a 'spending ministry' but instead they had to return to their hazard-based vision. It was not until the 1920s and 1930s initiatives with the quality grading and marketing of produce that a front-foot, positive and refreshed interpretation of the MAF's role emerged. Dale saw the principles of the MAF shifting from the question (in 1919) 'How can the State assist the farmer to produce?' to the question, 'Given a fair standard of production, how can the State ensure a living to the producer?'[115]

Despite this new direction for the MAF, there were internal divisions and personality clashes. An insight into this can be found in the biography of Sir Daniel Hall. When Hall joined the BoAF, first as Secretary (1917-19) and then as Chief Scientific Adviser (1919-27), he found a standoff between the veterinarians, led by Stewart Stockman, the CVO, and the administrators under Assistant Secretary Anstruther. The latter wanted full control, with the vets merely as technical advisers.

---

[114] Dale 1939; Savage 1987, 1996.

[115] Dale 1939, 15.

As a result, there was a 'mixture of dislike and contempt' between Stockman and Anstruther which held up policy development on livestock diseases.[116]

Harold Dale argues that it was Sir Francis Floud as Permanent Secretary of the MAF (1920-28) who built trust with the NFU. But regular changes of personnel at ministerial level throughout the decade and a half after the First World War led to weak leadership and a lack of vision. Civil servants were therefore able to make more of a mark than in the average ministry and their personalities and practices made inroads into policy and on the MAF's relations with other ministries and with the wider policy community interested in agriculture.[117]

While we can see from their actions that the institutional view of the civil servants of the MAF was undoubtedly pro-farmer, no such *formal* statements were ever made and it would be difficult to impute such motivations from the ministry's official publications. Even in their dealings with other ministries they were always careful to use neutral language of a suitably diplomatic and cooperative tone. This highlights one of the difficulties of using official reports and memos in policy research because more often than not candid opinions were reserved for confidential internal memos and face-to-face meetings.

Dale, as well as being a writer and lecturer on civil service matters was himself a career administrator and was involved with bTB policy as a principal assistant secretary at the MAF. Alongside him for this policy areas was John Blackshaw. Originally a dairy farmer and then Principal of the Midland Dairy College, Blackshaw was later a Superintending Inspector in the Dairy Branch of the BoAF and then an influential Dairy Commissioner in the MAF until his retirement in 1935, the same year as Dale's departure. Both have been classified as 'peripheral insiders' in bTB policy-making circles and they seem to have shared a similar brutally pragmatic and pro-farmer viewpoint that seems dissonant in the modern age of the precautionary principle.[118] Blackshaw and Dale were not themselves key decision-makers, but they represent a conservative and single industry-based view of the world that is very telling.

Although the MAF had data collection systems, including the

---

[116] Dale 1956.

[117] Savage 1996.

[118] Atkins 2010b.

annual agricultural returns made by individual farmers, they were not well informed about the views and needs of farmers. For this they came increasingly to rely upon the NFU, which had members everywhere, many of whom were enthusiastic local activists with strong opinions. The framings and rhetorical devices consistently deployed by the BoAF and the MAF and their fellow travellers in parliament increasingly came to mirror those of the NFU, to the exclusion of other interested parties:

1. The scientists do not agree, so who are we to interfere?

2. No-one in the farming industry wants action.

3. The public do not want to pay a higher price for their milk.

4. It would be too expensive to slaughter cattle and replace them.

5. Don't worry, trust me, there is little health risk and no need for public panic.

6. The public health lobby are eccentric extremists.

According to Gail Savage, the initial promise of the MH on its foundation in 1919 was not fulfilled between the wars.[119] She blames a recruitment system that staffed the ministry with no reference to expert specialism and instilled the broader Civil Service view that restraining expenditure was a greater priority than driving up standards for patients and other clients. This was partly a continuation of the 'do nothing, spend nothing' culture of the Poor Law administration that dominated health thinking in the predecessor LGB. The Permanent Secretary from 1920 to 1935, Arthur Robinson, bears much responsibility for the weakness and drift in our policy area, as does his favourite minister, Neville Chamberlain, who was three times Minister of Health: 1923, 1924-29, 1931. Chamberlain was responsible for a vast legislative programme of social reform, but driving through progressive change with regard to bTB does not seem to have been a priority for him.

Together Robinson and Chamberlain were browbeaten into accepting the penny pinching attitude of the Treasury. This did change, we must note, from 1933 onwards, but zoonotic disease control still looked then like an afterthought.[120]

---

[119] Savage 1996.

[120] Before this the Treasury had funded the Agricultural Rates Act (1923), the Land

Being a temporary creation of emergency conditions in both world wars, the Ministry of Food (MF) was somewhat of a novelty in Whitehall. From 1940 to 1943 it had a popular and high-profile minister, Lord Woolton, who has been credited with a number of successful policies.[121] But the MF was soon in conflict with the MAF. Winnifrith called them 'keen controversies', an example being debate about milk prices.[122] The MAF wanted prices to increase as an incentive to farmers but the MF wanted to hold them down to boost consumption among vulnerable groups.[123] Ironically after its duties with rationing ceased, the MF was merged in 1955 with the MAF, although many commentators saw this as a takeover by agriculture and a renewal of producer over consumer interests.[124] The latter group had not been well organized and they were only weakly represented in policy-making circles before the Second World War.[125] As a campaigning body with bTB on its agenda the PLH was a rarity but it was not a grassroots organization, being dominated by the clinical and public health elite. The Cooperative movement could reasonably claim to have been more representative but it made little impact in Whitehall with regard to zoonotic disease.

Drainage Act (1926), the Agricultural Credit Act (1928), the Agricultural Produce (Grading and Marketing Act)(1928), de-rating of agricultural land in the Local Government (Derating) Act (1929), and the Agricultural Marketing Act (1931).

[121] For a corrective view on Woolton's record see Oddy 2003.

[122] Winnifrith 1962, 38.

[123] Hammond 1954.

[124] Franklin 1994.

[125] Smith 1988.

CHAPTER 11.

POLICY PROGRESS, 1937 TO 1971

Introduction

Our conclusions in Chapters 9 and 10 were made without the benefit of a supporting literature in agricultural or veterinary history. As one of the most important problems facing agriculture in the 1920s, bTB rates no mention at all in Smith's short history of agricultural policy and very little in other publications.[1] This is true also of the area eradication policy initiated in 1937 and implemented in the 1950s. The present chapter therefore has little by way of historiographical precedent to build upon and no-one seems to have asked how it was possible for bTB policy to proceed so smoothly in the post-war era when every progressive measure in milk politics had been so fiercely resisted in the 1920s and 30s. Might the answer lie in the changed profile of the House of Commons? The Labour landslide in 1945 introduced a younger and more urban orientation and time-honoured vested interests were therefore disrupted. But there were also other forces at work. The strategic difficulties of food supply experienced during the Second World War had a major impact on government attitudes generally to farming and a fundamental rethink of agricultural policies seemed inevitable. The chapter will bring us up to the epidemiological threshold of 1971 when thinking about the spread of bTB in the UK entered a new era.

The Agriculture Act (1937) and the National Veterinary Service

In 1937 the policy log-jam did at last show some signs of shifting. The occasion was the IDC on Increasing the Productivity of the Soil in which the MAF put forward its ideas on reducing the toll of bTB.[2] Their new Minister, William Morrison, wanted the routine inspection of herds and was willing to contemplate the expense given that only

---

[1] Smith 1990.
[2] TNA: MAF 35/22.

£30,000 of the £750,000 set aside in 1934 to establish a 'pure milk supply' had by then been spent on the very slow start to attestation.[3] The IDC also recommended a TT survey of self-contained herds that would likely take two years to complete, and the attestation of all herds in six areas where bTB was low. Their estimates of costs were £250,000 for the TT survey, £400,000 for a state veterinary service, and £350,000 to cleanse six areas over four years.

As we saw in Chapter 10, the establishment of a State Veterinary Service had been debated between the MAF and the MH since 1933.[4] At last the Agriculture Act (1937) forced the amalgamation of the veterinary staff of the Diseases of Animals Branch and local authority veterinary inspectors to form a new Animal Health Division in the MAF. Centralised control gave greater standardisation of the inspection cycle but in reality this probably did little to reduce the amount of diseased milk reaching the consumer.[5]

Now, under the Agriculture Act, once a local public health department had detected bTB in its milk supply the investigation was handed over to the MAF. In some localities this led to delays at first because the vets were overwhelmed by the volume of work.[6]

A vital element of the Agriculture Act was the inclusion in Section 23 of the concept of area eradication, which was intended as a modest step towards ending the bTB problem. It was realised that test and slaughter for the whole national herd was impracticable logistically, as well as potentially very expensive in compensation. Starting with areas of low incidence, for instance where closed herds were common, was thought therefore to be a way to start, eventually extending to the more heavily infected areas. The farmer's individual incentive was admission to Attested herd status if the disease could be eliminated on the holding. The advantage nationally would be experience of conducting area-based campaigns and also the creation of a pool of TB-free herds as a basis for future breeding. The interruption of the Second World War delayed the implementation of extensive area eradication until the 1950s.

---

[3] TNA: MH 79/351.

[4] TNA: MH 79/367; Hardy 2003b.

[5] Wilson 1942.

[6] Jones 1939.

The 1937 White Paper and the Milk Industry Bills 1937-39

Meanwhile the promised White Paper on milk policy was published in July 1937 to general scepticism.[7] It was a partial attempt to put the Cutforth report into practice. *The Times* predicted trouble over its proposals for a Milk Commission.[8] The *Economist* complained that it was not the type of national policy that had been promised when Glasgow and Poole withdrew their Bills.[9] Local authorities were to be given powers to insist on pasteurization in their areas but there was to be no compulsion on them to exercise these powers. The *Economist* also objected to subsidies for farmers to clean up their milk production under the Accredited Herds Scheme and regretted that two of Cutforth's key recommendations had been watered down. These were, first, that power over fixing wholesale and retail prices of milk should be vested in a Milk Commission and, second, that the consumer should no longer bear the cost of dealing with seasonal milk surpluses.

The council of the NFU rejected the White Paper very quickly, as early as September 1937. This reflected the view of their 'Milk and Dairy Produce Committee' and also of local branches that the principles upon which they joined the MMS in 1933 were being 'dishonoured'. In a revealing letter to *The Times*, the General Secretary of the NFU, Cleveland Fyfe, said that his members were still 'sceptical about the commercial advantages of producing high grades of milk'.[10] The NFU's motivation was financial and, although they claimed to be serious about milk quality, they did not set up a Diseases of Animals Committee to collaborate with the MAF until just before the publication of the White Paper.

Following the set-back of farmer opposition, the milk policy was obviously in trouble but the government was committed to proceeding to a Milk Industry Bill incorporating at least some of the suggestions in the White Paper. The following is a summary of the issues.

> 1. Pasteurization. The public health lobby was in favour, supported by the MH. Producer-retailer members of the NFU were opposed but the nutritional argument against heat treatment was undermined by the

---

[7] *Milk Policy*, BPP 1936-7 (Cmd. 5533) xxi.699-706.

[8] *The Times* 2 August 1937, 15b.

[9] Anon. 1937b.

[10] Fyfe 1937.

definitive research at Reading.[11] The White Paper and the various drafts of the Milk Industry Bill sought powers for local authorities to compel pasteurization of milk retailed in their area. This proved to be one of the Bill's main sticking points.

2. Gallonage premia on designated milks to be increased to encourage the production of grades with low risk of *M. bovis*, including TT, TT (Pasteurized), TT (Certified), and Pasteurized. No opposition but represented only a niche market.

3. A Milk Commission to be in charge of strategy on production, marketing, and consumption. The version of the Milk Commission in the White Paper and the Bill was a mixture of Grigg's Joint Milk Commission and Cutforth's idea. It would also have taken over school milk and guaranteed continuity for the mother and infant scheme. From the outset the MH was sceptical about the ability of the Commission to look after public health matters, especially if commercial interests were represented on it.[12]

4. Uniformity between local authorities in their administration of the Special Designation Orders..

In June 1938 'pressure on parliamentary time' was given as the reason why preparations for the Bill were to be abandoned for the Session. As a result, for the third time a Bill extending the existing provisions for one year was brought forward and became Milk (Extension and Amendment) Act.[13]

The heat had been too much. The MMB and NFU had organized protest meetings, objecting particularly to the price fixing proposals and also to the idea of compulsory pasteurization.[14] The government had miscalculated. They had not even convinced their own backbench MPs.

Overall the government had bowed to the vociferous vested interest of the dairy farmers that they themselves had institutionalised in the MMB. This was a very clear and embarrassing defeat for the government and it would have surprised no-one that two weeks later the Minister of Agriculture, Morrison, thought that 'it is politically

[11] Milk Nutrition Committee 1937-39.

[12] TNA: MH 79/367.

[13] TNA: MAF 52/134.

[14] *The Times* Nov 26, 1938, 14c; Nov 28, 1938, 20c.

impracticable to proceed with those parts of the Bill that relate to the establishment of a Milk Commission, its organization of distribution, pasteurization Orders, and the financing of research, etc'.[15] The Ministers of Agriculture and Health met on 22 December 1938 with damage limitation in mind.[16] Morrison suggested dropping the Milk Commission but wondered whether some elements of the policy could go ahead in Scotland, where there was for instance less opposition to pasteurization. He also commented that private Bills on pasteurization would have to be allowed, now that the government had withdrawn its own proposals. Elliot predicted a

> battle royal on the floor of the House in regard to any private Bill containing pasteurization provisions. The government would have to make a statement and he assumed they would advise the house to let any such provisions go to committee ... At the committee stage they would have to submit a report and he assumed that this would not be hostile.

In the spring of 1939 there were still discussions in Whitehall about putting a revised version of the Bill to parliament and a new Milk Industry Bill was indeed published.[17] Morrison had by then been reshuffled and replaced by Sir Reginald Dorman Smith, who had been President of the NFU, indicating an entirely different attitude by Chamberlain as Prime Minister. But the revised Bill once again fell and was replaced by a much reduced Bill that became the Milk Industry Act (1939). This was merely a vehicle to continue the special premia for quality and welfare milks but Dorman Smith made it clear in the Second Reading debate that in future he intended to treat the matter of disease in the herd separately from matters to do with the overall structure of the milk industry.

Wartime policies

Wartime milk policy was much freer in the formulation and implementation than in the constipated period of the 1930s. Although Parliament still debated agricultural issues, a Milk Controller was appointed to replace decision-making by the MMB. Nevertheless the Board was kept as

---

[15] TNA: MH 79/368.
[16] TNA: MAF 52/156.
[17] TNA: MAF 52/130.

window dressing to prevent farmer disquiet and its full powers were not revived until 1954. Meanwhile the new MF oversaw strategy, taking over some duties from the MAF.

In a White Paper dated July 1943 the MAF undertook to implement an increase in herd inspections within the constraints of the wartime shortage of veterinary expertise.[18] In political terms this was less controversial than the stated intention of taking responsibility for milk hygiene away from local authorities and centralising it under the MH, who had already introduced a National Milk Testing and Advisory Scheme in 1942. At the same time a voluntary scheme, in collaboration with the NFU and NMVA, was also started where vets contracted with farmers to examine their animals at least four times a year in order to detect the major cattle diseases, including bTB. The MAF provided laboratory analyses where necessary.[19]

In 1942 the balance at last swung in favour of pasteurization with the publication of Graham Selby Wilson's book.[20] The text had actually been ready for publication in 1939 but was delayed by wartime paper shortages. It only came out after Wilson himself requested permission to publish it through the commercial house of Edward Arnold. The same year the MRC published a report by its 'Committee on Tuberculosis in Wartime', which encouraged the spread of pasteurization and deplored the use of raw milk in schools.[21]

Sensing an opportunity, in February 1943 a delegation went to lobby Woolton from the Royal College of Physicians, the Royal College of Surgeons, the National Association for the Prevention of Tuberculosis, the British Pediatric Association, the Joint Tuberculosis Council, and the PLH asking for more pasteurization of milk. Led by Professor Ralph Picken, Acting Chairman of the BMA, they stressed that 'there is no serious difference of opinion in the medical profession on the question of pasteurization; few questions in preventative medicine commanded so nearly complete unanimity'.[22] The PLH wanted compulsory pasteurization in towns of over 10,000 population and similar powers

---

[18] BPP 1942-43 (Cmd. 6454) xi.149.

[19] Anon. 1945c.

[20] Wilson 1942.

[21] Dawson of Penn 1942.

[22] Anon. 1943b, 265; Bryder 1988, 246.

available to smaller towns on application to the MH.[23] The Ministry of Food seems to have received this lobby favourably. Lord Woolton primed certain contacts to publish pro-pasteurization letters in the media[24] but this was to no avail and he was set back by a combination of opposition in the Cabinet and headlines in the Beaverbrook press.[25] The *Daily Express*, for instance, on 7 May 1943 ran a story entitled 'Don't do it Lord Woolton'.

This was followed in July 1943 by an announcement from the Minister of Agriculture, Robert Hudson, that he intended to take powers to specify areas in which the only milk that could be sold had to be in one of three categories: tuberculin tested, accredited, or pasteurized. Also, importantly, all bulked milk was to be pasteurized.[26] Defence Regulation 55G introduced these powers formally in January 1944[27] but no areas were designated until the 1950s.[28] The Lord President's Committee had agreed to limit the scheme to areas where rationalization was in force, but this meant that it would lapse after the Armistice. The MAF had over-reached itself and the backlash was less than subtle. An editorial in the *British Medical Journal*, entitled 'Milk is still unsafe', called this episode an 'extraordinary example of departmental bad faith' and reported that there had been a recent representative meeting of the BMA at which there had been a (satirical) call for 'for hanging on the nearest lamp-posts ex-Ministers of Health and their permanent officials'.[29]

Hammond, the official historian of Second World War British food policy, was positive about policy-making at the end of the War. His analysis showed that, despite the pre-war combatants once again jockeying for position as early as the end of 1943, the government was in a much stronger position after years of central control.

> Its knowledge was far greater; it need no longer rely on second-hand or partisan sources of information ... The aims of milk policy were no longer in dispute, nor did they differ between war and peace. The problem was less, therefore, one of decontrol than of providing

---

[23] People's League of Health 1943.
[24] Wellcome Contemporary Medical Archives Centre: SA/BMA/F108.
[25] North 1943a; Anon. 1943b.
[26] Anon 1945a.
[27] The Heat Treated (Prescribed Tests) Order.
[28] Anon. 1945a; Hammond 1956.
[29] Anon. 1945a.

permanent means for the Government to fulfil its social obligations regarding milk. It looked, in 1945, as if the 'milk enthusiasts' had entered into their kingdom at long last.[30]

In 1946 the Earl of Huntingdon, Joint Parliamentary Secretary of the MAF announced that government had decided to 'press on with the heat-treatment of milk'.[31] They intended to enable the designation of urban areas where only TT or heat treated milk could be sold, although this would be after a five year period to allow distributors to invest in the necessary equipment.

Corporatism in excelsis?

We saw in Chapters 7 and 10 that, from the moment of its inception, the NFU was an irritant in pre-war agrarian politics, acting as an effective counterbalance to the mercantile weight of the wholesale meat and milk trades. Respect for their negotiating muscle and persistence eventually brought them to the notice of government in the early 1930s at a time when Conservative politicians were looking for allies and for surrogates to help them carry out the restructuring of several commodity marketing systems that their radically reformist agenda required. The creation of the MMB in 1933 meant that the Minister of Agriculture, Walter Elliot, knowingly accepted an institution dominated by farmers. He ceded power to them and, despite some window dressing in the policy about reducing disease and dirt in milk, he in effect gave farmers a veto over any details they disliked.[32]

The NFU now became responsible for planning and running the MMB for England and Wales. They took on the mantle of saviours of an industry that had been in chaos, although from our point of view this is ironic because the NFU were deeply conservative in their thinking about the problem of bTB. It later took the rupture of the Second World War to create new conditions more favourable to real reform concerning this important disease.

The seeds of collaboration lay in a 1940 agreement between the

---

[30] Hammond 1956, 271-72.

[31] HL Deb 31 July 1946 vol 142 c1149.

[32] Interestingly there was no such warmth between the NFU and the MF, their brief wartime relationship being characterised by acrimonious disputes over prices. Smith 1988.

government and the NFU about guaranteed prices to boost national food output in wartime, subsequently institutionalised from 1943 to 1992 as the Annual Price Review in which farm incomes were supported where necessary by state subsidies. The relationship was not a cosy one, with friction particularly between the NFU and MF until the latter was disbanded, but it received a statutory basis in the 1947 Agriculture Act. The NFU was now in effect a full partner of the MAF and the expectation was that in return they would yield to efficiency measures, including the control of livestock disease.[33] The major post-war initiative on this front was the area eradication of bTB, and while it is difficult to find evidence of NFU enthusiasm for this policy, their lack of opposition to it was a key to its steady progress.

Despite these close ties, Martin Smith argues that the links between the NFU and the MAF were not full-blown corporatism as argued by some.[34] Regardless of the negotiations about commodity prices, the government remained in control of the formulation and implementation of policy. A better theoretical framework, he suggests, is that of the 'policy community' because in the British context departmentalism and clientalism was clearly visible in the actions of the MAF before and after the war.

Area eradication

As we have seen, the debate about the best approach to eradicating bTB continued in the 1930s but it became increasingly obvious that the Tuberculosis Order was not delivering enough in terms of the number of diseased animals (see Figure 9.1) removed from the milk supply, and the Attested herds scheme had a very slow uptake in its first two years. It was with this in mind that two changes were made in 1937. The first was to attempt to increase uptake of the attestation by the encouragement of Supervised Herds, where tuberculin testing was to be free. The second was the inclusion of area eradication in Section 23 of the Agriculture Act.

In 1939 it was decided to have a look again at the Attested Herds Scheme after the war, and gradually the idea emerged that 'area eradication

---

[33] The NFU also regained control of the MMB in 1954.
[34] Smith 1989.

is a probable development of the future'.[35] Then, true to this pre-war undertaking, plans were drawn up in May 1945, once hostilities in Europe had ceased.[36] From the outset of this new process, pragmatism dictated that the MAF try to guess the likely reaction of farmers. They knew that the pre-war Attested Herds Scheme had been only partially successful and that it had made no impact upon the majority of dairy farmers, particularly those in heavily infected areas. Early discussions favoured the abandonment of the milk bonus in favour of the more widespread slaughter of reactors with compensation. Technicalities under consideration included the possible branding of reactors to prevent them re-entering the dairy herd in a different district, and also the need to encourage farmers to breed their own herd replacements or buy only Attested animals. The spatial vision was one of self-sufficient cattle regions that had natural boundaries, with all of the necessary marketing and veterinary facilities to hand.

The predicted cost in 1945 was £50 million spread over twenty-five years equally divided between compensation for slaughtered animals and the cost of the tuberculin tests.[37] The bonus payments were not factored in at that stage. In the event the net cost of compensation was actually only £3.7 million from 1950 to 1960 (Table 11.1) and the tuberculin tests cost a further £19.7 million. Taking the broader period of 1945 to 1964 these figures were £5.2 million and £27.6 million respectively. Although this is less than the initial estimate, if we include the bonus payments and take the whole period of the Attested Herds Scheme from 1935 to 1964 inclusive, the sum jumps to £149.2 million, or in 2013 values, £3.35 billion. The area eradication figure for 1950-60 was the equivalent of £2.65 billion.

Entry to the Attested Herds Scheme was restricted in the war until mid-1944. In October of 1943 the quality premia had been increased, in the case of TT milk from 2¼d to 4d per gallon, and this encouraged more farmers to think of producing disease-free milk. The plans for area eradication, based on expanding the number of Attested herds, were under discussion from 1945 to 1950 by a group comprising officials from the MAF, the NFU, the NFUS and the MMBs. The NFUs

---

[35] Ritchie 1945, 182.

[36] TNA: MAF 35/487.

[37] Ibid.

Table 11.1 Cost of area eradication

	Animals Tested (000)	Slaughtered (000)	Attested herd bonus payments (£000)	Compensation, less salvage (£000)	Salaries, fees, travelling expenses, cost of tuberculin, less sales of tuberculin (£000)
1950	2,269	-	2,660	42	997
1951	2,828	-	4,321	32	1,468
1952	4,309	2	9,304	80	1,623
1953	4,604	2	10,484	85	1,486
1954	5,235	5	12,067	206	1,438
1955	6,111	11	9,949	385	1,581
1956	6,542	8	10,724	275	1,763
1957	6,648	11	7,734	383	2,148
1958	7,140	23	8,948	785	2,402
1959	8,111	26	8,487	819	2,421
1960	8,565	23	8,927	578	2,464
1961	9,361	15	7,760	544	2,442
1962	8,749	10	5,683	308	2,250
1963	8,700	6	3,907	190	1,455
1964	nd	6	2,078	184	1,645

Source: TNA: MAF 287/417.

and MMBs were compliant from the outset; indeed they urged speedy implementation of the concept.[38] Their negotiating stance was mainly about the financial details (valuation, compensation, salvage, expenses, bonuses, premiums) and terms that would engage the farmer. These post-war plans did not involve new thinking, just the political will to implement an expensive nationwide programme.

The 1945 plan was soon overtaken by a new scheme devised in 1948, because the former 'had been formulated under war-time conditions and was now considerably out-dated'.[39] Details were finalised in July 1950 and the plan was put into operation from 1 October, initially for a period of five years. Action under the new Tuberculosis (Attested Herds) Scheme (1950) started first with the easily dealt-with areas such the Isles of Scilly, Arran and Shetland (Table 11.2). They were the first Attested Areas declared, in February 1951.[40] On 1 April 1953 two groups of counties followed: Cardigan, Carmarthen and part of Pembroke, and Argyll, Ayr, Bute, Dumfries, Kirkcudbright, Renfrew and Wigtown.

These successes were achieved in a three-stage process. First, the Attested Herds Scheme provided financial incentives to farmers willing

---

[38] TNA: MAF 35/487; MAF 35/784.

[39] TNA: MAF 35/587; MAF 202/5.

[40] Ministry of Agriculture (1952) *Report on the animal health services* London: HMSO.

Table 11.2 Eradication Areas

Date of completion	Counties
1951	Scilly Isles, Arran, Bute (Great and Little Cumbrae), Shetland
1952	-
1953	Argyll (part), Ayr, Bute (part), Dumfries, Kirkudbright, Renfrew, Wigtown, Cardigan, Carmarthen (part), Pembroke (part)
1954	Carmarthen (part), Glamorgan (part), Pembroke (part), Dunbarton, Lanark, Peebles, Stirling
1955	Cumberland, Durham (part), Lancashire (part), Westmorland, Yorkshire North Riding (part), West Riding (part), Brecon, Radnor, Merioneth, Montgomery, Argyll (part), Clackmannan, Fife, Hebrides, Inverness (part), Midlothian, Selkirk, Kinross, Perth (part), West Lothian
1956	-
1957	-
1958	Berkshire, Buckinghamshire (part), Hampshire, Isle of Wight, Oxfordshire (part), Surrey, West Sussex, Yorkshire North Riding (part), West Riding (part), Anglesey, Caernarvon, Denbigh (part), Caithness, Inverness (part), Moray (part), Nairn, Orkney, Ross and Cromarty (mainland), Sutherland,
1959	Bedfordshire, Buckinghamshire (part), Cambridgeshire (part), Cornwall, Devon (part), Dorset, Durham (part), East Sussex, Essex, Gloucestershire, Herefordshire, Hertfordshire, Kent, London, Middlesex, Norfolk, Northamptonshire (part), Oxfordshire (part), Shropshire (part), Somerset, Suffolk, Warwickshire (part), Wiltshire, Worcestershire, Yorkshire North Riding (part), West Riding (part), Aberdeenshire, Angus, Banff (part), Berwick, East Lothian, Kincardineshire, Moray (part), Perth (part), Roxburgh, Flintshire, Denbighshire (part), Glamorgan (part), Monmouthshire
1960	Cheshire, Derbyshire, Durham (part), Huntingdonshire, Isle of Ely, Lancashire (part), Leicestershire, Lincolnshire, Northamptonshire (part), Northumberland, Nottinghamshire, Rutland, Soke of Peterborough, Staffordshire, Warwickshire (part), Yorkshire North Riding (part), West Riding (part), East Riding

Source: MAF, *Report on the animal health services.*

to subject their animals to tuberculin testing and the slaughter of reactors. Owners were compensated for any reactors removed at the market value of an untested beast, up to a maximum of £100.[41] The next TT was within sixty days and only when a herd had passed two tests without any reactors was the farmer able to apply to the Ministry's Divisional Veterinary Officer to join the Attested Herds Scheme. The herd then became a 'Supervised Herd' and had another test within sixty days, this time free of charge. If again there were no reactors the farm could join the Register of Attested herds. Bonus payments to Supervised Herds were 2d per gallon for four years, then 1d for a further two years, or £2 per head for beef animals for four years, and then £1 per head for two years. In addition many of these farmers qualified for the TT premium for superior hygienic quality, again at 2d per gallon for four years. Second, 'free-testing areas' were declared where the Attested Herds Scheme had made progress and more than seventy per cent of farms were engaged. Here, usually for six months,

---

[41] An 'untested' animal was worth about 75 per cent of the value of an 'attested' one. TNA: MAF 35/785.

farmers could have their cattle tuberculin tested by ministry vets at the cost of the state. Third, Eradication Areas were then established, each usually comprising two or three average-sized counties. They were as self-contained as possible to minimise movement from outside, but with licensed stock marketing facilities to allow the continuation of trade. Testing was now compulsory and there were no gallonage payments for the farmers forced into the scheme at this late stage. The movement of all cattle was restricted. Imports were licensed and new animals had to be tuberculin tested, including Irish stores. Farm buildings were cleaned and disinfected.

In the event, farmers were quicker to pick up on the Attested bonus than expected, with thirty per cent more in the scheme in 1953 than had been anticipated in 1949. Indeed the area eradication of the 1950s seems to have been largely uncontroversial. The NFUs were fully consulted throughout and their sensitivities, particularly about bonuses and compensation, are the main topic in the relevant Ministry papers along with the need to placate the Treasury about the size of the overall spend. Other considerations included a shortage of veterinarians to carry out the tuberculin tests and the disruption to cattle markets while a county was being subjected to area eradication.

One key point that is rarely mentioned in the history of area eradication is that throughout the 1950s the meat of slaughtered animals continued to enter the human food chain. This was after the lesions were trimmed from the carcase. One wonders how many consumers would have approved of this process if they had known but it was perfectly legal and indeed this is what still happens in abattoirs around the country.[42]

Attestation was finally declared for the whole of the UK on 1 October 1960, although this was more a matter of political convenience than a reality on the ground. Slaughterhouse data showed that as late as 1959 tuberculosis was still rife. Cardiff, for instance, had eleven per cent of its carcases showing evidence of the disease even though South Wales was attested that year. The following decade, 1961-70, saw another 56,847 reactors slaughtered.

---

[42] But note here that some reactors are over thirty months and animals beyond that threshold have not been allowed into the human food chain since 1996 as a precaution against BSE.

The situation now was that after area eradication the problem of bTB was concentrated in a few regional hotspots. However, at the national level the policy makers and administrators were able to pigeon hole the issue and move on. They had several other nationwide veterinary priority issues on their minds, such as brucellosis, and the tone of the MAF archive for the 1960s was that the bTB campaign had been a great success and that the residue of disease was containable.

Conclusion

The MAF/MAFF has had a relentlessly bad press for their close relations with the NFU, especially in the policy area of livestock disease. Richardson and colleagues, for instance, labelled them the MAFFia[43] and Donaldson and his team were equally damning:

> The FMD crisis was a revelation ... First, the crisis revealed the complacency in the ways that animal disease issues had come to be approached and managed within the farming industry. Sloppiness in precautionary disease control measures were compounded by the effects of changes in the farming industry, which led to higher stocking densities and many more animals being moved about, more frequently, and over longer distances.[44]

Personally I am sceptical of the corporatist literature that stresses so heavily the MAF being in the pocket of the NFU. In my view it is more profitable to think of the coincidence of interests and deployment of resources and this helps to explain the step change in the success of bTB policy from before to after the Second World War. Before 1939 the degree of overlap of interests fluctuated from issue to issue. As we saw above, the MAF narrative was fundamentally pro-farmer but we might reasonably ask pro which farmer? There were many different farmer interests and even within the dairy sector there were slippages between the small producer-retailers and the larger capitalised farms supplying wholesalers.

The historiography of twentieth century agriculture in Britain is somewhat ambivalent about the role of interest groups and the rise of policy networks. The majority view seems to be that the fading of the

[43] Richardson et al. 1978.
[44] Donaldson et al. 2006, 5.

CCA and the rise of the NFU was a challenge to successive governments but not a great sway on policy. This was the influential view of Self and Storing and it has been further developed with nuanced variations by Cooper, Martin, Smith, and Bromund.[45] With regard to the admittedly rather narrower fields of milk and meat, our argument here is that, on the contrary, the NFU played a crucial role in the politics and the restructuring of the livestock industries.

With specific reference to the postwar MAFF/NFU relationship as a model case study, political scientists have used the label 'corporatist', implying close ties with a high level of continuity and shared aims. But if we look closely at the historical detail there was actually nothing inevitable about the MAFF/NFU relationship. Consider that the industry was comprised (mostly) of small producers of a perishable product and therefore not did not have inherent strength. These were producers who had been disorganized and exploited in the 1920s. They were scarcely candidates for a partnership with government and the closeness was a complex creature that evolved through time, always path dependent. It was never a symmetrical arrangement, nor one of everyday consensus on the minutiae of policy decisions, but it nevertheless suited both parties to a degree that a mutual dependence developed.

The NFU's collective will to power has certainly been extraordinarily consistent over the century of its existence. One reason is that it scores highly on many of the criteria for policy community inclusion listed by Maloney: organizational capacity and cohesion, strategic economic significance, size of membership, technical expertise, political sophistication, and ability to engage with policy implementation.[46] It was not until the 1980s that their close relationship, *unter einer decke*, with the MAFF began to fade.[47] The salmonella in eggs fiasco in 1988/9 was a major blow and soon after the ministry was reeling from its inability to deal satisfactorily with cattle diseases such as BSE and FMD.[48] Indeed the latter catastrophe in 2001 proved to be the last breath of the MAFF and in 2002 it was merged into Defra.

The raison d'être of the NFU being the furtherance of the interests

---

[45] Self and Storing 1962; Cooper 1989; Martin 2000; Smith 1989; Bromund 2001.
[46] Maloney et al. 1994.
[47] Jordan et al. 1994.
[48] Grant 1997.

of their members, their policy-making has always been about reducing costs and maximising profits. At various points in the last one hundred years they have sought to prevent the imposition of government regulations about bTB where they seemed to be too bureaucratic, too interventionist, or too costly to the individual farmer. The pocket book populism of this approach has undoubtedly slowed the passing of progressive measures with regard to this disease and, arguably, in the long term it has been against the interests of the livestock industry as a whole. Having said that, farmers were not the only group seeking to prevent radical policy initiatives. Indeed we seek to show that their role as pantomime villains in the bTB story is both unfair and inaccurate. This is not least because interests-based understandings of the policy process fall short of providing even a partial explanation.

Nowadays the NFU elected leaders and researchers are well informed and sophisticated in their arguments but in their policies they continue to be drawn to the lowest common denominator because of the economic and psychological plight of so many of their members. Milk producers in particular have had their livelihoods challenged by the low prices offered in recent years by wholesalers and supermarkets. Since the demise of the MMB in 1994 competition in the sector has been fierce and one senses that morale has also been dented by the devastating cattle diseases in recent decades: first BSE, followed by FMD and now bTB. It is understandable that farmers want to deflect criticisms of their biosecurity on to wildlife reservoirs of disease, especially badgers, but this does not mean that their use of the science is accurate. Chapters 12 and 13 will return to the science-based arguments surrounding bTB and we will see that the material slipperiness of *M. bovis* leaves room for uncertainty and controversy about its epidemiology and interventions that are appropriate.

CHAPTER 12.

EPIDEMIOLOGICAL UNDERSTANDINGS OF BOVINE TUBERCULOSIS

Introduction

This chapter represents a change of gear. Here we will switch from a national-level policy history to the type of epidemiological analysis that in future may provide one of the scientific evidence-based foundations for controlling and then eradicating bTB. There are a couple of points to make here by way of context. The first is that, although work on the epidemiological variables associated with the disease has a pedigree of about 100 years, the most relevant and advanced research is relatively recent. Much of it has been state-sponsored in countries such as the UK, RoI and New Zealand which together have had the greatest exposure to risk in their livestock industries. To illustrate this, Table 12.1 shows the funding for bTB research in the UK in the last twenty-five years. Note that there seems to be a cycle of interest among politicians. The recent surge in projects peaked in 2012 and the challenge is to maintain the research momentum from one parliament to the next.

Table 12.1 Defra-funded projects on bovine tuberculosis, annualised 1990-2015

	Projects	Funding (£)		Projects	Funding (£)		Projects	Funding (£)
1990	2	305,708	1999	37	4,031,394	2008	27	5,869,124
1991	3	475,308	2000	25	3,226,390	2009	28	6,192,802
1992	11	1,871,641	2001	26	3,214,939	2010	30	6,611,041
1993	11	1,871,641	2002	31	4,633,668	2011	27	6,220,862
1994	14	2,056,656	2003	29	4,580,558	2012	30	8,287,129
1995	20	2,702,677	2004	28	4,643,924	2013	29	6,408,325
1996	15	1,312,206	2005	34	7,297,124	2014	25	5,820,550
1997	17	1,455,076	2006	22	5,584,627	2015	13	4,902,394
1998	24	2,078,279	2007	20	5,164,902			

Source: Defra

The second, linked, point is that the results of epidemiological research of the last few decades have been complex, with findings that at times appear to be inconclusive or even contradictory. This is presumably because the situation is so multifaceted and intricate that it is difficult to capture factors that vary both regionally and through time.[1] Given the constraints of funding and manpower, detailed questionnaire-based work, for instance, has been limited usually to individual localities, although in the UK the government-sponsored TB99 and CC2005 studies were broader. Geo-referenced multivariate statistical modelling has also made an important contribution, although fieldwork has again necessarily been circumscribed. Overall it has been very difficult to arrive at definitive epidemiological generalizations about bTB in cattle, and we are in need both of more field-based data collection and also more modelling of the large existing cattle-based databases that are now available to help us through the maze.[2]

The susceptibility of cattle to bTB can be studied at several scales. The animal-level risk varies with age, gender, breed, body condition, immune status, and genetic resistance.[3] At the herd level the history of previous breakdowns is a crucial factor, along with herd size, enterprise type and management regime. Whether diagnostic tests are performed is important, and also whether new animals are brought into the herd. The movement of animals seems to be a disease risk, as does contact between members of the herd. Other herd factors include the abattoir inspection of carcases, exposure to wildlife reservoirs of disease, and the persistence of *M. bovis* in the environment.[4] Regional-level risks encompass environmental factors such as climate, and land use type.[5] Strategic risks include long-term regulatory policies such as test and slaughter, culling of wildlife, and control of regional trade in live cattle.

This chapter then is about the identification of the epidemiological risk factors of bTB and the difficulties and uncertainties that continue when attempting to make causal statements. This is illustrated by variations in opinions at the national level. When required by the European Commission to state the reasons for the persistence of bTB in cattle at the local level, the governments of the UK and the RoI

---

[1] Vial et al. 2013.

[2] Such as Skuce et al. 2011, 2012.

[3] Goodchild and Clifton-Hadley 2001; Humblet et al. 2009.

[4] Ibid.

[5] Ibid.

provided rather different figures. The RoI estimated that fifteen per cent was due to residual infection in cattle herds, nought to twenty per cent was the result of contiguous spread between neighbouring farms, and nineteen to thirty-nine per cent due to infection from wildlife.[6] The UK on the other hand ascribed fifty per cent of cattle TB to badgers in high-risk areas and about 6.6 per cent overall to bought-in cattle.[7] What is the significance of these differences? There are national- and regional-scale ecological differences that are part of the answer. In addition, there are variations of analytical and political approaches. When put together with the materiality of *M. bovis* we have a situation that is best understood through what we will call 'political ecology'.

Epidemiology

Although *M. bovis* is an ecotype of the *M. tuberculosis* complex with a clear host preference for cattle marked by molecular differences, it nevertheless has amongst the widest ranges of any known pathogen.[8] Francis gives a detailed account of its prevalence among farm and domestic animals, wild mammals and even reptiles.[9] The pool of disease amongst badgers and deer is especially troublesome to control and this is often cited as an explanation for the continued infection of dairy cattle.[10]

M. bovis is flexible, opportunistic, adventitious and astonishingly successful, but how does it spread? The first route is airborne, with mycobacteria attaching themselves to particles of dust or moisture. Francis showed that they can survive in cough droplets, for instance, for up to eighteen days, on the clothing of a herdsman or milker for several weeks, and in dust for three to eight days.[11] The second pathway is faecal-oral. This was probably more important in the past but still remains a risk today. *M. bovis* is an obligate parasite and cannot therefore grow outside a body but it is nevertheless remarkably resilient on its

---

[6] European Commission 2014.
[7] European Commission 2012.
[8] Smith, Kremer et al., 2006; O'Reilly and Daborn 1995.
[9] Francis 1958; Thoen et al. 2009.
[10] Zuckerman 1980, Dunnet 1986, Krebs and the ISG 1997.
[11] Francis 1958, 17.

own in the environment. It seems to survive in manure, soil, on grass and possibly even in water.

Estimates suggest that about twenty-five to forty per cent of tuberculous cows emit live mycobacteria in their manure.[12] The availability of nutrients and moisture in the soil are limiting factors to bacterial survival, along with temperature and acidity, but in the cool, shady, moist conditions common in Britain it has been suggested that *M. bovis* excreted by cattle or badgers or spread in slurry can remain viable for between six months and two years.[13] There is strong evidence of a heightened risk on pastures spread with slurry, especially if grazing recommences too soon or the slurry has not been held long enough for the mycobacteria to die.[14] Using a molecular technology (Polymerase Chain Reaction), fragments of the DNA of *M. bovis* have also been found in and around abandoned badger setts and latrines, hinting at widespread and persistent environmental contamination. There is recent, ominous evidence of the ability of mycobacteria to penetrate amoebae but anyway they can survive in running water for 400 days and so provide another vehicle for their survival outside of mammal bodies.[15] Survival in direct sunlight is not possible though, because the mycobacteria are speedily desiccated, within hours or days.[16]

The infection of cattle by mouth at pasture is possible, then, but is a lower risk than other routes.[17] We know this because experimentally it has been shown that a 100-1,000 times greater dose of *M. bovis* is required orally for infection than through inhalation by aerosol.[18] By the latter route only one mycobacterium is enough to infect a calf.[19]

---

[12] Williams and Hoy 1927; 1928; 1930; Christiansen et al. 1992.

[13] Wray 1975; Kelly and Collins 1978; Morris et al. 1994; Ghodbane et al. 2014.

[14] Griffin et al. 1993; Menzies and Neill 2000; Scanlon and Quinn 2000; Reilly and Courtenay 2007; Ramírez-Villaescusa et al. 2010; McCallan et al. 2014.

[15] Phillips et al. 2000; Young et al. 2005; Courtenay et al. 2006; Mba Medie et al. 2011.

[16] Maddock 1933; 1934.

[17] Maddock 1936; Morris et al. 1994.

[18] Collins and Grange 1983; Griffin and Dolan 1995; O'Reilly and Daborn 1995.

[19] Neill et al. 1988.

Intensive farming systems: farm, herd and animal risks

Global-level studies have found that bTB is clustered in regions of intensive dairy systems, particularly where production is concentrated in a small number of large production units.[20] It is here that the conditions for airborne transmission are optimised.[21] Stocking density, both on pastures and in cowsheds, are associated variables and are claimed to be significantly correlated with bTB in some analyses.[22] It is therefore no surprise (Figure 12.1) that both the historic and the recent spatial patterns of bTB have been correlated with densely stocked regions such as the North West of England up to 1960, and South West England and South Wales since 2001 (Figure 12.2).

The epidemiological literature on bTB has emphasised both farm/ herd level and sub-regional spatiality. This has yielded important insights and has provided the basis of our understanding of the spread of the disease and of the relationship between the disease in cattle and in the

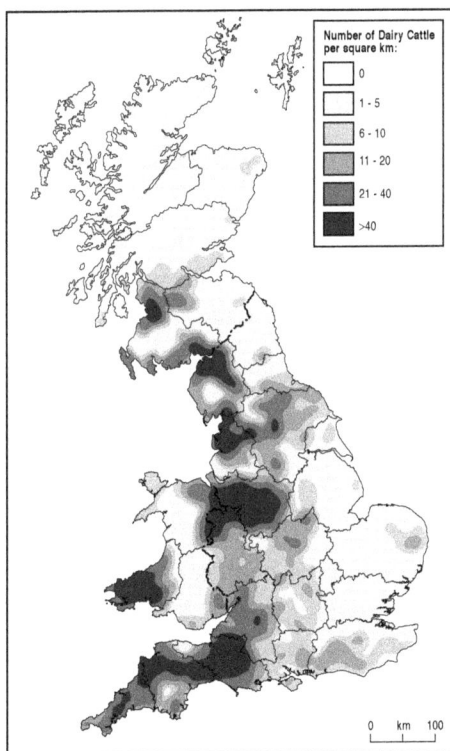

Fig 12.1
The regional density of dairy cattle
Source: RADAR 2008

---

[20] Brittlebank 1929; Van Arendonk et al. 2003; Humblet et al. 2009.

[21] Menzies and Neill 2000.

[22] Neill et al. 1989; White and Benhin 2004; Humblet et al. 2010.

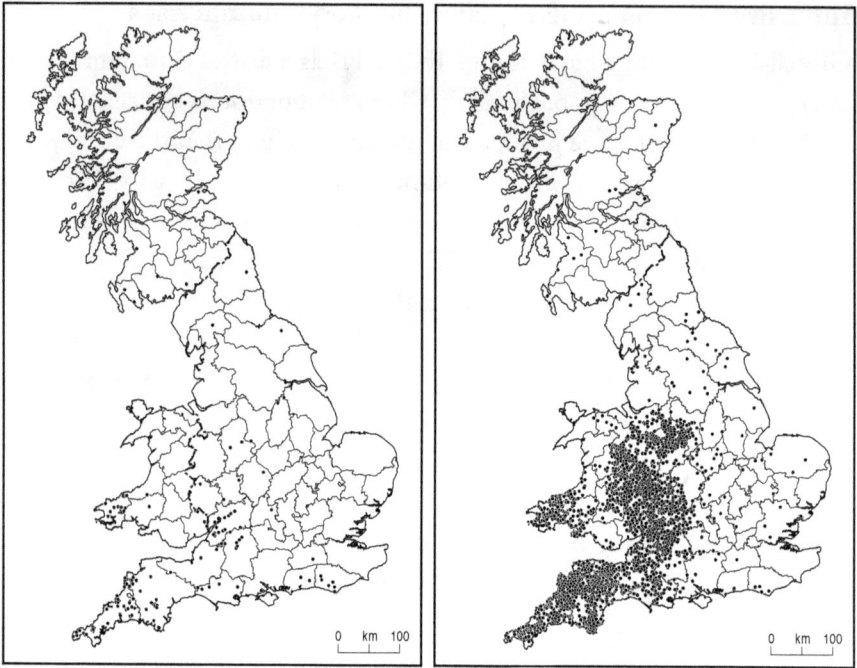

Fig 12.2 The recent spread of bTB
(Source: Animal Health and Veterinary Laboratories Agency, UK)

wildlife reservoir. But the large literature on herd and individual animal risks has so far not generated a convincing consensus. The reason for this may well be that the principal explanatory factors vary with region and with environmental and agronomic context. In other words there is no one-size-fits-all model that we can use to plan a simple set of policy responses. The following list of nine variables is not exhaustive, nor is it intended to be in priority order of significance, but it does draw together some of the headlines in the literature.

(1) Beef or dairy

As far as we can tell, dairy cows have always been more susceptible to bTB than the cattle population in general (Table 12.2). Animals in the breeding and feeding areas in the UK were - and still are - kept on the whole on open pastures and when butchered at two to three years of age they have always showed less evidence of infection than their milking sisters.[23] In the late nineteenth and early twentieth centuries dairy cows were different for three reasons. First, they were housed for

---

[23] Francis 1958.

a number of months every winter and the incidence of tuberculosis in cattle pens or in sheds seems to have increased by approximately 7.5 per cent each year until roughly forty per cent were infected with bTB at five to six years old.[24] A relationship between age and level of infection has frequently been confirmed, although whether this is due to exposure to infection or a function of long-term latency is unclear.[25] Second, the life of a dairy cow is shorter nowadays in the UK, at about two to three milking years, than used to be the case. At the turn of the twentieth century it was said to be an average of seven lactations, falling in the 1930s to 4.5, and after the Second World War to three.[26] Third, dairy cows are milked twice or three times a day and therefore more frequently come into close proximity with each other than in beef grazing systems.[27]

Table 12.2 New breakdowns in England by herd type, 2013

Risk zone	Herd type	Herds	Breakdowns	Breakdowns per 100 herds
High risk area	Beef	18,190	2,032	11.2
	Dairy	5,836	1,403	24.0
	Other	486	25	5.1
Edge	Beef	6,491	180	2.8
	Dairy	1,305	136	10.4
	Other	105	4	3.8
Low risk area	Beef	17,615	70	0.4
	Dairy	3,470	35	1.0
	Other	0	0	0
England	Beef	42,296	2,282	5.4
	Dairy	10,611	1574	14.8
	Other	805	29	3.6
All	All	53,712	3,885	7.2

Source: AHVLA 2014a
Note: the high risk, low risk and edge areas will be defined and discussed in Chapter 14.

(2) Herd size

The most fundamental herd-level risk is herd size itself (Tables 12.3 and 12.4).[28] This is, first and most obviously, because the more animals there are in a contact group the greater is the probability that one

---

[24] Francis 1947, 1958.
[25] Griffin et al. 1996; Pollock and Neill 2002; Green et al. 2012.
[26] King 1901; BPP 1933-4 (Cmd. 4591) ix.540; Francis 1947.
[27] Humblet et al. 2009.
[28] Brooks-Pollock and Keeling 2009 suggest that increasing herd size may be a false scale economy as far as the risk of a bTB breakdown is concerned.

with an infection will pass it on to the others.[29] This includes infection across boundaries because large holdings have more neighbours and more opportunities for cattle to interact where fences or hedges are inadequate. In addition, herd size may be a function of complex husbandry practices including cattle purchase criteria, housing type and grazing systems, all of which are themselves known bTB herd risks. It is also usually positively correlated with variables such as farm area and number of farm parcels, which have also been reported in some studies to be associated with confirmed breakdowns.[30]

Table 12.3 New bTB breakdowns in England, 2013

Herd size	Herds	Breakdowns	Breakdowns per 100 herds
1-10	11,943	134	1.1
11-50	14,636	528	3.6
51-100	8,356	629	7.5
101-200	8,267	948	11.4
201-300	3,930	616	15.6
>300	4,832	1,003	20.8
All	53,607	3,885	7.2

Source: AHVLA 2014a

Table 12.4 New bTB breakdowns in England by herd type, 2013

Herd type and size	Herds	Breakdowns	Breakdowns per 100 herds
Beef			
1-10	11,030	120	1.1
11-50	13,557	489	3.6
51-100	7,039	526	7.5
101-200	5,645	600	10.6
201-300	1,851	260	14.0
>300	1,625	262	16.1
Dairy			
1-10	613	9	1.5
11-50	819	34	4.2
51-100	1,228	97	7.9
101-200	2,551	338	13.2
201-300	2,053	353	17.2
>300	3,188	740	23.2
All	53,712	3,885	7.2

Source: AHVLA 2014a

---

[29] Some statistical studies argue that herd size disappears as a factor once other herd-related variables are allowed for. Karolemeas et al. 2011; Green et al. 2012.
[30] Mill et al. 2012.

The importance of herd size has almost certainly increased. Since the 1980s the cattle economy has been restructured so that average herd sizes have become larger, with heightened animal to animal risk of disease transmission.[31] If the time spent in a herd is taken into account, the bTB incidence per 100 years is now 1.7 for small herds of ten animals and under, and 29.5 for herds over 300.[32]

(3) Previous herd history

A herd's previous history of infection is another major factor, particularly because many herd breakdowns are recurrent.[33] For instance, in Britain over half of OTF-W (Official Tuberculosis-Free status Withdrawn) breakdowns occur in herds which have been subjected to government-imposed movement restrictions in the previous thirty-six months.[34] The length of breakdowns and the number of animals involved is increasing.[35] The average length of restrictions for British herds was 179 days in 1990, 208 in 2000, and 319 in 2013; more than thirty-five per cent continue for 240 days or longer.[36] In the so-called High Risk Area (HRA) of the South West this is greater in counties such as Cornwall (358 days), Avon (330), and Gloucestershire (319). Duration of OTF-W breakdown by herd size varies from a mean of 171 days for herds of under ten animals, up to 427 days for herds over 300. The percentage of incidents with more than one reactor has also increased, from 35.8 per cent in 1990, to 52.5 per cent in 2000, and to 67.9 per cent in 2013.[37]

In 2014 Defra admitted that sixty per cent of herds in the HRA have had a breakdown in the last ten years. In Devon, Cornwall and Gloucestershire, less than five per cent of dairy herds with fifty or more cattle have remained TB-free since 1990, according to figures published by the BovineTB.info website following a freedom of information request.

---

[31] House of Commons, EFRA Select Committee 2007, Evidence, Q.12, J. McInerney.

[32] AHVLA 2014a.

[33] Kelly and More 2011.

[34] Conlan et al. 2012.

[35] Goodchild and Clifton-Hadley 2006.

[36] Karolemeas et al. 2010; AHVLA 2014b.

[37] AHVLA 2014b.

The HRA in England has experienced an increasing risk of recurrent OTF-W breakdowns, up from forty-four per cent in 2006 to fifty-eight per cent in 2013. The main reason for recurrent breakdowns is that between eight and twenty-one per cent of such herds are still harbouring infection even when they are given the all-clear and movement restrictions are removed. This will be no surprise to those who believe either that environmental contamination is to blame or that a local wildlife reservoir is the source of infection. But there is another possibility. As mentioned above, it increasingly seems plausible that infection may persist both in animals that are anergic to the skin test for various reasons and in those that have temporarily resolved a lesion but remain at latent risk of its reactivation.[38] In the work of Conlan and colleagues, for instance, up to half of recurrent breakdowns can be attributed to infection missed by tuberculin testing.[39] Some of this may be for technical reasons to do with the tuberculin or its method of application but a portion is likely to be due to transient anergy.

Within-herd persistence was the strongest likely explanation of the sixty per cent of breakdowns recurring in Great Britain at a test six months after a previous one.[40] According to Karolemeas, 'the imperfect sensitivity of the SICCT test, together with potential reactivation of latent states, could create a bank of residual infection in the herd'.[41] The fact that inconclusive reactors are associated with further breakdowns seems to bear out this persistence hypothesis, but it is only relatively recently that the British authorities have come into line with the EU Directive 64/432/EEC requiring the removal of such animals after one retest rather than two and so this particular problem may now at last be alleviated.[42] At the time of writing [July 2015] herd movement restrictions can be lifted only following a clear test after sixty days for unconfirmed reactors that do not become a breakdown and 120 days for confirmed breakdowns.[43] Despite the inevitable disruption of trade,

---

[38] Pollock and Neill 2002.

[39] Conlan et al. 2012.

[40] Karolemeas et al. 2011.

[41] Karolemeas et al. 2011. Wolfe et al. 2009 found for the RoI that persistence was greatest in herds with breakdowns of eight or more reactors.

[42] Ramírez-Villaescusa 2009; Karolemeas et al. 2011.

[43] Restricted cattle can, however, be sold to an Approved Finishing Unit or sent direct to slaughter.

it is arguable that even tougher movement restrictions would yield dividends of reduced disease in the long term.

(4) Neighbourhood effect

Another important herd risk, the bTB status of contiguous herds, is statistically significant in some studies, although the mechanisms may vary.[44] The sale of animals over short distances is one, followed by the hiring of bulls, and another is cattle coming into contact across boundaries.[45] A study in the RoI, for instance, found that seventy-nine per cent of boundary fences there were not able to prevent direct animal contact.[46] Research in Northern Ireland has found similar contiguity transmission between herds.[47] The other factor in local transmission is the possible existence of a wildlife reservoir of the disease.

(5) Cattle movement

Is infection brought in with purchased cattle? From 1953 attested cattle were ear-tagged in Britain, legitimizing a concept that had long been used as part of bTB control in other countries, for instance Canada.[48] The logical extension of the idea, that detailed and sustained surveillance of the whole national herd was necessary, took longer to be accepted and it was not until 1998 that Britain's Cattle Tracing System was established to satisfy EU requirements following the BSE crisis of the 1990s. In 2001 statutory authority was acquired to force the logging of details about the births, movements and deaths of all cattle.[49] It has been said that the CTS is inefficient, with up to ten per cent of cattle 'lost' at any one time, and in its early days, during the FMD emergency the MAFF reported one million cattle movements in February 2001 but then later

---

[44] Griffin et al. 1996; Denny and Wilesmith 1999; Gilbert et al. 2005; Olea-Popelka et al. 2006, 2008.

[45] Denny and Wilesmith 1999.

[46] Ibid.

[47] Menzies and Neill 2000.

[48] MAF 1953. The *Annual Report* of the CMO in 1935 reported a system of permanent marking of each animal with an identification number. Presumably this had been introduced at the beginning of Attestation.

[49] Gilbert et al. 2005; Mitchell et al. 2008; Vernon 2010.

had to double its estimate.[50] The CTS currently records fourteen million cattle movements each year across the UK.[51] This is supplemented by the VetNet database,[52] which among other things records skin and blood test results, and in 2005 these databases were joined by the Rapid Analysis and Detection of Animal-related Risks system (RADAR), which collects veterinary surveillance data. From these sources together it is possible to recreate the life histories of most animals.[53]

The analysis of these databases and farm-level surveys in order to draw reliable conclusions about cattle movement and other factors in the spread of disease requires skill and precision. Ramírez-Villaescusa and colleagues, for instance, reflected that the creation of their particular dataset on herd and individual animal risks involved 'a large amount of data manipulation' and 'a very careful step by step process when creating queries in the relational database'. This was for them 'a significant challenge ... in terms of developing variables that are revealing in ... showing groups of cattle with higher risk of reacting, and meaningful in terms of interpretation'.[54]

Once compiled in a Geographical Information System, these data become useful for statistical epidemiology.[55] A space-time analysis of herd breakdowns, for instance, found them to be clustered, one group at a scale of less than four kilometres and another at more than twenty.[56] The former clustering seems to back the suggestion that *M. bovis* is mainly localised and that it also seems to be, relatively speaking, spatially stable over time.[57] It is common to claim that tight spatial patterning is proof that cattle movement is not a factor in the spread of disease because, if it was, one would have expected there to be more mixing of spoligotypes between regions.[58] But three alternative explanations need to be borne in mind.

---

[50] Donaldson et al. 2006.

[51] House of Lords Secondary Legislation Scrutiny Select Committee, *Inter-authority Recoupment (England) Regulations 2013.*

[52] Replaced 2011/12 by the Sam database.

[53] National Audit Office 2003; Green and Kao 2007; Vernon 2011.

[54] Ramírez-Villaescusa et al. 2009, 2010.

[55] Epidemiological network modelling seems to have potential in analysing such geo-referenced databases. Vernon and Keeling 2009; Volkova et al. 2010; Vial et al. 2011.

[56] Green and Medley 2008.

[57] Smith et al. 2006b, Skuce et al. 2010.

[58] Spoligotypes are strains of bTB. For an explanation see below.

First, consider the structure of cattle trade: 36.3 per cent of cattle movements in Britain are direct to slaughter, 26.5 per cent farm-to-farm, 24.8 per cent farm-to-farm via market, 9.5 per cent to slaughter via market, and 2.8 per cent other. The bTB hotspots are often also areas of high levels of cattle movement, either via markets or directly from farm to farm, a situation exacerbated by the closure of many slaughter-houses in recent decades.[59] The hotspots are co-located with or close to nodes of intensive livestock enterprise where specialisation in different enterprises - rearing, beef, dairy - inevitably leads to trade. Much of this is within a radius that broadly corresponds to the 'spoligotype' zones that will be discussed later. For dairy cattle the most frequent movements are nought to twenty kilometres farm-to-farm and to a lesser extent twenty to forty kilometres farm-to-farm via market.[60] Although there are also long distance cattle movements, the CTS and other data suggest a local experience for most animals.

The biggest disruption to this local geography came in 2001 with the FMD epidemic. The cattle markets were temporarily closed and there were bans on the movement of animals.[61] Later, because many whole herds were slaughtered, restocking was necessary and this frequently involved long-distance transfers of cattle. Research on this period indicates that the restocking was responsible for the migration of spoligotypes of *M. bovis* well beyond their home ranges and that, unsurprisingly, the greatest risk was from importing cattle from herds that have previously been infected.[62] There is statistical justification for the hypothesis that the risk from brought-in cattle is minimized if they have recently been cleared by a tuberculin test, thus giving support for the policy of pre-testing commenced in 2006.[63]

Related research on endemic areas in South West England found that farms with no history of a breakdown could maintain that status for long periods if not restocked with cattle from herds with a history of

---

[59] EU hygiene regulations have led to the closure of some smaller slaughterhouses but there has also been competition from the supermarkets, who make their own arrangements.

[60] Wint et al. 2004; Mitchell et al. 2008; Skuce et al. 2011.

[61] Carrique-Mas et al. 2008.

[62] Green et al. 2012.

[63] Szmaragd et al. 2013.

bTB. In other words, the farm effect can be one of positive momentum as well as negative.[64]

Second, the fact that many breakdowns at the present day still involve only one reactor per herd is sometimes used as an argument that cattle-to-cattle transmission is unlikely. But it is possible that many herds have a pool of infected, sub-clinical non-reactors; and there is no reason to deny that their infective work may well be done in the cowshed or in close proximity at pasture.[65]

The third alternative scenario is that environmental factors may explain the pattern in Figure 12.2b. This may reflect the regional and seasonal variations of temperature and rainfall that in turn may affect the persistence of *M. bovis* in slurry, in moist shade, or even in water courses, and certainly influence local suitability for pastoral husbandry.[66] But it might also be that the regional ecology of a wildlife reservoir of *M. bovis* explains heightened risk to cattle and vice versa through a cycle of infection. Evidence for the latter is abundant in that the strain of the disease found in badgers is often identical to that found in cattle nearby.

In Belgium and in some studies of the RoI, cattle movements do not seem to be a major contributor to heightened risk.[67] But they clearly are in several regions of the UK.[68] What may differ between these regions is the nature of the marketing economy. In the South West of England and in some parts of Ireland North and South there is rapid turnover of cattle as a result of the local livestock husbandry context.[69] Breeding and feeding regions that harbour disease are a risk in the onward movement of animals. If farms that are naïve of bTB bring in animals from such areas they are knowingly raising their risk profile. A series of reports from 1972 to 1988 claimed that eight to ten per cent of confirmed herd breakdowns in South West England were the

---

[64] Ramírez-Villaescusa et al. 2009, 2010.

[65] Denny and Wilesmith 1999; Phillips et al 2003

[66] Wint et al. 2002; Jin et al. 2013.

[67] Only seven per cent of breakdowns in the RoI are attributable to infected incoming cattle. Clegg et al. 2008; Skuce et al. 2011.

[68] Griffin 1993; Griffin et al. 1996; Denny and Wilesmith 1999; Munroe et al. 1999; Carrique-Mas et al. 2005; Gilbert et al. 2005; Johnston et al. 2005; Gopal et al. 2006; Reilly and Courtenay 2007; Clegg et al. 2008; Carrique-Mas et al. 2008; Green et al. 2008.

[69] O'Mairtin et al. 1998a.

result of the purchase of infected stock. For the rest of the country the figure was fifty to sixty-four per cent.[70] This suggests that something is different about the South West - local persistence in cattle or a reservoir of infectious wildlife are the most frequently cited causes. In their study, Green and his colleagues concluded that seventy-five per cent of *M. bovis* infections in high-risk areas were due to local factors and overall only sixteen per cent could be attributed to cattle movement.[71]

Researchers have frequently pointed to the need for improved movement controls, both within hotspots and from heavily infected areas to regions naive of the disease.[72] In studies by Ramírez-Villaescusa and colleagues, it was argued that pre-movement testing would be beneficial and this was indeed introduced in England and Wales in 2006, a year after Scotland.[73] Cattle in the areas where herds are tested annually must have had a tuberculin test within sixty days and in Scotland there is also a post-movement test. Some reactors will be found that would otherwise have escaped detection, so boosting the headline slaughter statistics but it will be surprising if the impact of these additional tests is not positive in the medium and long term.[74] Pre-movement and/or post-movement tuberculin testing may reduce this risk but some will remain because of the inefficiencies of the test and the existence of anergic animals and latent infections.

In addition to pre- or post-movement testing, there are other ways to reduce the risk of infection travelling with cattle. An obvious one is the operation of a truly closed herd, using artificial insemination or embryo transfer rather than bringing in bulls, calves or heifers. Another is the quarantine of purchased animals for three to four weeks.[75]

Cattle movement from farm to farm may explain breakdowns but they may also occur in closed herds where there is one or more animal with sub-clinical disease and if there are a number of them in a

---

[70] Goodchild and Clifton-Hadley 2001. According to AHVLA/APHA data, up to eighty per cent of breakdowns in low risk areas of the UK are now the result of cattle movements from higher risk farms. Bovine TB Risk-Based Trading Group 2013.

[71] Green et al. 2008.

[72] Gilbert et al. 2005; Green and Cornell 2005; Johnston et al. 2005; Gopal et al. 2006. See also Green et al. 2008; Clegg et al. 2008.

[73] Ramírez-Villaescusa et al. 2009 and 2010; Christley et al. 2011.

[74] The Defra prediction from modelling was that from 2010-2015 pre-movement testing would prevent 1,500 confirmed new breakdowns in high TB incidence areas.

[75] Skuce et al. 2011.

locality this may represent a ghostly reservoir of infection from which reactors are occasionally identified. Risk-based trading might be a way for purchasing farmers to minimise their exposure to disease.

(6) Buildings

With regard to risks associated with buildings there seems to be a spectrum of opinion. Unless there is incontrovertible proof that the policy will work, many farmers resent being told to improve their buildings' ventilation, or make them inaccessible to wildlife, or create stock-proof fencing, but epidemiologists are reluctant to give any such guarantees. The evidence is ambiguous, although immediately after the Second World War researchers such as John Francis were in no doubt that the principal context of infection was the cowshed, citing the circulation of bacteria-laden aerosols in confined and congested spaces.[76] Today's situation is different. Fewer cattle in advanced countries ever reach this stage of being a high risk to their peers and, anyway, the conditions of cattle housing have improved, particularly with regard to ventilation. The hazard remains but the risk has been reduced.[77] Nevertheless the ISG did find that in South West England a confirmed breakdown was 5.06 times more likely on farms where covered yard housing was used.[78]

(7) Animal risk factors

Undernourished or malnourished cattle and those with a compromised immune system are more susceptible to bTB infection and progression of the disease than better fed animals. We can see at the present day this in some African cattle and their patterns of disease may well be a model for the situation as it was in Europe and North America in the late nineteenth and early twentieth centuries, when knowledge of bovine nutrition was at an early stage and many small farmers were unable to provide their beasts with a balanced diet.[79]

Skuce and his colleagues have reviewed the bTB risks as they

---

[76] Francis 1947, 1958.

[77] Griffin et al. 1993; Costello et al. 1998.

[78] ISG 2004; Johnston et al. 2005.

[79] Griffin et al. 1993; Humblet et al. 2009.

affect individual animals.[80] Transmission from cow to calf is possible through the vertical route (congenital) and through milk if the udder is diseased.[81] In addition there is the beast's age, gender, breed and physiological state (pregnancy, lactation, parturition), and any stress – metabolic or behavioural. Enterprise type is also important. As we have seen, dairy cattle are especially susceptible because they live longer and spend more time in confined spaces. The animal's immune status is important, depending on viruses, and any other concurrent infection.

Another factor to consider is the possibility that a relatively small number of cattle are super-spreaders of bTB, having the ability to affect many others without necessarily being detected themselves. Identifying and dealing with such animals is a priority.[82]

(8) Silage

The use of silage has also been identified as an issue, particularly in those areas where it has grown in popularity as a winter feed over recent decades. In order to reduce labour costs, there has been a tendency to introduce group feeding of silage with its attendant heightened risk of airborne infection and stress for the animals.[83] Because silage sometimes causes loose faeces, there may be some splashing and the aerosolization of any mycobacteria present.[84] In addition to grass silage, there is now also maize. From almost nothing in the UK before 1960, maize has become an important forage and grain crop, with farmers in the South West of England the most enthusiastic innovators (Figure 12.3). Since maize is also nutritious and palatable for badgers, its presence may be an important new explanatory variable, especially on farms where biosecurity is weak and badgers can gain access to storage clamps.[85] The badgers may interact with cattle whilst in the farm buildings or they might urinate and defecate in the feedstore, again with potential risk to the cattle.

---

[80] Skuce et al. 2011. See also Phillips et al. 2002 and Humblet et al. 2010.

[81] Skuce et al. 2012.

[82] O'Hare et al. 2014.

[83] Griffin et al.1993; Goodchild and Clifton-Hadley 2001.

[84] Goodchild and Clifton-Hadley 2001.

[85] Phillips et al. 2003; Reilly and Courtenay 2007; Roper 2010.

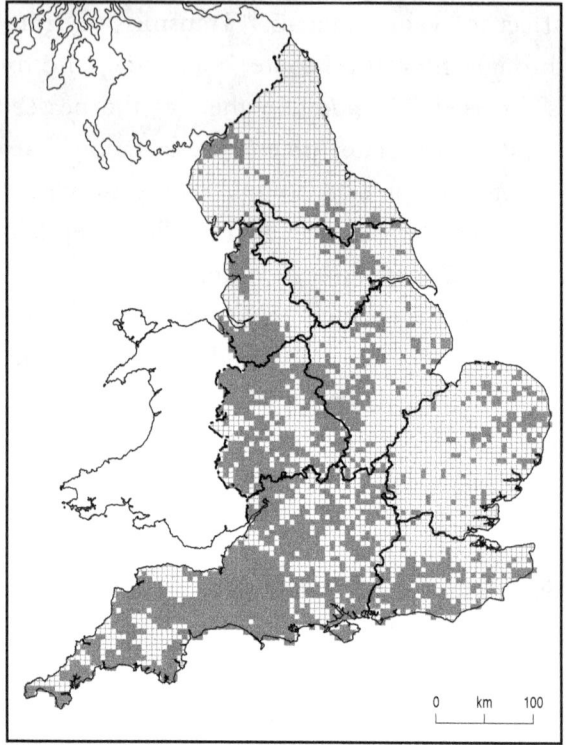

Fig 12.3
England, principal areas of
maize production, 2010,
5 km² grid
(Source: Defra)

(9) Molecular epidemiology

It is possible to identify points of susceptibility and resistance within the bovine genome, and it may be that the switch to high yielding but less resistant breeds, such as Holsteins, may have been a contributory factor in the recrudescence of disease in the UK since the 1970s.[86] There is also research suggesting genetic variations of response by breed to the skin test so that some herds are less likely to react when they are infected.[87] The reverse side of this coin is that it should be possible for breeding to reduce susceptibility to bTB, and the selection of bulls with resistant genes will begin in the near future.[88] Because we know that *M. bovis* strains vary in their immunogenicity,[89] tuberculin doses could then be varied or the skin test results interpreted differently according to a herd's genomic profile.[90]

---

[86] Driscoll et al. 2011; Bermingham et al. 2009; Bermingham et al. 2011; Tsairidou 2014.

[87] Amos et al. 2013.

[88] Driscoll et al. 2011; Le Roex et al. 2013.

[89] Ritz et al. 2008.

[90] Goodchild et al. 2003; De la Rua-Domenech et al. 2006; Wright et al. 2013.

Not only is there a genetic difference between *M. tuberculosis* and *M. bovis* but within both there are sub-strains that can be identified. It has been shown, for instance, by spoligotype and the profile of Variable Numbers of Tandem Repeat (VNTR), that *M. bovis* genotype frequencies and sublineage makeup vary from region to region.[91] These differences allow the investigation of the development of local pockets of genetically distinctive infection and may possibly help us eventually to understand the movement of a sub-strain from one area to another.[92]

The sub-strains tend to be anchored for decades to specific locations. Over eighty are found in cattle in the UK and about forty-four per cent of reactors are infected with either genotypes nine or seventeen. Figure 12.4 depicts this pattern clearly, although bear in mind that this is generalised and leaves out the many minor spoligotypes that are found in cattle around the country.

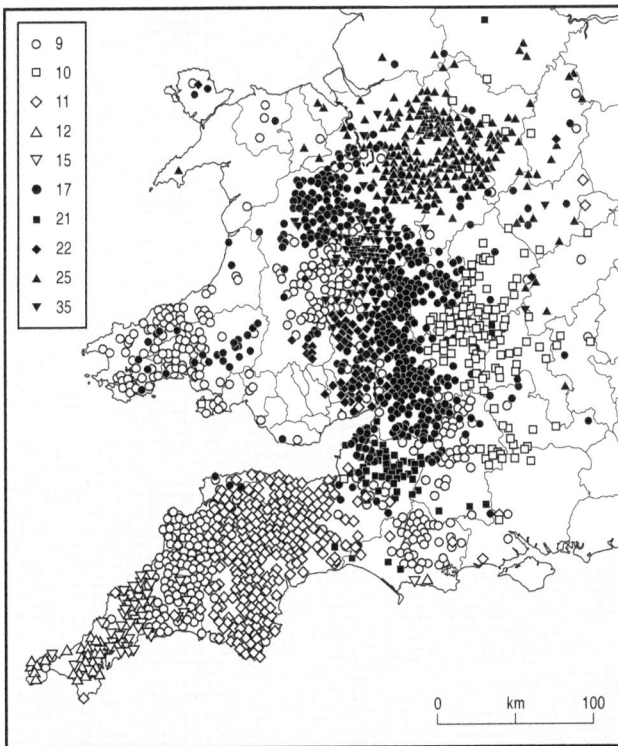

Fig 12.4 The main bTB spoligotypes identified from 2013 samples
(Source: AHVLA 2014b)

---

[91] Harris 2006.
[92] Smith and Upton 2012; Allen et al. 2013.

Conclusion

In Chapter 1 we introduced the notion of an onto-political ecology. This sees material objects, such as *M. bovis*, as playing a key role in environmental issues facing society, and therefore having political leverage. As we have seen in the present chapter, bTB may no longer pose much of a zoonotic threat but a study of its epidemiology shows that it has many options for exploiting the weakly defended boundary between society and nature. At one level we can see it as the most troublesome and costly of the livestock diseases. But another perspective is that *M. bovis* is now so closely interwoven with the agro-ecology of UK farming that it has become part of it, not something separate. A response therefore demands a new type of politics, working with and through the ecological possibility spaces that the mycobacterium has created for itself and has had created for it by society.

One way to approach this new politics is from a foundation of dynamic analysis, looking at the emergence of patterns of infection through time. But an extraordinary feature of the literature reviewed in this chapter is its indifference to past patterns of bTB. None of the papers cited can account for the macro-scale patterns in Figures 4.1 and 9.2 for instance.[93]

A second conclusion through the lens of political ecology is that the relationship between *M. bovis* and the environment may be more complicated than hitherto imagined. There may well be avenues of spread that have not so far been quantified, and possibly interactions between variables that are spatially contingent in ways that may at least partially explain the local dimension to bTB that we have mentioned. By way of example, one recent study based upon a sophisticated multivariate analysis of 193 variables has revealed some unexpected results. It found first that areas subject to flooding seem to be at risk in a way not previously considered, hinting at a new mechanism of spread. Second, the study found that the best-fit statistical explanation for bTB prevalence in particular localities involved a total of 16 different variables.[94] In other words, the search for one or even a small cluster of causal factors is doomed to failure because the epidemiologi-

---

[93] But see Atkins and Robinson 2013a.
[94] Brunton 2014; Brunton et al. 2015.

cal pathways of *M. bovis* are a complex patchwork. Inevitably we must therefore be wary of interventions that are seeking national or even regional eradication of the disease through action based upon lowest common denominator epidemiological variables. If cost effectiveness is to be a driver of policy resources then a spatially differentiated approach is likely to yield the best results.

CHAPTER 13.

M. BOVIS *AND WILDLIFE RESERVOIRS*

It is uncontroversial to claim that successive badger control policies have failed.[1]

Introduction

Everything changed in 1971 when tuberculosis was identified in a badger carcase in Gloucestershire and the conclusion was drawn by many observers that this was evidence of a wildlife reservoir of the disease, thereby helping to explain why bTB recurred in herds that would have been expected otherwise to have progressed to OTF status.[2] The carcase had been collected in April of that year and the disease identified by the Central Veterinary Laboratory in June. The MAFF's archives suggest that a badger link was suspected well before 1971, however, including a note by the Berkshire Pest Officer that in the period 1941-47 all of the setts in his county had been gassed even though this was illegal at the time.[3]

Since 1971 it has become clear that wildlife reservoirs of bTB are by no means unusual. The possum in New Zealand, wild boar in Spain and white-tailed deer in the United States are just three among a long list of species capable of harbouring the disease and thought to pass it on to economically valuable domestic species such as cattle.[4] The present chapter will consider both the complex inter-species ecologies that are implied by wildlife reservoirs in the UK and the attempts that have been made to intervene, through culling and other measures, to minimise the risk of bTB to cattle. Not only does the culling of badgers raise controversial issues about animal welfare in connexion with this most iconic of wild animals, it also underlies an extraordinary disintegration

---

[1] Macdonald et al. 2006, 269.

[2] Murhead et al. 1974; TNA: MAF 145/21.

[3] TNA: MAF 131/170; MAF 257/6.

[4] Palmer et al. 2012; Hardstaff et al. 2014; Drewe et al. 2014.

of the former policy consensus among the five nations that occupy the British Isles: the four in the UK (England, Wales, Scotland and Northern Ireland), and the Republic of Ireland. Each now has its own distinctive policy (Table 13.1) and the background to this will require some explanation.

Table 13.1 Policy with regard to badgers and bTB, in place 2015

- England - experimental culls organized by the private sector.
- Wales - vaccination of badgers.
- Scotland - no cull.
- RoI - 12,000 badgers to be snared and shot 2015-16.
- Northern Ireland - test and vaccinate or remove.

Wildlife and bovine tuberculosis: transmission scenarios

Since the 1970s there have been several official reports finding compelling 'evidence that badgers were a significant source of infection in cattle'.[5] Few scientists would disagree that this circumstantial evidence exists and yet the trapping data indicate that eighty-five per cent of badgers never contract bTB, that only about five per cent become infectious, and that a mere two to three per cent are super infectious.[6] Moreover it seems likely that the disease hazard is limited mainly to two or three channels.

The first is cattle coming into contact with badger-infected urine, faeces, sputum or wound exudates. Urine is the most likely given that *M. bovis* is found in greater concentrations there than in faeces.[7] Badgers urinate in more locations than they defecate and cattle are less able to avoid the resulting contaminated pasture than they can badger latrines, which tend to be on the edges of fields. Early work suggested that cattle were reluctant to eat grass contaminated with badger excreta due to its odour.[8] However, subsequent evidence suggests that whether or not contaminated grass is avoided depends on the nature of the grazing

---

[5] Krebs and the ISG 1997, 6. See also Griffin et al. 2005a and 2005b; Donnelly et al. 2006.

[6] Woodroffe et al. 2006; Woodroffe et al. 2005; Bourne et al. 2007; Society for General Microbiology 2008.

[7] Griffin et al. 1992.

[8] Benham 1985; Benham and Broom 1989; Benham and Broom 1991. But Hutchings and Harris 1999 demur.

regime.[9] If grazing pressure is high - for example because of cattle numbers or because most of the good grass in a pasture has already been eaten - cattle become less fussy and consumption of contaminated grass is possible.[10]

The problem with this badger shedding hypothesis is that there is overwhelming evidence that cattle become infected through the respiratory route.[11] In the modern era they seem predominantly to inhale the mycobacteria rather than ingesting them (see Chapters 4 and 12). It is possible that cattle, in disturbing the grass while they eat, may aerosolise some bacteria but there is no convincing evidence that this happens.

The second scenario is that badger waste may be deposited in farm buildings as they forage for grain or silage and is later ingested by unsuspecting cattle.[12] As we saw in Chapter 12, maize clamps are particularly attractive to badgers and that this crop is concentrated in the south west of England where cattle bTB is also mostly found.

A third idea is that encounters between badgers and cattle are more common than used to be thought likely.[13] This may be because the cows highest in the herd hierarchy are also the most inquisitive about badgers and, in addition, have the greatest level of contact with other herd members.[14] They are therefore in a key position as potential spreaders of infectious disease. The most recent, detailed fieldwork seems to show, however, that, while contacts do happen, they are more likely to be indirect than direct.[15] Indeed in Ireland badgers are said to avoid any contact with cattle wherever possible.[16]

Badger ecology

European badgers (*Meles meles*) are burrowing animals that are nocturnal and omnivorous by habit. They are Britain's largest wild mammal and

---

[9] Hutchings and Harris 1997; Smith et al. 2009.

[10] Ward et al. 2010.

[11] Phillips et al. 2003.

[12] Garnett 2002; Garnett et al 2002; Ward et al 2008; Tolhurst et al 2009.

[13] ISG 2007.

[14] Böhm et al. 2009; Scantlebury et al. 2006.

[15] Bohm et al 2009; Drewe et al. 2013.

[16] Mullen et al. 2013.

are distributed all over the country, being particularly abundant in the South West of England. This is the result of the availability of preferred foods such as earthworms,[17] which abound in permanent or rotational grasslands close to woodland edges.[18] The density of badgers in this region can reach more than twenty individuals per square kilometre.[19] We cannot be sure, however, that their present regional distribution truly reflects their ecological potential because historically badgers have been targeted in some areas by gamekeepers, arable farmers and sett diggers. As a result, in regions such as East Anglia there are fewer than might be expected.[20]

Badgers live in groups of three to ten animals, with an upper limit of twenty-five in the most favourable conditions.[21] Their setts are complexes of tunnels and chambers, sometimes substantial in spatial extent and longevity of use. These underground habitats are humid and stable in temperature from day to day and lacking in ultra-violet light. These are the ideal conditions for the survival of *M. bovis* over long periods.[22]

It is not difficult to imagine the underground exchange of bacteria-laden air between individual badgers in the confined and enclosed spaces of the sett and several studies confirm that their respiratory system is the main locus of infection.[23] In addition, bTB is spread through infected bite wounds and by post-natal maternal transmission to cubs. This is not to say that proximity guarantees infection because the occupation of setts seems to involve some separation or zonation as dictated by the aggression of the dominant boars.

In Britain at the micro scale there is no clear correlation between badger population density and bTB infection.[24] This is partly because, at the highest densities, badgers are super-territorial and migration is

---

[17] Kruuk and Parish 1982.
[18] Clements et al. 1988; Wilson et al. 1997; Delahay et al. 2006.
[19] Delahay et al. 2003.
[20] Cresswell et al. 1990.
[21] Neal and Cheeseman 1996; Delahay et al. 2000.
[22] White and Harris 1995; Moore and Roper 2003; Courtenay et al. 2006, 2007.
[23] Cheeseman et al. 1989; Gallagher and Clifton-Hadley 2000.
[24] Delahay et al. 2003. But Woodroffe, Donnelly, Wei et al. 2009 found that social group size is a negative correlate of bTB infection in badgers.

rare between neighbouring groups.[25] The degree of clustering is such that it is not unknown to have a highly infected group living next to one with no disease.[26] Thus for the infection of badgers it seems that population density is less important than the status and dispersal of diseased individuals.[27]

By far the most important finding in recent years about the behaviour of badgers is that disturbance by humans can cause perturbation. This is particularly relevant where the culling of badgers has been localised or incomplete and has disrupted their socio-spatial organization. In consequence individuals range more widely, resulting in contact between groups that would not otherwise have occurred.[28] There is solid evidence from British studies that culling with perturbation presents an unrivalled opportunity for disease diffusion that would otherwise not be present in high density areas.[29] Ironically then, if culling is not comprehensive enough and efficiently undertaken, the surviving members of disturbed groups will escape into the surrounding countryside, taking any infection with them to naive badger communities and possibly to new cattle herds.

Evidence of co-location of badger and cattle tuberculosis

Badger numbers are increasing, especially in England. A survey in the years 1985-88 indicated 37,490–46,298 social groups in the UK, growing to 45,914–54,568 in a survey undertaken between 1994 and 1997.[30] The most recent field research (2011-13) found 66,400–76,900 social groups, suggesting an increase of about seventy per cent over twenty-five years.[31] Equivalent surveys in Scotland (1994-97 and 2007-09) also found a substantial increase in occupied setts, but in Northern Ireland (1990-93 and 2007-08) there was no significant change.

It is not possible to say what percentage of badgers is infected with

---

[25] Woodroffe et al. 1995; MacDonald et al. 2006; Böhm et al. 2009.

[26] Cheeseman et al. 1981; Cheeseman et al. 1985; Delahay et al. 2000; Delahay et al. 2001.

[27] Vicente et al. 2007; Weber et al. 2013..

[28] Carter et al. 2007; Pope et al. 2007; Bielby et al. 2014.

[29] Donnelly et al. 2007; Woodroffe, Donnelly, Cox et al. 2009.

[30] Cresswell et al. 1990; Wilson et al. 1997.

[31] Judge et al. 2014.

bTB in each region. The best we can do is to refer to Figure 13.1, which is an approximation for the period from 1972 to 1990. Since about a fifth of the adult badger population is killed each year in road traffic accidents (RTAs), it was known that there would be carcases to test for clinical signs of the disease. Members of the public were therefore encouraged to collect and hand in road kills for post mortem checking. This was a valuable source of data, although it is immediately obvious from the map that the distribution of RTAs is not fully representative of the national pattern of badgers. This is partly because members of the public reporting carcases were more aware of the need for testing in some parts of the country than others, but there are also reports that the testing laboratories rejected some carcases, presumably because of their limited processing capacity.[32]

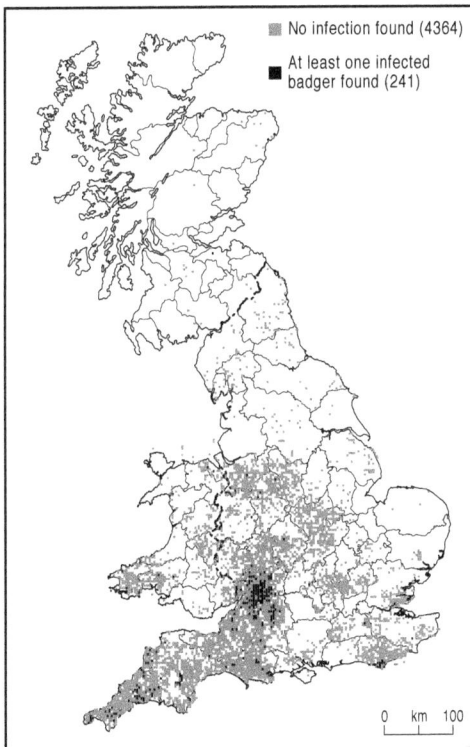

No infection found (4364)

At least one infected badger found (241)

0   km   100

Fig 13.1
Badger RTAs 1972-1990
(Source: Krebs and the ISG 1997)

In those regions with data we can show the location of tuberculous badgers in relation to those without the disease. Despite scepticism in some quarters, it has been claimed that RTAs *are* informative indicators

---

[32] Cheeseman et al. 1989; Krebs and the ISG 1997; Abernethy et al. 2003.

of the prevalence of bTB in the badger population, although they cannot be taken as definitive evidence.[33] There have been suggestions of bias in the database towards tuberculous animals, presumably because they might be less nimble in crossing roads, or a bias against them because they are less likely to venture away from the sett. From her experience, however, Woodroffe thinks such biases to be unlikely because 'it is a pretty random assortment of animals that get killed on roads'.[34]

Figure 13.1 shows a large cluster of badger bTB in Gloucestershire, Herefordshire, Somerset, Wiltshire and Worcester, with some hot spots in Cornwall, Devon, Dorset, East Sussex and South Wales. This closely mirrors the distribution of cattle breakdowns at the time and such co-locations have usually been taken to imply a pathway of cattle-to-badger infection. There are two riders, however. First, there were large swathes of the country where plenty of badger carcases were handed in but most were not diseased. This has important implications that we will investigate further. Second, some tuberculous RTA badgers were found where there was no detected bTB in cattle.[35] This seems to suggest that bTB can sometimes be self-sustaining in badgers without there necessarily being implications for other species.

Similar to the epidemiological reasoning in Chapter 12, a number of statistical studies have concluded that the presence of infected badgers *is* the most likely explanation of the clustering of bTB in cattle herds.[36] At the local scale this has been strengthened by the typing of individual *M. bovis* strains known as spoligotypes, often found to be co-located in cattle and badgers.[37] From the annual reports published by the APHA and its predecessors it is clear that over time the clusters of each strain have reproduced themselves in relative isolation, within radii of only ten to fifty kilometres (Figure 12.4).[38] Any outliers beyond these

---

[33] Goodchild et al. 2012.

[34] House of Commons, Select Committee on Agriculture, *Fifth Report*, Session 1998-99, Q.242.

[35] Krebs and the ISG 1997.

[36] Griffin et al. 1996; Reilly and Courtenay 2007; Murphy et al. 2011; White et al. 2013.

[37] See Chapter 12.

[38] Skuce et al. 2005; Smith, Marion et al. 2006; Jenkins et al. 2007.

distances are probably the result of long-distance cattle movements.[39] Given that the cattle tracing system shows that most sale movements are also within twenty kilometres of the farm of origin, we now have two separate confirmations of the granularity of the overall spatial pattern.

The spoligotypes of bTB in cattle are closely mirrored by the same spoligotypes in badgers.[40] Again badgers stay within a narrow radius. In the absence of perturbation they range only a few kilometres from their home setts and a wave diffusion of badger-to-badger infection is therefore unlikely to move any faster than at a glacial pace across the countryside. Modelling indicates rather that it is the association between *M. bovis* infections in badgers and cattle that is the most important one in providing a spatial explanans of the epidemiological structure of the disease. At present it is not possible to say whether this is the result of badgers infecting cattle or vice versa but the literature seems to assume the former. One possible indicator is that the increase in badger populations that we commented on earlier is correlated with areas where the recrudescence in cattle disease is focused.[41] Again this is not proof of a causal direction but it is certainly more than a statistical nudge.[42]

Long term infection of badgers?

Insights into the relationship between bTB in badgers and the disease in cattle have depended upon behavioural ecology and ecological modelling, approaches which between them exhibit an ontological tension. One method is observational and the other virtual but they co-exist in many projects because statistical models require field data for calibration and the estimation of parameters. Yet the scientific styles remain at variance.

By way of example, we noted above the lack of support from ecological fieldwork for the commonly assumed positive correlation between badger group size and bTB infection.[43] But ecological models, particularly those employing multiple simulations, tell a different story.

[39] Gopal et al. 2006.
[40] Woodroffe et al. 2005b; Jenkins et al. 2007.
[41] Wilesmith 1983; Menzies et al. 2011.
[42] It may eventually be possible to assess the direction of infection using phylodynamics. Allen et al. 2011.
[43] But see Allen et al. 2011.

Anderson and Trewhella found badgers to be a possible maintenance host of bTB on the basis of a model that predicted an equilibrium prevalence of about eighteen per cent after thirty to forty years.[44] By an extension of this logic, White and Harris found persistence in ninety-five per cent of their simulation outcomes over a 100 year period. Overall they concluded that bTB 'has the potential to persist in the badger population for a long time, even at small group sizes and at low prevalences, without any reinfection being required'.[45] By 'small group' they meant six adults and yearlings, although eight adults and yearlings were required for a higher probability of intragroup infection and disease persistence. Others have drawn similar conclusions and according to Smith, 'when social group size drops below about 6.3 adults and yearlings disease extinction may occur within 50 years'.[46] Large groups tend to be found in Type I habitats: low to medium altitude with woodland interspersed with good agricultural land, as seen in classic badger study sites such as Wytham Woods, Oxfordshire, and Woodchester Park, Gloucestershire.[47] Type II habitats, low to medium altitude, primarily pastoral farmland with limited woodland, and Type III, medium to high altitude with upland vegetation, are less likely to facilitate disease persistence or spread, because they have mean group sizes of 5.1 (with cubs) and 3.5 respectively.

Even within the modelling community there are divisions between the deterministic and stochastic approaches and between aspatial and GIS-based models. As a result, the analysis of the spread of FMD in 2001 descended into bickering about whose models should be used as the basis of government slaughter policy.[48] Due to such professional disagreements, we are still not clear whether badgers are maintenance hosts or spillover hosts of bTB. In a maintenance host a disease persists due to the circulation of an infection among a group of individuals, sometimes for lengthy periods. Spillover hosts in contrast require occasional re-infection from outside for disease persistence.[49] A third

---

[44] Anderson and Trewhella 1985.
[45] White and Harris 1995, 404.
[46] Smith et al. 1995; Hardstaff et al. 2012; Smith et al. 2001, 530.
[47] Feore and Montgomery 1999.
[48] Bickerstaff and Simmons 2004; Law and Moser 2012; Atkins and Robinson 2013b.
[49] Corner et al. 2011; Nugent 2011.

possibility is that bTB has maintenance status in some regions but is otherwise only a spillover disease.

Consider the following points made with historical spatial patterns in mind. First, given the heavy concentration of bTB at the present day in both the cattle and badgers in the South West of England, South Wales, and a few other localities, it seems hard to justify the claim that the disease is 'endemic in many badger populations *throughout* England'.[50] Woodchester Park in the Cotswolds, where much work has been done on badger ecology, has among the highest badger densities anywhere in Europe and care is therefore needed in extrapolating the work done there beyond its regional context.

Second, a point opaque to homogeneous spatial thinking is that the highest peak of bTB in cattle before 1960 was to be found in Cheshire, in North West England, in a part of the country where bTB in badgers has since been found by the RTA exercise to be low (Figure 13.1).[51] This means either that (a) badgers were not involved in the first half of the twentieth century, when the disease would therefore have been spread cattle-to-cattle; or (b) that badgers were involved in previous decades but somehow the disease did not persist amongst them in the way usually assumed.[52] Either way, this historical disjunction of the maps of bTB poses a major challenge to any simplistic assumption that somehow the South West of England was always fated by its ecological context to be the major hotspot of the disease in the UK for either badgers, cattle, or both.

A short history of badger culling

The MAFF acted speedily to explore the new badger threat that arose in 1971. By 1973 there was a Badgers Act on the statute book that both improved the general protection of badgers and also enabled the issue of licences for killing them. Although individual farmers and landowners were now to be allowed to trap and shoot badgers, it was recognised that progress would be slow, so the government took powers

---

[50] Anderson and Trewhella 1985, 374, emphasis added; Fisher et al. 2012.

[51] Francis 1948; Atkins and Robinson 2013a.

[52] It would have disappeared sometime between the end of area eradication in 1960 and the beginning of the RTA collection in Cheshire in 1976, not long according to the timescales usually assumed by the modellers.

in the Conservation of Wild Creatures and Wild Plants Act (1975) and Section 9 of the Agriculture (Miscellaneous Provisions) Act (1976) for strategic culling. By August 1975 this had commenced in Dorset, with Gloucestershire and Avon following in December 1975, and Cornwall in 1976. Over the next four years badger setts in 166 areas averaging seven square kilometres each were gassed with hydrogen cyanide.

It is important to note that gassing was not new. It had been used since 1900 for rabbit control and was specifically legalized by Section 4 of the Prevention of Damage by Rabbits Act (1939) and the Agriculture Act (1947). The Universities Federation for Animal Welfare (UFAW) had even encouraged and developed the technique from 1935 in order to minimize the problems of animal welfare, and the Scott-Henderson Committee's report on cruelty to wild animals (1951) thought gassing to be 'undoubtedly the most effective and humane method of killing badgers'.[53] It was also used extensively across Europe in the 1960s and 1970s as part of programmes of rabies control.[54]

Despite the various legislative and regulatory frameworks, comprehensive culling has not been carried out frequently in the UK. Thornbury (Avon) was one example, from 1975 to 1981, resulting in a significant reduction of bTB in cattle there for fifteen years afterwards. Other examples are Steeple Leaze (Dorset, 1974-84) and Hartland (north Devon, 1984), again both with claims of a long-term and sustained reduction in the disease in cattle.[55]

It was immediately obvious in the early 1970s that culling badgers would be a contentious policy, with strongly held views from farmers on one side and conservation groups on the other. A Consultative Panel on Badgers and Tuberculosis was therefore created by government in 1975 to seek the views of experts and interested parties.[56]

By the late 1970s the topic had become so controversial that an enquiry was ordered in 1979 by Peter Walker, the Minister of Agriculture. He chose Lord Zuckerman as chair, who had been the government's Chief Scientific Advisor and was at the time President of the Zoological Society. His scientific credentials and reputation as a Whitehall insider

---

[53] Scott Henderson 1951; TNA: MH 118/48.
[54] Griffiths and Thomas 1997.
[55] TNA: MAF 459/26.
[56] TNA: MAF 459/3.

made him a safe political choice. Zuckerman conducted extensive enquiries and seems to have been deeply and personally engaged with the topic. In his report in 1980, he concluded that badgers were indeed vectors of bTB, especially in the South West of England, where the density of both badgers and pasturing cattle was high.[57] He commented that their distribution seemed to correlate with dairy and cattle breeding areas because they feed to some extent on pastures. In these areas bTB infection rates were high in both species and when setts were gassed he observed that the disease in cattle declined.

Zuckerman therefore recommended the resumption of gassing, using improved techniques where possible.[58] He also asked for research on the prevalence of bTB in badgers, such as post mortems on animals killed in RTAs, and the publication of annual reports on the control programme. Finally, he asked for a further review after three years. All of these recommendations were accepted by the Minister.

In July 1982 the Consultative Panel considered the various options for controlling badgers. Shooting and digging were thought to be 'highly unsatisfactory' and were dismissed out of hand. Cage trapping was thought to be promising, possibly supplemented by snaring in difficult terrain. Poison baiting and gassing needed further research.[59] The Chemical Defence Establishment at Porton Down had already reported that the technique of blowing the powder, Cymag (hydrogen cyanide), into setts where it released gas on contact with moisture in the air, was ineffective in the furthest reaches of the network of underground tunnels. It seemed possible that cubs might be orphaned or badgers die slowly underground. As a result, gassing ceased nationwide in June 1982 and was replaced by live trapping.

From 1982 to 1985 a 'clean ring' strategy operated, in which social groups of badgers on and around a breakdown farm were identified, trapped and a sample of carcases from these groups was examined. Where infection was found, all badgers in the social group were removed. The ring was extended outwards until groups with uninfected badgers were found. Trapping took place in the cleared area for a further six months to keep the area 'clean'.

---

[57] Krebs and the ISG 1997.

[58] It had been suspended in 1979 upon the commencement of his enquiry.

[59] TNA: MAF 459/3.

At Zuckerman's own suggestion, a review was commissioned in 1984, known in Whitehall as the 'Son of Zuckerman'.[60] Professor George Dunnet was appointed and delivered his report after two years. This recommended an 'Interim Strategy' of continued badger control until further detailed research could be completed and a test developed for bTB in live badgers.[61] He wanted only tuberculous animals to be killed and for culling to take place only on the farm where a cattle breakdown had occurred. The reason for this was partly to do with the cost of the clean ring approach. Michael Jopling, the Minister of Agriculture, accepted Dunnet's recommendations in April 1986 and noted in a press release that this new approach would mean less disturbance of badgers.[62] It was a significant threshold because the initiative for action was now passed by the ministry back to individual farmers.[63]

Dunnet's Interim Strategy has subsequently been judged to be the weakest of the culling methodologies used to that date.[64] Although it was only intended as a stop-gap, it actually lasted for an uneasy ten years. In that time further protection for setts came in the Badgers (Further Protection) Act (1991) and the Protection of Badgers Act (1992), making this the most protected of wild species in Britain.[65] After that any culling had to be licensed. In 1993 the Consultative Panel made further recommendations, including the need for the development of a badger vaccine; a blood test alternative to the traditional skin test in cattle; the monitoring of disease in badgers killed in road traffic accidents; and the need for research on badger movements when disturbed by culling.

Krebs and the Randomised Badger Culling Trial

Following the rising numbers of reactors being identified in the early 1990s, Professor John Krebs was appointed in 1996 'to review the

---

[60] For the background to this, see TNA: MAF 459/22.

[61] This was not released for trials until 1994 and then proved to have poor sensitivity.

[62] TNA: MAF 459/20.

[63] Spencer 2008.

[64] House of Commons, Select Committee on Agriculture, *Fifth Report*, Session 1998-99, Q.415.

[65] Badgers are also protected under the Council of Europe's Bern Convention on the Conservation of European Wildlife and Natural Habitats, although culling for disease reduction is allowed.

incidence of TB in cattle and badgers and assess the scientific evidence for links between them'.[66] His Group speedily produced a report that is a model of its kind: a clear and concise statement of existing knowledge with a proposed way forward based upon a scientific experimental design. Using their ecological and statistical expertise, the Krebs group suggested a large-scale field-based trial in which badgers were to be culled and the effects of this monitored on the incidence of bTB in cattle. It was to be the largest such trial ever attempted, with costs to match, and it is perhaps a little surprising that government so readily accepted the proposition.[67]

Krebs recommended the establishment of what came to be called the Independent Scientific Group (ISG). This new group was to oversee field work in 100 km² blocks arranged in triplets (Figure 13.2) in ten hotspot areas in the South West of England. Each triplet was to have a zone of 'proactive' (repeated, annual) culling across the whole area, one

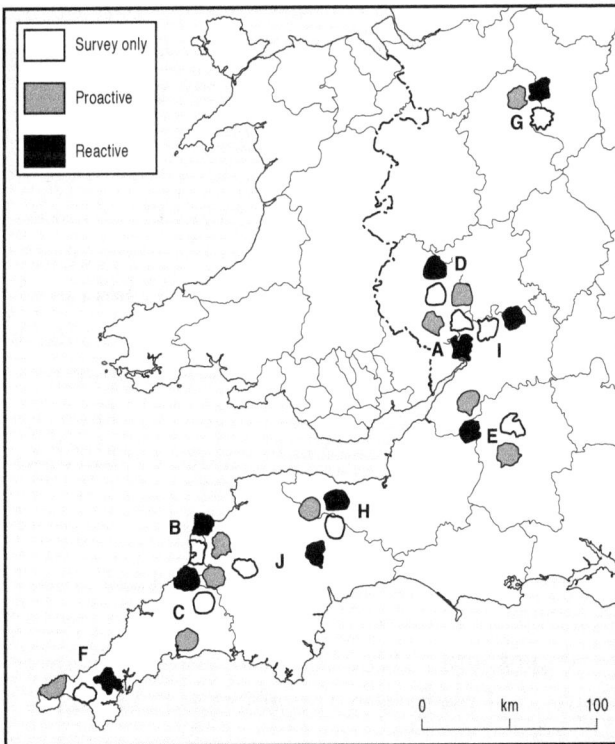

Fig 13.2 The triplets in the RBCT (Source: Donnelly et al. 2006)

[66] Krebs and the ISG 1997.
[67] It cost £50 million.

of 'reactive' culling in localized areas where there were tuberculous cattle, and a control 'no cull' or 'survey' area.[68] This controlled experiment approach in their view was the best way to settle once and for all the issue as to whether the culling of badgers reduces the risk of infection for cattle. It was designed to guarantee the political neutrality of the project and by controlling for chance it was planned to yield results of a greater statistical significance.

In 1998 the ISG was appointed under the chairmanship of Professor John Bourne, and with the support of Defra the triplets were established. The project was known as the Randomised Badger Culling Trial (RBCT) and it ran until 2007 with 11,000 badgers being killed.

One of the limitations of the RBCT was that some of the badger trapping was disrupted by animal welfare activists and a number of landowners refused access. In addition, an enforced long pause in work during the 2001 FMD outbreak was an inconvenience. A final embarrassment came when the reactive culling part of the trial was stopped ahead of schedule (in 2003) by the government because of indications that it was causing an upsurge of bTB in cattle. There is also a question as to whether the farming community were ever really signed up to the trial. Many farmers objected because there would be no culling of badgers outside the triplet areas while the trial was in progress and it was reported that some took matters into their own hands.[69]

In 2005 the ISG was prevailed upon by Defra to issue some interim results. They are said to have been reluctant to do this because their analysis was incomplete and they were no doubt wary of the way any material might be used by the politicians. There was certainly disquiet when Defra soon after issued a public consultation on culling badgers.[70]

The ISG produced a series of six reports, the final one being in 2007, and its individual members have also published numerous papers on the technicalities of the trial and the detailed results. This body of work is complex and written in the careful and nuanced style one expects of a group of professional scientific researchers. It is difficult to

---

[68] Donnelly et al. 2006.

[69] House of Commons, Select Committee on Agriculture, *Fifth Report*, Session 1998-99, Qq.416-18, 565.

[70] Wilkinson 2007.

reduce to a number of headline findings but the following points have been those most commonly debated.[71]

1.In areas of high incidence of bTB in cattle there was a correlation between cattle and badger disease.

2.The relationship between host density and disease transmission is not linear.

3.The contribution of badgers to spreading bTB among herds in the RBCT areas is about half, with a robust lower bound of thirty-eight per cent.[72]

4.The reactive culling, far from reducing the incidence of TB in cattle, actually increased it, on average by twenty-seven per cent. As a result, the reactive cull was suspended in 2003.

5.The proactive culling reduced cattle TB in the culled areas more than in the survey-only areas: by thirty-two per cent by the end of the trial, and by twenty-eight per cent five years after the trial ended. However, during the RBCT the incidence of TB in cattle increased, by about twenty-four per cent on average, within a two kilometre band around the outside of each culled area.[73] This increase in cattle TB outside the culled areas more or less cancelled out the decline within the culled areas, so that the net effect of proactive culling was too small for culling to be cost effective. This was the 'perturbation effect' caused when badgers that had been disturbed migrated to new areas.

6.A technical point is that culled areas soon see badgers moving in from surrounding areas to exploit the opportunity. This encourages the mixing of previously separate groups and maximises the chance of disease transmission. Areas with natural barriers such as rivers, mountains, coasts, or human-made barriers such as motorways, are the only ones spared this recolonization.[74]

---

[71] Drawn from Donnelly et al. 2003; Donnelly et al. 2006; Donnelly et al. 2007; Jenkins et al. 2008; McDonald et al. 2008; Jenkins et al. 2010; Defra 2011; Donnelly 2012; Donnelly and Nouvellet 2013.

[72] This compares with a previous study suggesting that badgers were implicated in approximately 90 per cent of cattle tuberculosis breakdowns in South West England and another for Northern Ireland where the figure was said to be closer to 40 per cent. Clifton-Hadley and Cheeseman 1997; Denny and Wilesmith 1999.

[73] The risk was 6 per cent lower in this band between 1.0 and 3.5 years after the last cull. Donnelly et al. 2007.

[74] House of Commons, EFRA Select Committee 2007, vol. 1, Q.18, R. Woodroffe.

7. It is possible from the RBCT results to calculate the effect of culling by area targeted. For example, assuming a herd density of 1.25 per km^2 and eight confirmed breakdowns per 100 herds, it would be necessary proactively to cull the badgers in 330 km^2 in order to see a benefit of a ten per cent reduction in breakdowns.

8. Overall, the conclusion was that 'you cannot eradicate the TB in the badger by culling' and that 'badger culling can make no meaningful contribution to cattle TB control in Britain'.[75]

The ISG's final report was academic in style: thorough, cautious about making claims from the evidence, and it had taken nine years. None of these are characteristics admired by politicians. Moreover the ISG's conclusion was so comprehensively negative about culling that in a sense they gave the wrong answer because politicians dislike the closing of options.

It is important to note that it is not only farmers who are in favour of badger culling. The views of vets are similar, as expressed through the British Veterinary Association (BVA), the British Cattle Veterinary Association, and even some outspoken members of the State Veterinary Service (SVS).[76]

Gordon Brown becoming Prime Minister in June 2007 has been linked with a shift in the policy mood.[77] The Defra ministers were all moved on apart from the pragmatic Jeff Rooker, who was said to have been open to a cull. In July the government's Chief Scientific Advisor, Sir David King, was brought in to assess the findings of the ISG. Sir David and his small group of experts rejected the RBCT's principal finding and put badger culling back on the policy agenda. It is said to have taken them only a day and a half of meetings to come to this conclusion.[78]

Professor Bourne is reported to have 'reacted angrily' to Sir David's report, calling it 'hastily written' and 'superficial'.[79] He and other former members of the ISG pointed to six major concerns with the science in the King report and a stinging editorial in the leading scientific journal,

---

[75] Ibid. Q.19., R. Woodroffe; ISG 2007.

[76] Ibid. Q.141, T. Lawson.

[77] Spencer 2008, 2011.

[78] Ares 2014a.

[79] *Guardian* 25 October 2007; Lodge and Matus 2014.

Nature, criticised Sir David for 'the mishandling of the issue' and called his reworking of the ISG report 'an example to governments of how not to deal with such advice, once it has been solicited and received'.[80] A meeting between the ISG and Sir David in December 2007 seems to have been a stand-off with neither side giving ground. It took the EFRA Select Committee in 2008 to extract a consensus between the ISG and Sir David that culling could be effective, but that 'it must be done competently and efficiently; be coordinated; cover as large an area as possible (265 km² or more is the minimum needed to be 95 per cent confident of an overall beneficial effect); be sustained for at least four years; and be in areas which have "hard" or "soft" boundaries where possible'.[81]

Ultimately Sir David's intervention was of no consequence because, in a further twist of the politics of the New Labour government, in July 2008, the Secretary of State for Defra, Hilary Benn, accepted the recommendation of the ISG that the culling of badgers should be abandoned.

This shift in policy was not followed by the devolved Welsh government.[82] Following the Welsh Assembly Elections in 2007 and the appointment of Elin Jones, a Plaid Cymru assembly member, as Minister for Rural Affairs in the Welsh coalition government, a non-selective cull was authorised. This was opposed in the courts by the Badger Trust and in 2010 the Court of Appeal ruled against the Welsh government and their cull was dropped.[83] Soon after, in 2011, a change of government and a new Labour administration in Wales instead formulated a badger vaccination policy with field operations starting in the summer of 2012. Over 4,000 animals were vaccinated to the end of 2014 at a cost of about £660 each.[84]

---

[80] Bourne et al. 2007; *Nature* 450, 2007, 1-2.

[81] House of Commons, EFRA Select Committee (Fourth Report Session 2007-08, *Badgers and cattle TB: the final report of the Independent Scientific Group on Cattle TB*, 27 February 2008.

[82] Enticott and Franklin 2009.

[83] Enticott and Lee 2015.

[84] Chambers et al. 2014; *Veterinary Record* 176, 2015, 32.

The Coalition badger cull, 2013-15

In September 2010 Jim Paice, a Defra minister, issued a consultation on badger culling. This policy had been in the manifesto of the Conservative Party but not that of their new coalition partners, the Liberal Democrats. The decision to move forward with two pilot culls was then announced in December the following year and areas in the South West of England were identified in January 2012. In order to qualify cull zones had to satisfy a number of criteria:

- They had to be larger than 150 km², and the average was planned to be 350 km². Four year licences were to be issued by Natural England.

- Applications were only accepted from limited companies – groups of farmers – who were responsible for hiring trained contractors to perform the cull. The companies to bear the cost, depositing a sum in advance.

- Culling had to be on seventy per cent of the designated land and reduce the badger population by 70 per cent, thresholds suggested by the ISG.

- The plan was to roll out culling nationally but with no more than ten new areas added per year.

- Hard boundaries (rivers, coastlines, motorways) had to be identified to minimise the risk of badger 'perturbation'.

- Additional cattle controls and biosecurity were to be compulsory in the cull zones.

- The companies had to liaise with the local police in order to minimize the risk to public order.

The cull was intended to start in 2012 but it was postponed to the summer of 2013 because the number of badgers in each area was said to be more than expected and it was thought unlikely that sufficient numbers could be dispatched in the limited time available before the shooting season finished in the autumn.[85] Despite this slow start, the cull proceeded in the 2013 and 2014 seasons but the results were disappointing and the originally intended roll out to other regions was cancelled. From the culling companies' point of view they underperformed in the number of animals they were able to shoot or

---

[85] Ares and Hawkins 2014.

trap in the trial areas of Somerset and Gloucestershire. Nevertheless the new Conservative administration elected in 2015 has promised to continue with culling and to revive the idea of rolling it out to new areas.

One simulation study has shown that the resource-intensive nature of badger culling means that in the British context it will always cost more than the economic benefits of fewer cattle breakdowns.[86] Nevertheless a return to gassing might improve the efficiency of large-scale culls. Cyanide was banned as inhumane in 1982 but alternatives, such as carbon monoxide or nitrogen oxide-laden foam, are possibilities for the future.[87]

The first step in another policy avenue was taken in 2012-14 when the government began subsidising badger vaccination. Projects were eligible for the loan of equipment and advice from vaccination experts. Each scheme had to cover a minimum of fifteen square kilometres. This was very small scale but has the potential for expansion, especially if and when an effective bait-based vaccine becomes available.

Culling and its discontents

Pro-badger enthusiasts acted locally until 1986 when nineteen groups joined together to form the National Federation of Badger Groups. This was necessary to find a national voice in the culling debate that by then had been going on for over a decade. In 2008 the name was changed to the Badger Trust, now representing over fifty groups and having a membership of 5,000 but significantly more weight than those numbers suggest.

There seems to be an assumption that badgers have a positive image with the British public and that, as a result, killing them in the name of disease control will inevitably cause a political backlash. Certainly the qualitative research on the cultural background of badgers seems to bolster the view that the 'good badger' of Wind in the Willows outweighs the 'bad badger' that eats live hedgehogs and chickens.[88] The true public mood at present is, though, quite difficult to judge. The

---

[86] Wilkinson et al. 2009.

[87] Ares 2014b; Carrington 2014.

[88] Cassidy 2012.

public consultations and opinion polls that have been conducted over the last decade are mostly contaminated by the interests of those who commissioned them or by the tactics of large-scale activism. So too are the series of e-petitions against culling, which are an interesting new form of protest. The most significant one attracted 304,253 signatures in 2013, one of the largest ever, and there was another of 10,257 in 2014.[89]

There was a public consultation in 2005-6 in which the Labour government asked for views about badger culling. There were 47,472 responses received by letter and email and there were also 13 related petitions against a cull containing 12,100 signatures and 10,000 text messages. This astonishing return was largely orchestrated; 68 per cent of responses were from campaigns run either by wildlife or by farming groups (Defra 2006a). Although ninety-six per cent of these contacts were against a cull, the citizens' panels designed to be a representative 'demographic' were divided more evenly.[90] A second consultation by the new government in 2010 was also impressive. This time there were 59,540 responses, of which sixty-nine per cent expressed opposition to culling.

The bioethics of culling badgers have been examined in the context of evolutionary ecology. Although ethics were certainly considered by those organizing the 2013/14 culls and were mandatory by the terms of their licences for those carrying them out, nevertheless the actual killing was not carried out in a humane way.[91] This was the conclusion of the government's own Independent Expert Panel appointed to monitor the practical details for the 2013 season.[92] Between 7.4 and 22.8 per cent of badgers that were shot were still alive after five minutes and therefore likely to have suffered acute pain and the Panel commented on the unwillingness or inability of the contractors to follow the best practice guidelines that were designed to protect animal welfare.

Lodge and Matus have looked at British newspapers from 1986 to 2013 and found 854 actor arguments in 728 relevant articles on

---

[89] http://epetitions.direct.gov.uk/petitions/38257 and 54685.
[90] Spencer 2008.
[91] Crozier and Schulte-Hostedde 2014; Defra 2014a.
[92] Munro 2014; Defra 2014a.

bTB and badgers.[93] They identified thirteen actor groups and found stability in the positions they adopted, with some polarization towards the end of the study period. The justifications became more technically sophisticated, for instance the deployment of the perturbation argument by the anti-cull side. The authors found, however, that the different strands of arguments did not coalesce into collective action. On the anti-cull side, for instance, the Badger Trust, the animal welfare groups, Brian May's 'Team Badger', and a number of vociferous scientists all spoke independently. They remained in a loose alliance as is often the case with such advocacy but, while there was one spectacular success in the cancellation of the Welsh badger cull, they could not replicate the strength of the relationship between the MAFF/Defra and the NFU. Indeed the then Secretary of State of Defra, Caroline Spelman, claimed at a NFU Conference in February 2012 to have 'one of the most farmer-centred ministerial teams ever'. In the same speech she also announced that the first two cull areas were chosen 'from a short list proposed by the farming industry'.[94]

What are we to make of the NFU's involvement in this policy? It seems to me that the NFU bears a heavy weight of responsibility for its selective use of the available science, for instance in calling for culls of badgers when they know very well that they cannot meet the exacting conditions for success indicated by the members of the ISG. Conservative and Liberal Democrat politicians know that sections of *rural* opinion are in favour of killing badgers and that Defra cooperation with the NFU is therefore a requirement of re-election for some of their MPs, but they also know that the cull cannot be shown scientifically to have worked, even if numbers of bTB reactors fall, because the necessary funding was not made available for properly controlled research. Some of the indicators imply a failed cull 2013-14, along with the inability of the contractors to meet satisfactory standards of animal welfare.

Preventing contact between badgers and cattle

The biosecurity approach is attractive in principle to government, because the cost of implementing it would be relatively small by comparison

---

[93] Lodge and Matus 2014.
[94] NFU 2012.

with policies such as badger culling or vaccination and because the responsibility for implementing it could be passed on, at least partly, to farmers rather than resting entirely with the government. Unfortunately, however, biosecurity measures are presently hard for farmers to justify owing to the fact that we are uncertain how transmission occurs. For example, if we knew for sure that badgers transmit TB to cattle when they go looking for food in and around farm buildings, then it would be worth making the relevant buildings more secure. Or, if we knew that cattle troughs were a significant locus of transmission, then we could find ways of preventing badgers from climbing into them. But because of the uncertainty there is a disconnect between the top-down biosecurity rhetoric and the reality on the ground.

Enticott and colleagues have looked into biosecurity and biocontainment. Not surprisingly, they encountered different 'versions' of disease according to the interviewee being questioned.[95] This is partly due to enactments in the sense of Mol - the disease appearing or retreating according to the circumstances of measurement and perception.[96] It was also a matter of the context in which individuals found themselves, so farmers who have experienced bTB breakdowns or who live in high risk areas have a different viewpoint from those without that everyday exposure. Beyond this, Enticott's work on biosecurity is helpful because he is able to explore the idea of preventative measures in the public health literature, with rich insights in terms of 'living with disease'. The differentiation of what works in particular localities or with the enterprise mix of individual farmers means that biosecurity cannot be a matter of centralized instruction but must rather be organized pragmatically according to situated context.[97] Such conclusions will seem vague to those imbued with a neoliberal sensibility of regulation but their ideas about bTB regulation do not work according to the abundant evidence available. As Enticott pithily remarks, 'living with disease may be essential to one day live without it'.[98]

Defra has financed research into ways of preventing badgers from gaining entry to farm buildings: for example, by installing electric

---

[95] Enticott et al. 2012a.

[96] Mol 2002.

[97] Enticott 2008a.

[98] Ibid. 336.

fencing or by badger-proofing the gates of cattle sheds.[99] This research shows that it is indeed possible, often at relatively modest cost, to make farms more biosecure. However, the research also suggests that because every farm is unique, exclusion measures need to be tailor-made for the individual circumstances. This makes it difficult for Defra to issue generic advice or prescriptions to farmers about biosecurity measures. In addition, the same research has shown that individual farms differ enormously in the extent to which they are visited by badgers but we have failed to discover why this is so. Consequently, there is no way of determining which farms are most at risk and which, therefore, stand to gain most from enhanced biosecurity.

Conclusion

There are three points that can be raised from the material in this chapter. The first is that a web of conclusions about badger-cattle interspecies relations has been drawn from largely circumstantial evidence of heterogeneous association. Nose-to-nose encounters may take place but we have only the merest traces of them. Much of the research using tracking devices has been about recreating that landscape of imagined risk – making it present. At an even more basic level we might say the same about badger behaviour and infection, which has often been inferred rather than directly observed. This is indeed knowledge acquired from an oblique angle.

Second, matching our ecological and behavioural knowledge of badgers has proved difficult to correlate with disease in cattle. The RBCT evidence was valuable but in a negative sense with regard to badger culling and many politicians, farmers and veterinarians found this difficult to accept. The tension remains, partly at least because the various groups approach bTB as in effect different diseases according to their particular understandings.

One element missing from the debate is dissonance of scale. While maps of the spread of bTB in the last two decades have concerned policy-makers at the regional scale, most of the ecological literature is pitched, rather, at the local scale. The value of an intermediate vision of scale is encapsulated by one group of researchers who see bTB

---

[99] Tolhurst et al. 2008.

as 'a series of [separate] mini epidemics', based upon the molecular geographies of *M. bovis* genetics.[100] More Defra-sponsored work is now proceeding on the home ranges of these bTB genotypes and it seems that each local variety has found expression in the bodies of both cattle and badgers.[101] As a result, the inter-species pooling of infection is now more certain than ever, although Goodchild and colleagues found that over short distances genotype dissimilarity is greater in cattle than in badgers and they conclude, as a result, that this is 'evidence that cattle were exposed to other sources of infection', presumably other cattle.[102]

Third, from this chapter one might think that such an overwhelming portion of the British public is against widespread badger culling that the only way for it to happen is through the lobbying of the NFU, aided and abetted by the Conservative party. Such an impression would be grossly reductive, however. Instead of focusing just on the high profile of farmers' representatives, it is important to take a step back and be aware of the lay knowledge, culture and practical experience of ordinary farmers. Their views have been marginalised or ignored in the debate about bTB policy and yet they have to bear much of the burden of implementation and cost. The present writer would argue that no bTB policy can be successful without farmer input and buy-in.

Brian Wynne's work on the lay ecologies of the countryside, and particularly his research on sheep farming in Cumbria in relation to nuclear fallout, stands as a warning to scientists and policy-makers not to patronise or suppress local knowledges.[103] Qualitative work with farmers suggests a wide range of views, not just related to their self interest but informed by their experience of bTB breakdowns and their nuanced understandings of what practical measures work best in particular agro-ecologies.[104]

But what epistemological perspective is appropriate in gathering the views that will make a difference in reducing bTB? Naylor uses visual vignettes, Vanclay and Enticott try script theory, and Maye employs telephone interviews that are based on a biographical narrative approach.[105] None of these is as effective as 'insider' technique used by

---

[100] Allen et al. 2011, 11.

[101] Olea-Popelka et al. 2005; Woodroffe, Donnelly, Cox et al. 2009.

[102] Goodchild et al. 2012, 8.

[103] Wynne 1996.

[104] Warren et al. 2013.

[105] Vanclay and Enticott 2011; Enticott and Vanclay 2011; Naylor et al. 2014; Maye

Robinson, a vet turned researcher, who interviewed farmers from his standpoint of experience and applied scientific knowledge.[106] Using local dialect he was able to create a bond of trust and elicit insights into the farmers' plight as they saw it. These were small and medium-sized farmers in Northern Ireland whose very livelihoods are at risk from the everyday depredations of an unpredictable disease. They feel that the authorities are imposing unreasonable and costly biosecurity measures on them and many feel that badgers are the most likely source of the problem. It is arguable that the epidemiological balance of risks has not been fully explained to them and under such circumstances it seems not unreasonable that they should blame the badger, which by law has been taken out of their control.

The work of Fisher on trust and distrust shows that farmers absorb biosecurity messages from certain contacts but on the whole are sceptical of the motives of government.[107] Although this is standard fare for rural sociologists, the point here is that bTB is such a complex and fugitive disease that for once the authorities would do well to take seriously the social and cultural lenses through which farmers understand it. If farmers are discontents with regard to crude top-down regulation, whether it be tuberculin testing, cattle movement, farm biosecurity, or wildlife culling, then the policies will not work effectively. They have to believe that the measures are in the general interest and not just picking them out in order for politicians to appear to be active.

Enticott's research clearly shows that trust is complex and multidimensional and that relational distance between regulating agencies and their client farmers is crucial to the likely acceptance and implementation of bTB policies.[108] Overly scientistic messages about disease that ignore scale and social context cannot command farmers' full confidence. Farmers tend to have somewhat general views and beliefs about bTB that match their understandings of nature, for instance thinking that the spread of the disease may be the result of there presently being 'too many badgers'. Enticott also found a degree of fatalism about the disease in those he and his team interviewed.[109]

---

et al. 2014.

[106] Robinson 2014.

[107] Fisher 2013.

[108] Enticott et al. 2014.

[109] Enticott 2008b.

CHAPTER 14

1971 ONWARDS: M. BOVIS *FIGHTS BACK*

Introduction

One of the most shocking aspects of the history of bTB in the UK cattle herd is that it seemed to be on the brink of eradication in 1960 but has since come back to haunt the very authorities that withdrew testing resources in the 1960s and 1970s. Other than close neighbour the RoI, no other high income country has a problem of this particular zoonotic disease even approaching that of the UK. Together the UK and the RoI have eighty-nine per cent of the infected herds in Europe that have been tested.[1] Although this does not represent much of a risk to milk or beef consumers, it is surely a national humiliation that successive UK governments have been unable to find a workable framework of control.

This chapter then is about the recrudescence of bTB. It begins with a descriptive statistical introduction, bringing the story up to the time of writing with data from the latest Defra publications. It then reverts to a discussion of the official methods of disease testing, the initial history of which was set out in Chapter 4. There are several problems with the available tests and we will look briefly at how they might be improved. These difficulties in veterinary products and implementation are not sufficient alone, however, to explain the present spread of *M. bovis*. In Chapter 13 we looked at the suggestion that there is a wildlife reservoir that requires elimination and here we will investigate recent measures to reduce the risk of cattle-to-cattle infection. In addition, two other dimensions are under discussion for possible future roll-out. One is improved biosecurity on affected farms and the other is the possibility of vaccinating cattle against catching the disease. Both are expensive options and it remains to be seen if either government or the farming community have the stomach for them.

---

[1] EFSA 2014.

The recrudescence

As we saw in Chapter 11, Britain as a whole was declared attested on 1 October 1960. Technically this meant that in all of the Eradication Areas a substantial majority of herds had been attested but it did not necessarily mean that all herds had been individually attested or that the disease had been defeated. Indeed the annual number of reactors slaughtered did not fall below 5,000 nationwide until 1965 (Figure 14.1). The areas that persisted with a higher than average numbers of reactors were concentrated in the South West of England and a few other regions for reasons that were not immediately apparent at the time.

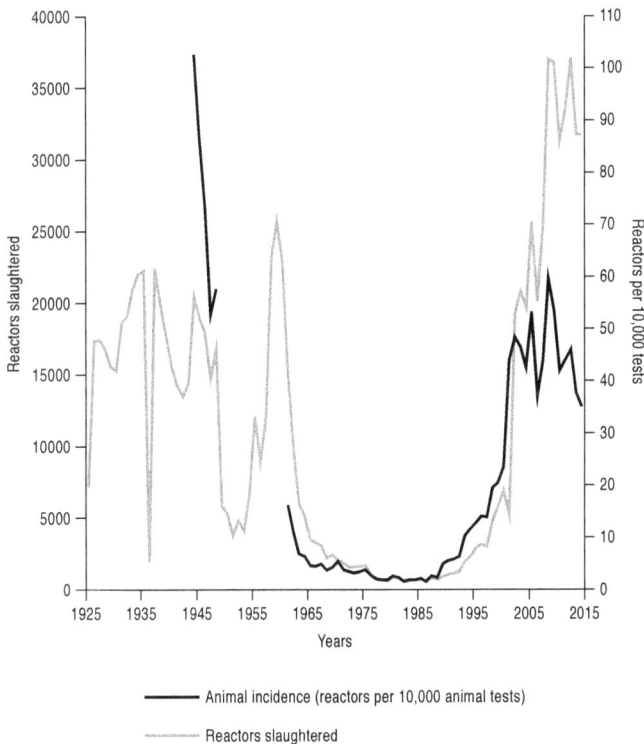

Fig 14.1 Tuberculous cattle slaughtered annually, Great Britain, 1925-2014
(Source: MAFF; Defra)

From October 1964 the Milk (Special Designation) Regulations (1963) withdrew the category known as TT Milk because all milk by then came from Attested herds and so by definition all of the cows in them were tuberculin tested. Tuberculin testing continued beyond the Attested Herds Scheme but by the late 1960s in the eyes of all stakeholders it had become a low-profile, routine procedure. In order to save veterinary inspection resources for other bovine diseases, for instance brucellosis, the MAFF decided to reduce the frequency of testing. In the South West of England where bTB remained, the testing remained annual or biennial, but elsewhere it slipped in most parishes to once in every four years. There were 9.2 million tests in 1961, 7.5 million in 1965, and 5.8 million in 1969, but then a steep fall to 3.9 million in 1970 and 3.0 million in 1975. In the late 1970s and 1980s the numbers continued to fall, the low point being 1.8 million in 1989.[2] But since the number of bTB reactors and their contacts had begun to increase again in numbers since 1982, alarm bells rang in Whitehall and annual testing gradually returned to those parishes with herd incidents.

As can be seen in Figure 14.1, the bTB recrudescence was well under way by the turn of the millennium but the events of 2001 were catastrophic for containment efforts. In that year FMD affected many farms in the UK and, because whole herds were cleared out by the government's ruthless slaughter policy, extensive restocking was needed. Unfortunately some of the purchased incomer cows seem to have been responsible for the spread of disease, to completely new areas in a few cases or to individual farms without a previous history of infection. Since then the number of reactors has accelerated remarkably, although in some parishes this may be an artefact of greater intensification of testing, which uncovered an already existing problem.[3] In 2002, immediately after the FMD crisis, the number of tests was 4.0 million for Britain as a whole, and this has increased gradually, year on year, to a peak of 9.0 million cattle tested in 2014. It is interesting to note, however, that this still does not match the level of 1961 (9.2 million).

The number of animals slaughtered (reactors and dangerous contacts) in the UK was lowest in 1982 at 614, rising to 8,123 in 2000. Then after the FMD epidemic of 2001 these numbers ran out of control. There were 29,231 in 2005, 39,007 in 2008, and 31,732 in 2014. There are two striking aspects of this second wave of disease. First, in spatial distribution it bears no resemblance at all to the map of bTB in the decades before 1960. Second, it does nevertheless have

---

[2] The reason was financial. At the present day the average cost of a routine herd test is £350 to farmers and £770 to taxpayers. Defra 2014b.

[3] Green and Cornell 2005.

a legible geographical structure, hinting at some of the epidemiological explanatory variables that have already been explored in Chapter 12.

Testing types and protocols

Two versions of the intradermal test are used globally at the present day, both measuring 'a delayed-type hypersensitivity' response to the animal's immunologically generated antibodies.[4] The first, the Single Intradermal Test (SIT), measures swelling at the caudal fold. In the second, in the Single Intradermal Comparative Cervical Test (SICCT) two injections of 0.1 ml of antigen are made with two tuberculins, bovine and avian, in order to compare the immune responses. The SICCT was officially adopted in the UK in 1947, the RoI in 1954, and Northern Ireland in 1958, and it has proven to be both economical and practical for routine testing.[5] Although it is less specific, the advantage of the SICCT over the SIT in British conditions is that it avoids a large number of false positives caused by environmental mycobacteria. Between eight and twelve per cent of apparently non-tuberculous cattle in the UK react positively to the SIT but not to the SICCT because of sensitization to these other mycobacteria, such as *M. paratuberculosis* subsp. *avium* and *M. hiberniae*.[6]

After seventy-two hours the two injection sites in the SICCT are checked and the swellings measured with callipers.[7] The animal passes if there is no swelling at the bovine site or if there is a swelling at both sites of the same size. In the latter case the animal is assumed to have been exposed to *M. avium* and is cross-reacting with *M. bovis*. Under the 'standard interpretation', if the swelling at the site of the bovine antigen exceeds the avian one by more than four millimetres the animal is said to have failed. A smaller comparative swelling indicates an 'inconclusive' and the animal has to be retested within sixty days at the higher threshold of the 'severe interpretation'.[8] A failure is now said to

---

[4] Monaghan et al. 1994.

[5] Anon. 1947a; Anon. 1947b; MH Circular 28 October 1947; MAFF 1965; Pritchard 1988; Monaghan et al. 1994, 111; De la Rua-Domenech et al. 2006; Westergaard 2007.

[6] Good and Duignan 2011.

[7] West 1988; Good and Duignan 2011.

[8] Green and Cornell 2005; Westergaard 2007.

occur when the comparative swelling is more than two millimetres. The severe interpretation is also used when a breakdown is confirmed by abattoir or laboratory evidence, the test now being extended to the rest of the herd and contacts.

One problem with the SICCT is that it is not always enacted as recommended. Enticott has shown that the methods employed by private veterinarians are not as standardised as one might expect given that the testing protocol is in theory well established and clear. He argues that in practice the implementation is rather informal and situated.[9] The ontological slipperiness of the object of measurement is a factor, partly the result of the inevitable variations of conditions in the field, but partly also, Enticott's ethnographic work in Wales has shown, due to the attitudes and practices of the vets. There is in effect what he calls a 'culture of testing'. This is borne out by a consultancy report for the Welsh Government:

> Deviations from the procedures are common – in some aspects almost universal ... Non-compliance with the TB test procedures may result in some inconclusive reactors being missed, but ... it was most unlikely that it would result in missing a reactor.[10]

Tuberculin testing is physically demanding, sometimes dangerous, and frequently stressful. It is a story of actions in the real world of measurement and heterogeneous relations and the impossibility of reproducing in field the scientifically controlled conditions of a laboratory. As far as we can tell, there is no reason to think that the test would have been conducted any more scrupulously fifty years ago. Indeed, anecdotal evidence suggests the reverse.

Since October 2013 government-employed, Official Veterinarians in England have been subjected to an enhanced quality assurance programme with regard to their bTB testing procedures and skills.[11] The same issue has been identified in the RoI, where researchers have looked at the relative effectiveness of testers by comparing their testing results with abattoir lesion findings.[12] As a result it has been possible to

---

[9] Enticott 2011, 2012a, 2012b, 2014.

[10] DNV 2006, 17.

[11] *Official Veterinarian* 9, 2014, 9.

[12] Clegg et al. 2015.

produce a league table of Irish vets from the most to the least effective testers.

The treatment of inconclusives in Britain changed in January 2010. Before that they were slaughtered if not resolved after two retests. Now one negative retest means a condemnation but the AHVLA (Animal Health and Veterinary Laboratories Agency) data suggest that this happens in only a minority of cases, partly because many of the animals are sold out for slaughter anyway. Inconclusives are nevertheless problematic and controversial.

In addition to skin or blood testing, all slaughtered cattle are checked for lesions of bTB. This is particularly important for reactors, to see if they were genuinely diseased. But other animals, apparently healthy before slaughter, are occasionally also found to have had the disease. Slaughterhouse checks find more than half of the bTB incidents that occur in the low risk areas and so are vital in detecting the disease there.[13] But not all reactors show visible signs of disease at slaughter. The most likely reason for this is the difficulty of precision post-mortem screening in the busy conditions of commercial slaughterhouses.[14] In other words, the tuberculous lesions may be there but the time and resources are rarely available to find them.[15]

Tuberculin sensitivity, specificity and anergy

The immunological response to bTB in humans, cattle and wildlife is complex and can be thought of as a spectrum from subjects at one end showing good cell-mediated immunity and little or no antibody formation and, at the other end, poor cellular responses and abundant antibody production.[16] There is therefore a proportion of infected cattle that remains anergic to the skin test and beyond the reach of eradication procedures unless they can be identified by a blood test or some other means.

Immediately after being infected with *M. bovis*, cattle are mildly infectious themselves for a limited period, although the numbers of

---

[13] The figure nationwide is ten per cent. Krebs and ISG 1997; Green and Cornell 2005; Mitchell et al. 2006; Frankena et al. 2007.

[14] De la Rua-Domenech et al. 2006.

[15] Shittu et al. 2013.

[16] Lenzini et al. 1977; Neill et al. 1994; O'Reilly and Daborn 1997.

mycobacteria shed are small.[17] Then gradually their bodies mount an immune response which peaks at eight to sixty-five days following the infection.[18] In most cattle a reaction to tuberculin is possible within twenty to thirty days of infection, but in some it is delayed to fifty days.[19] This occult period may actually last for months or even years and it seems somehow to depend on the size of the initial infective dose of bacteria.[20] Such animals may later on re-emerge as communicators themselves of the disease.[21] It used to be thought that cattle did not harbour residual infection in the way that *M. tuberculosis* can lie dormant in the human body and then reactivate, but recent questioning of that knowledge may represent an important threshold in the understanding of bTB.[22] Anergic animals may be far commoner than thought hitherto and their switching on and off of reactions to the skin test may help to explain why statistical epidemiological modelling has at times struggled to identify clear patterns.

The final stages of generalized bTB may also not be picked up by the skin test, although by then there may be clinical symptoms of the disease. In addition, the tuberculin test may produce false positive reactions when an animal is infected with Johne's disease or with avian tuberculosis.[23] Poor responders to tuberculin also include animals with a confined infection of the udder, periparturient cows, and those infected with the common helminth parasite, *Fasciola hepatica*.[24] The final confounder is that some animals become densensitized to the SICTT if it is repeated within six to eight weeks, especially around the site of the injection.[25] This can lead to false negatives and inconclusive results.[26]

We can see from this list of exceptions that there is good reason

---

[17] McCorry et al. 2005.

[18] Phillips et al. 2003.

[19] Neill et al. 1994; Good and Duignan 2011.

[20] Skuce et al. 2011; Green et al. 2012.

[21] Pollock and Neill 2002; Cassidy 2006. It seems that some cattle can overcome the infective challenge of *M. bovis*, maybe when the dose of mycobacteria is small. Menzies and Neill 2000.

[22] Kelly and More 2011.

[23] Ritchie 1945; Francis 1958; Monaghan 1994.

[24] Ritchie 1959; Good and Duignan 2011; Claridge et al. 2012.

[25] An interval of at least 42 days between consecutive tests is normally recommended but 6-20 months of desensitization seems possible in regularly tested cattle. Barlow et al. 1997.

[26] Coad et al. 2010.

why the skin test cannot deliver perfect accuracy. The SICCT has a high specificity of 99.9 to 99.99 per cent; in other words it falsely condemns to be slaughtered only one in one thousand to ten thousand animals tested.[27] But the same cannot be said for its sensitivity, which is poor, in a range sixty to ninety-five per cent with a likely average of about eighty per cent.[28] So, about one in five test results incorrectly indicates that an animal is free of tuberculosis.[29] This beast then remains undetected and potentially infectious for others in the herd or, worse still, it may be moved and infect a entirely new herd or locality. According to Costello and colleagues the worse news is that sensitivity is still only 90.9 per cent for animals later found to have visible lesions.[30]

The cost of a breakdown

At the present day a herd breakdown in England involves a median of three reactors but nearly a third of breakdowns have six or more animals.[31] Bennett and Cook found in a 2003 survey of 450 cattle farms that, although the majority made a loss on each breakdown: the compensation did meet most of their costs.[32] A later Defra-sponsored research project found that the average cost of a herd breakdown is £34,000, shared between the state and the farmer in the approximate ratio of two-thirds to one-third.[33] But Bennett's recent survey of 151 breakdown farms found costs ranging from £229 to £104,000 per farm.[34] The average for dairy farms was £18,500 and for beef enterprises £11,500. The farmer is faced with reduced income from milk and meat production, increased costs of feed, and the inability to sell cattle. Animal welfare might also be at risk in cramped conditions as the herd grows in numbers through the birth of calves. And then there is the cost of replacements for the reactor cattle.[35] In addition, the cost of insuring against such losses is prohibitive in high risk areas, if it is available at all.[36]

---

[27] Goodchild and Clifton-Hadley 2001.
[28] Clegg et al. 2011b; Szmaragd et al. 2012.
[29] Ritchie et al. 2011.
[30] Costello et al. 1997.
[31] AHVLA 2014a.
[32] Bennett and Cook 2006.
[33] Defra 2014b.
[34] Bennett 2014.
[35] Butler et al. 2010; Szmaragd et al. 2013.
[36] House of Commons, Select Committee on Agriculture, *Fifth Report*, Session 1998-99,

Such financial costs do not tell the full story of bTB. In 2009 the Farm Crisis Network interviewed sixty-eight farmers who had had a herd breakdown. Their report is a sobering account of the stress, anxiety, physical and mental illness and relationship problems that seem to go with this kind of unpredictable and difficult-to-control livestock disease.[37] Farmers commonly seem to have a sense of hopelessness and frustration with regard to bTB, as expressed by Mark from Cornwall: 'one of the worst things with TB is that you have no control over it... . Living with TB on your farm is really depressing. Losing cows you have cared for and bred for fantastic pedigrees is soul destroying.'[38] He takes his 'biosecurity seriously but it just doesn't seem to be enough. I see badgers here in the yard at night and there's nothing I can do. I am forced to watch my cattle get killed while I know the cause is walking around.'

The UK's changing test regime since 2005

The various changes that have taken place in bTB policy since 2005 amount, in the view of some commentators, to three fundamental ideological shifts. First, starting in 2005 with the removal of the State Veterinary Service from direct Defra control, there has been a retreat by government from the front-line veterinary public health. Responsibility has been 'agencified' so that ministers are no longer involved in routine decision-making. One example of the implications is the removal of expertise on livestock disease from the centre, with the result that such advice can be ignored by politicians more easily.[39] The second ideological shift is the adoption of the neo-liberal agenda of 'cost and responsibility sharing'. In short this means that farmers are increasingly expected to bear the burden of bTB control.[40] They are not necessarily opposed to this but demand in return a greater say in strategic policy-making and in practical details such as a legal context in which they can reduce risk from the wildlife reservoir of disease. Any politician with an eye on the popular vote is likely to be wary of granting such a carte blanche. Third, neoliberal management of animal disease amounts to the harmonization

Qq 438, 482.

[37] Farm Crisis Network 2009.

[38] http://www.tbfreeengland.co.uk/home/ [accessed 2 February 2015].

[39] Enticott et al. 2011; Enticott, Lowe and Wilkinson 2011; Maye et al. 2014.

[40] Enticott 2014; Maye et al. 2014.

and globalization of biosecurity practices. This last dimension has a long history stretching back to restrictions on international trade during epidemics in the nineteenth century.

Decisions about whether to tighten the policy of test and slaughter in cattle are a matter of balancing the costs against the risks. In 2005 it was decided that the costs of compensation for slaughter were no longer sustainable and therefore policy changes were required. Routine tuberculin testing is expensive and requires complex logistical planning. As a result, in Britain in the first decade of the present century, despite its heavy burden of bTB, roughly seventy to eighty per cent of cattle were not skin or blood tested during their lifetimes.[41] One possibility was that more cattle testing, although expensive in the short term, might contribute to a lowering of the burden of disease.

In the UK there are two types of testing: routine surveillance tests on all animals over six weeks and those associated with disease control.[42] The latter are used with suspect herds and their contiguous neighbours and also on the herds from which infected cattle were purchased. Routine tests are annual in areas of high and medium risk but every four years where the risk is low. There are some exceptions. In herds which are geared to fattening rather than breeding, cattle are exempt from testing altogether if they are destined to go straight to slaughter. And in herds belonging to producer-retailers of unpasteurised milk, or bull hire and heifer rearing herds the testing is annual even in the low risk regions.

When an animal in a herd naive of bTB reacts to tuberculin it is isolated and its milk cannot be used for human consumption. The rest of the herd is then tested and all reactors slaughtered. Their carcases are checked at the slaughterhouse and tissue samples from any visible lesions are cultured in the laboratory for possible *M. bovis*. If any is positive for the mycobacterium, the herd breakdown is said to be 'confirmed' and the herd, now OTF-W, is restricted until there have been two clear tests at sixty-day intervals. The first of these tests uses the severe interpretation of the skin swelling. If it is 'unconfirmed' a clear test at forty-two days will remove restrictions.[43] Only when OTF status is restored can milk be sold raw.

---

[41] Mitchell et al. 2008; Amos et al. 2013.

[42] Mitchell et al. 2006.

[43] Szmaragd et al. 2013.

In 2005 the authorities' patience ran out with farmers who failed to arrange their tests according to the required schedule. Since then such a herd's OTF status has been suspended and the Single Farm Payment reduced. In 2012 there was a further toughening when compensation levels for reactors were also hit.

In 2006 compulsory pre-movement tuberculin testing was introduced for cattle due to move out of herds in the high risk areas and gamma interferon was added as a supplementary test, for instance in culture and/or lesion positive breakdowns in non-endemic areas. This has proved to be an important way of detecting disease, with 7.6 per cent of all breakdowns in Britain being found this way in 2013.[44]

The gamma interferon blood test has been allowed since 2002 by Council Directive 64/432/EEC for parallel use with tuberculin but not for primary testing. The experience gained encouraged its further roll out in parishes with a biennial testing regime and since 2014 it has been used in areas of intermediate risk for all OTF-W breakdowns. Gamma interferon has been shown in the RoI to detect a higher proportion (eighty-seven per cent) of reactors that have visible lesions than the SICCT (seventy-five per cent), and together they can detect ninety-six per cent.[45] This very encouraging result of co-testing begs the question why is gamma interferon not used more widely. The answer is that it is not cost-effective for large-scale routine testing.[46] A skin test costs £3 but the blood test is £30 plus transport to the laboratory.[47]

In January 2010 there began a switch in the spatial resolution of British testing policies from the traditional parish to the county. Although this means a simplified map and a cruder scale of policy geographies, one incentive was that the EU awards OTF status to regions and provinces, not to smaller units. Italy has already presented itself in this way and the success of Scotland in gaining that status in October 2009 was a significant fillip.

Also in 2010 an official HRA was identified in the South West and West Midlands of England in which annual testing was now to be the

---

[44] At the time of writing [July 2015] all movements of cattle from annually tested herds must be backed by a clear test within sixty days beforehand.

[45] Gormley et al. 2014.

[46] Pfeiffer 2013; Schiller et al. 2011.

[47] House of Commons, EFRA Select Committee 2013, vol. 1.

norm throughout the whole zone, and this was buffered by a biennial testing region. The boundaries of these two areas were later modified and in 2013 there was a further major departure: England was in effect been split into three zones, each of which was to have its own bTB strategy. The HRA was expanded, as was the buffer zone, which now became known as the Edge Area.[48] And the third region beyond the Edge was to be called the Low Risk Area (LRA)(Figure 14.2). Both the HRA and the Edge now have annual testing and the LRA remains on a four year plan, which is the minimum specified by the EU for countries that do not have OTF status. The former two-year and three-year testing regimes have disappeared. For the first time since the 1970s the majority of herds in England are now being tested annually.[49]

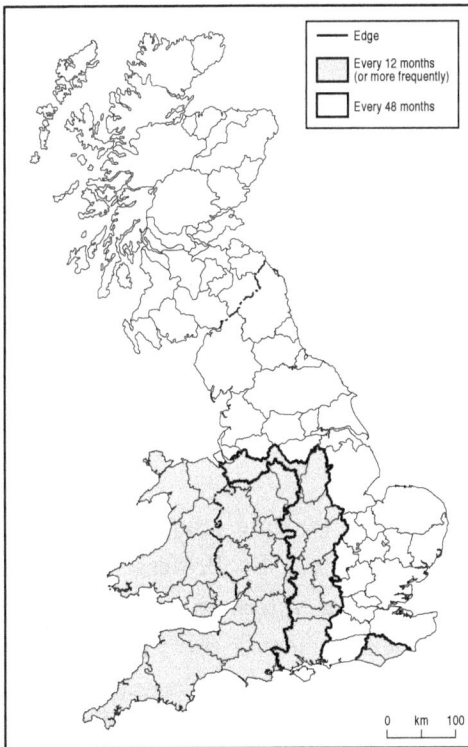

Fig 14.2
Skin testing intervals in 2014
(Source: Defra)

Meanwhile, the devolved administrations have developed their own policies. All of Wales is on annual testing, as if it were in the HRA. Scotland, now having OTF status has moved to risk-based testing, with

---

[48] AHVLA 2014a.
[49] Ibid.

low-risk enterprises exempt from routine testing. Northern Ireland has had annual testing since 1983.

When a herd breakdown happens in the LRA in England, surveillance commences for neighbouring herds within a three kilometre radius. This means an immediate test followed by further tests at six and twelve months, and pre-movement tests for any animals sold on. These herds have also become part of the pre-movement testing scheme where animals are tested within sixty days prior to movement.[50] In addition, there is a ban on new cattle being brought in to join a breakdown herd until all of the cattle have been tested, and a thirty day window for the disposal of reactors. In most cases the APHA remove these reactors to a slaughterhouse and arrange for full compensation at the current market price, which is geared to the animal's pedigree status, whether it is dairy or beef, and other factors. The salvage value of the carcase is retained by the authorities.

Each change of UK government seems to require a new BTB committee. The UK Zoonoses, Animal Diseases and Infections (UKZADI) Group was formed in 2008 by the amalgamation of the UK Zoonoses Group (UKZG) and the Surveillance Group on Diseases and Infections in Animals (SGDIA). It is chaired in rotation by the UK CMOs and CVOs in the Devolved Administrations. BTB is only one of many diseases discussed. In addition there is a Cross-Government Working Group on *M. bovis* that has representatives from Defra, the APHA, Public Health England, the Department of Health and the Food Standards Agency.

Also in 2008 the Labour government set up a limited life Bovine Tuberculosis Science Advisory Body, chaired by Professor Quintin McKellar, Principal and Dean of the Royal Veterinary College. Some points in its 2009 report were used when the new Conservative/Liberal Democrat Coalition government's TB Eradication Programme was published in 2011. The resulting Animal Health and Welfare Board for England (AHWBE) first met in November 2011, with a mission 'to bring external experience and perspective into the heart of the decision-making process'. The claim was that the Board represented a break with the traditional Whitehall model, bringing independent persons[51] with

---

[50] Animal Health and Veterinary Laboratories Agency (2012) *Official Veterinarian* 7.

[51] They were said to have 'the confidence and support of major stakeholder interests.'

relevant knowledge and skills together with senior government officials under an independent chairman, becoming 'the principal source of Departmental advice to Defra Ministers on all strategic animal health and welfare policy matters relating to kept animals.'[52] Representation is half from the farming industry and half civil servants from Defra.[53]

The Tuberculosis Eradication Advisory Group (TBEAG) is a sub-group of the AHWBE. It was set up in July 2013, the inspiration coming from New Zealand where the industry pays more of the costs of disease control. One driver for restructuring is that as things stand forty per cent of breakdown costs are incurred dealing with just ten per cent of breakdown herds. The TBEAG advises on matters such as husbandry best practice, policies such as pre-movement testing, biosecurity, risk zoning and frequency of testing, risk-based trading. Its membership in October 2014 was three farmers and a NFU representative, two vets, a NGO farm manager, an academic and four civil servants.

The Conservative/Liberal Democrat Coalition government that was in power 2010-15 was responsible for a number of technical changes in the regulation of bTB, along with strategic changes in policy. In the long term these will be seen as a paradigm shift in the framing of the problem of bTB. Beginning with the England Advisory Group that reported in 2010 on 'Responsibility and Cost Sharing for Animal Health and Welfare' there was a significant shift in governance structures for livestock diseases such as bTB. The Radcliffe Report, as it is generally known, suggested that a new Partnership Board should be established. By granting greater powers to the industry, ministers would also be requiring them to shoulder more of the costs and agree to a new system of compensation. The NFU immediately made its view known when it called these proposals 'a sham'.[54] They wanted it to be fully independent and so 'depoliticize' the bTB debate.

In November 2013 a voluntary risk-based trading scheme led by the NFU was launched, with farmers encouraged to provide three pieces of information before selling an animal: the date of its last pre-movement test; the date of the last whole herd test; and whether the herd has ever

Defra 2014c, 67.
[52] Ibid.
[53] European Commission 2012.
[54] *Farmers' Guardian* December 2010/January 2011.

had bTB and, if it has, when it last came off restrictions.[55] The idea behind risk-based trading is to enable farmers to think about the relative disease risk of the animals they purchase, and so make better informed decisions.[56] In theory they will be able to take responsibility for managing their herd risk in a way that hitherto has not been practicable. In 2013 the Reilly Committee recommended a comprehensive, accessible database to be used by farmers, vets and auctioneers to 'facilitate access to a range of TB risk factors such as movement history, testing history, background endemicity and also include an overall risk rating at the herd level'.[57] There are, however, significant challenges in the establishment of the nationwide computer system with all of the necessary information on farms and animals. If farmers do not engage, it seems likely that the policy will be tightened to a statutory one, with reduced slaughter compensation if necessary for those unwilling to cooperate.

The situation in the UK in 2015

Membership of the European Union has added a layer of administrative scrutiny of bTB in all of the constituent states. On the whole this seems to have been beneficial because of the high standards of public health protection aspired to in Brussels. In 2000 the EU set up a Task Force for monitoring animal diseases eradication and a sub-group on bovine tuberculosis followed in 2008, with a view to making a cost-benefit assessment of EU policy.[58] That same year a Reference Laboratory for TB was designated at the University of Madrid.

A new EU veterinary vocabulary has also been added, with some previously unfamiliar terms now common in the literature. A small number of these are relevant to our discussion. Examples include labels used for herd breakdowns, such as 'OTF-S' - Officially Tuberculosis Free Status Suspended, and 'OTF-W' - Officially Tuberculosis Free Status Withdrawn. OTF-W is used for a herd when a reactor or an inconclusive is linked to a slaughterhouse identification of visible lesions

---

[55] *AHVLA Briefing Note* 05/13.

[56] Hitherto cattle passports have not been available until after a sale.

[57] Bovine TB Risk-Based Trading Group 2013, 4.

[58] European Commission 2013.

or a positive culture of *M. bovis.* An OTF-S herd has had a reactor or two inconclusives but no confirmation from the slaughterhouse.

In 2014 the UK government launched a new bTB strategy, with a twenty-five year prospect.[59] The policy aims for OTF status for the north and east of England by 2025 and for the whole country by 2038.[60] In order to achieve this efficiently, an increasingly risk-based approach will be adopted. The control principles articulated are again a significant departure from the somewhat lax attitude of the past. In terms of risk, for instance, there will be a continuation of the spatial differentiation introduced in 2010, where England and Wales was divided into three zones with their own strategies calibrated to regional risk profiles. By 2011 the AHVLA had prepared the ground for a risk rating for every herd in the country individually. This will be used to incentivise farmers to reduce their risk.[61] The 100 per cent compensation policy introduced in 1998 will be changed, with variations according to their engagement with farm biosecurity and their willingness to be involved in a risk-based trading system.

With regard to research, the strategy seeks a start to cattle vaccination/DIVA (Differentiating Infected from Vaccinated Animals) test field trials in 2015. In 2017 (at the earliest) subject to successful field trials, negotiations with the EU and regulatory work will begin on permitting the use of a cattle vaccine and a validated DIVA test. In 2019 it is hoped to follow this up with deployment of the vaccine for cattle not intended to enter intra-EU trade and of an oral badger vaccine. Full deployment of the cattle vaccine is unlikely before 2023.

A recent revision of measurement methodology has provided new insights into the incidence and prevalence of bTB in British herds. Herd prevalence is now said to be the percentage of herds that were not OTF due to a bTB incident, and herd incidence is the number of breakdowns per 100 herd years at risk, with a supplementary measure of breakdowns in OTF-W herds. Herd incidence was 0.7 breakdowns in 1996, rising to 4.4 in 2005, then falling back before rising again to 6.1 in 2015. As pointed out by the APHA, the most recent rise is probably the result

---

[59] Defra 2014b.

[60] Ibid.

[61] Defra (2011) *Bovine Tuberculosis Eradication Programme for England, July 2011* (PB 13601).

of increased testing and time will tell whether taking out more reactors will eventually cause this headline figure to decline.[62] The HRA has the most breakdowns, with an incidence of 17.1 per 100 herd years at risk in 2014. This rises to 23.2 in Gloucestershire, 22.5 in Wiltshire, 21.0 in Devon and 19.3 in Avon.[63] Though having lower incidence overall, the Edge Area is a current cause for concern because the detection of disease is accelerating. By comparison, national herd prevalence has diminished, from a peak in 2008 of 5.6 herds under restriction to 4.3 in 2015.

Vaccination: the future?

At first sight, the vaccination of cattle seems preferable to the vaccination of badgers for a number of reasons. It is far easier to vaccinate the larger animals and to conduct research on them. In addition, more of the kind of background knowledge needed to develop a vaccine, such as the host's immune system, is available for cattle than for badgers. But since no vaccine is ever completely effective, vaccinated herds would still have to be monitored. As things stand the present-day tuberculin test would classify a vaccinated cow as a reactor. So mixing the two is impossible unless a new DIVA test can be developed. EU Council Directives 64/432 and 78/52 currently forbid the vaccination of cattle, the main reason being that the Organisation Mondiale de la Santé Animale advises[64] against it where trade is protected by tuberculin testing.[65] Negotiation with the EU would therefore be necessary before a vaccination policy could be widely implemented and there would be at least a ten year period of testing before vaccinated animals would be allowed into international trade.[66]

Field trials of cattle vaccines will begin in 2015 or 2016. Currently the most promising candidate is BCG, the vaccine that has been used for

---

[62] APHA 2015a

[63] APHA 2015b

[64] OIE 2009.

[65] The UK's trade in livestock and their products is too valuable to sacrifice. With other European countries in 2011 exports amounted to £496,000 for live cattle, £490m for meat and £1.2bn for dairy produce. EFRA Select Committee 2013 Report, vol. 1, 8.

[66] Defra 2014b.

decades in humans.[67] This has been thoroughly studied at a molecular level and acknowledged as safe, not just in humans but also in other species. But BCG gives complete protection to only fifty per cent of cattle and partial protection to a further thirty per cent. It would have to be injected annually and might be a way forward where transmission is mainly cattle-to-cattle but it is less likely to be effective where badgers are an agent of infection.[68] To get around this, research under way on a possible 'prime-boost' strategy in which BCG would be combined with some other vaccine, possibly providing complete protection to about seventy per cent of cattle and partial protection to a further twenty per cent.[69] This is the level of improvement required to make vaccination economically worthwhile.

For badgers the most promising candidate vaccine is again BCG, and again its effectiveness is limited to a sixty to seventy-five per cent reduction in disease. It has already been shown to be safe in badgers and to limit disease progression in artificially infected animals under laboratory conditions. Following the licensing of a vaccine in 2010, a 'Badger Vaccine Deployment Project' was set up to begin field testing, targeted towards cattle farms and their immediate surroundings. Initially it was intended to cover six trial areas, but this was reduced to one to save money. The protocol was capture and inject because an oral vaccine was not at that point available even for field trials. In the long-run it will be too slow and expensive to trap and inject all badgers.[70] Rather, an oral form of the vaccine, to be delivered in bait, will be required. This has to be palatable to badgers but not other species, and ideally it would not all be consumed by the greediest individuals. The vaccine also has to be able to survive in the acid conditions of the badger's stomach.

Conclusion

The present book's theme of uncertainty has come to the fore again in this chapter. We saw in Chapter 13 that 1971 was the year when a major new explanation of the epidemiology of bTB in cattle was initiated

---

[67] Chambers et al. 2014.

[68] House of Commons, EFRA Select Committee 2013 Report, vol. 1, 11.

[69] Vordermeier et al. 2014.

[70] Defra estimates £2000-4000 per km². EFRA Select Committee 2008, vol. 1.

– the wildlife reservoir. Here we have seen that this was followed by an extraordinary recrudescence of the disease in England and Wales that was unforeseen and was at least partly due to the withdrawal of the testing vigilance that had been so strict in the 1950s and 1960s. The uncertainty runs far deeper than this, however. On reflection it is a fundamentally ontological indeterminacy that stems from the character-istics of *M. bovis*. This is a bacterium that has proven to be beyond our ability to find a way of knowing it under field conditions. It eludes the standard tests and some conjecture that it can remain dormant in the bovine body for periods that were not previously suspected. Although there is scientific progress with tests and vaccines, the pay-off still seems to be at least ten years away. Even then most commentators think that bTB will take further decades to bring under control in the UK.

Policy changes since 2005 have been positive, although their impacts on the national statistics so far have been minimal. The introduction of pre-movement testing and the tightening of other technical aspects of the testing regime were arguably long overdue. A significant improvement was the move from a parish-based geographical strategy to one that is tuned to regional risks. At last this represents a recognition that the spatial complexity of the disease needs to be considered if testing resources are to be used efficiently. Perhaps the main change in this period, though, is government's insistence that greater responsibility be taken by farmers. This existential shift is double-edged because, on the one hand it means the farmers themselves taking the initiative on matters such as risk-based trading, but on the other hand they have also been allowed to take charge of badger culling. This is an ideological change that bears obvious political risks.

The UK government has strategic plans to win OTF status for the whole country by 2038. While this may seem far off to some, in the present author's opinion it is sensibly in line with the very considerable challenge facing both the public veterinary authorities and the private interests of the livestock sector. The large-scale vaccination of cattle is unlikely before the mid to late 2020s and accomplishing the necessary widespread reduction in disease in ten years after that is a very tight timetable. Much more likely is that a number of regions will achieve OTF status, with the most 'difficult' areas joining by 2050, the bicentenary of the date chosen for the start of this book. Even then one suspects that bTB will persist for decades in small pockets because of *M. bovis*'s powers of survival and regeneration.

CHAPTER 15.

IS UNCERTAINTY THE FUTURE?

It's hard to make predictions, especially about the future. Danish proverb.

Introduction

A considered answer to the question in the title of this concluding chapter will require the discussion of six themes. First, we will ask what lessons the historical geography of bTB has for us. The answer to this is far from straightforward because of various elements of uncertainty. Second, we will reflect on the relationship between policy and problems of an indeterminate nature that cross and then redefine the border between environment and society. This leads us then into the issues of the relationship between policy and expertise, so-called 'wicked' problems, and lay knowledge. The concluding remarks touch on the need to come to terms with the uncertainty and indeterminacy of a disease that will be with us for decades to come.

Spatial uncertainty and the ghosts of the past

Although never stated in deterministic terms, one can readily gain the impression from the now extensive UK-based epidemiological literature on TB in cattle that the South West and West Midlands of England, along with South Wales, are the areas *most* likely regions to have reactors. The reason usually given is that the likelihood of infection is greatest where there is an abundant badger population. A probability style of risk calculation seems to point in this direction and, stretching the same logic back in time, there are reasons to believe that this link would have been the same in the past. First, the distribution of badgers would have been broadly similar because the ecological niches available in the South West were the most favourable. Second, as we saw in Chapter 13, bTB is thought to be self-sustaining and long-lasting in the large badger communities that develop where optimum feeding opportunities are found. From these two premises a kind of presentism has developed which assumes that the disease distributions seen today can be projected into the past and into the future. It is therefore not surprising that policy makers are drawn to interventions that have static spatial structures embedded within their foundational thinking. In the 2013-14 badger culls, for instance, there was (initially) the idea that if the interventions worked well in Gloucestershire and Somerset, the methodology could then be rolled out to other areas in the expectation that it would have universal application. It is understandable that politicians and their advisers seek to construct simplicity from complex situations but here the associated claim to be making informed policy decisions is misleading.

The lesson of the present book is that there is no justification for thinking that bTB is so straightforwardly spatially predictable or that policies which work in one region will be necessarily be appropriate elsewhere. This is not what politicians want to hear, of course, because the heightened uncertainty quotient we are indicating makes one-size-fits-all policies irrelevant. The present review suggests that success requires more complex and spatially nuanced interventions than have hitherto been on the agenda.

As we saw in Figures 4.1 and 9.2, the map of infection before 1960 was very different from that of today. Cattle bTB was concentrated, not in the South West of England but in the North West, with the dairy county of Cheshire at the very peak. In 1938 there were on average 130 reactors per thousand head tested in Britain as a whole, with over 300 per thousand in eight counties and a peak of 416 per thousand in Cheshire. One knowledgeable commentator observed that the true figure for Cheshire was actually probably 600-800 tuberculous dairy cows per thousand and for Derbyshire over 500.[1] The data behind Figures 4.1 and 9.2 are different from each other but the spatial patterns are strikingly similar and there is further corroborative evidence of these ghostly traces in the map (Figure 3.1) of human bTB. The argument for adding this third strand of evidence is that, apart from a few large cities, infected milk was consumed locally within regions.

The spatial disjuncture between bTB at present and before 1960

---

[1] Francis 1947.

poses an important question. How is it that there is little evidence of continuity in wildlife disease in those regions where cattle in the past were so heavily infected? One would have expected a proportion of badgers in, say, Cheshire still to have been tuberculous in the 1970s and 1980s, within ten to twenty years of the eradication of bTB in cattle in that county (1960). Why then is it that only one of 389 badgers collected from RTAs in Cheshire 1972-90 proved to be tuberculous (Figure 13.1)? At the moment there is no clear answer as to why the present-day map of bTB should be so different from that before 1960 but here are two speculative scenarios.

Scenario #1. With regard to Cheshire, the wildlife reservoir may never have been a major factor in infection in that county because it may well have been cattle-to-cattle infection that was largely behind the high levels of disease there before 1960.[2] Following on from this, it could be that bTB in badgers is a spillover rather than an endemic disease in most regions and does not persist over lengthy periods.[3] Maybe the reproduction of bTB requires an average badger group size that is larger than that present in Cheshire and can only be achieved in a relatively few favourable ecological niches.[4] And despite the statement above about heightened risk of bTB in the South West of England, we must remember that at high densities badgers are territorial and therefore unlikely to pass infection from group to group.[5] In the view of some commentators the likelihood of bTB passing between badgers and cattle is greatest in this region when the perturbation of the former causes wider ranging than would otherwise occur, or where infected cattle are moved, thus posing a disease challenge to naive badger groups.

Scenario #2. Another possible explanation of macro-spatial differences between the 1930s and the present may relate to farm practices. Herd sizes and cattle density have increased, for instance, both acknowledged risk factors for bTB,[6] although not necessarily connected to the wildlife reservoir. It is true that during the twentieth century there was a gradual intensification of cattle husbandry in the west

---

[2] Atkins and Robinson 2013a.
[3] Corner et al. 2011; Nugent 2011.
[4] Allen et al. 2011.
[5] Böhm et al. 2009.
[6] Brooks-Pollock and Keeling 2009.

of England as against the arable eastern counties, but the South West did not benefit disproportionately vis-à-vis the North West.[7] Second, from almost nothing before 1960, maize has become an important forage and grain crop, with farmers in the South West of England the most enthusiastic innovators. Since maize is both nutritious and palatable for badgers, this may be an important new factor, especially on farms where biosecurity is weak and badgers can gain access to storage clamps.[8] Third, cattle marketing has changed, facilitated in recent years by electronic communications. Since 2001, movements have been recorded in the British Cattle Movement Service's Cattle Tracing System database and this shows that the greatest concentration of on-movements is currently in the South West and Midlands of England, and in South West Wales.[9] According to Robinson and colleagues, Britain's cattle network is becoming more cohesive with the result that risk of disease spread is enhanced, and it is generally agreed that cattle-to-cattle transmission is important in the spread of bTB.[10]

Conclusions from this discussion are that notions of continuity of spatial pattern are misplaced and that there is likely to be a great deal more regional and sub-regional complexity in the present-day epidemiology of bTB than is normally contemplated. The policy lesson that follows is to take spatial differentiation seriously. The present use of three risk zones in England and Wales is a move in this direction though somewhat crude in its boundary drawing. Our inclination, admittedly impressionistic from the historical analysis, is that a finer spatial grain of risk-based policy is desirable in the Edge Area and the HRA, though not a return to the former parish scale, which had no functional meaning.

Policy disasters or a 'reluctant state'?

Environmental and technological risks with potentially global unintended negative consequences are sometimes thought of as recent phenomena.[11] But complexity and wide spatial reach are certainly not

---

[7] RADAR 2008.
[8] Roper 2010.
[9] Mitchell et al. 2005.
[10] Robinson et al. 2007; Gilbert et al. 2005; Green et al. 2008.
[11] Giddens 1991; Beck 1992.

new in cattle diseases. Consider the rinderpest epidemics (cattle plague) of 1709-20, 1742-60, 1768-86 and 1865-66 that spread around Europe to devastating effect and FMD in 1841-52, 1861-66, 1967 and 2001. In addition there were enzootics such as contagious bovine pleuro-pneumonia, brucellosis, Johne's disease, and bTB. These widespread diseases were disruptive and costly and frequently crossed borders in shipments of live animals and dead meat. For 200 years now the dairy and grazing industries have had to be alert to the threat of occasional epidemics coupled with the constant risk of the common cattle diseases. Forming effective policy to counter these threats has been a long-running challenge to find scientific consensus on aetioliogy and epidemiology, to arrange for the logistics of response, and also to decide who should bear the risk.

According to the late Thomas Dormandy, the slow pace of dealing with bTB was 'Britain at its dilatory worst'.[12] But how can we explain such a sluggish development of policy? We have made two proposals so far. In Chapters 9 and 10 we used convention theory to suggest that the contrasting worlds of performance of the MAF and the MH amounted to different framings of the problem and so led to friction between (and to some extent within) ministries. In Chapter 11 we added the further thought that is was the alignment of interests and actions between the MAF and the NFU that was ultimately the key to the successful roll out of the area eradication policy in the 1950s. Without farmer cooperation this would have been impossible, irrespective of the political colour of the party in charge or the persuasiveness of civil servants. The NFU were willing and enthusiastic participants in a post-war deal offered to them in the shape of subsidies and price support and agreeing to clean up bTB was a sacrifice they recognised they had to make.

There is far more to bTB in the UK than an interests-based explanation, however. Historians of public policy seem to have concluded that it was more to do with a failure of governance. With regard to the grotesque cost in the last three decades of dealing with outbreaks of BSE, FMD and bTB, the conclusion has been that government response was poor, particularly that of the responsible ministry, the MAFF. In the constructivist tradition of unintended consequences, Abigail Woods in

---

[12] Dormandy 1999, 330.

her history of FMD, for instance, calls it a 'manufactured plague'.[13] And on BSE Van Zwanenberg and Millstone on the first page of their book claim that government policy was 'profoundly flawed', having 'neither scientific nor democratic legitimacy'. To them BSE was 'a paradigm of policy failure'.[14] While both sets of authors develop nuanced arguments, they are nevertheless clearly in the 'policy disaster' school of thought.

Patrick Dunleavy is even more gloomy when he claims that 'Britain now stands out amongst comparable European countries, and perhaps amongst liberal democracies as a whole, as a state unusually prone to make large-scale, avoidable policy mistakes'.[15] He proposes a number of reasons for Britain's exceptionalism: (a) the risk inherent in large-scale centrally-driven policy decisions, partly due to the lack of a regional tier of government; (b) swings of policy due to the election cycle that goes with a first-past-the-post electoral system; (c) politicians gain preferment by radical initiatives; (d) Whitehall is run by highly talented generalists who are good at making a case but whose policy decisions are often superficial in terms of evidence and expertise; and (e) there are ineffective checks and balances.

Of Dunleavy's list only points (d) and (e) are really relevant to bTB in the long run, and anyway I am candidly wary of catastrophist reasoning that seeks the headline rather than interrogating the admittedly drier empirical detail. It is surprising to me how many academic commentators have felt comfortable with making highly critical retrospective judgements, particularly of BSE, so close in time to the events.

There have been attempts to enrol bTB into this hall of infamy of 'policy disasters'. The disease certainly raises serious issues of biosecurity, disease surveillance and regulatory competence but in the present author's opinion bTB cannot be said to be an 'intractable' problem as claimed by Wyn Grant.[16] It is under control in Scotland which had a major, widespread infection up to the 1950s. It has also been reduced to a minimum in other European countries, such as Denmark and Germany, where the scale of the livestock disease in the late nineteenth and early

---

[13] Woods 2004b.

[14] Van Zwanenberg and Millstone 2003.

[15] Dunleavy 1995, 52.

[16] Grant 2009.

twentieth centuries was as great if not greater than in the UK. Decisive action coupled with political will brought bTB to the point of extinction in most of England and Wales too in the 1960s but at that point the cost of continued vigilance was considered too great and every aspect of policy was relaxed. This error was then compounded by the one-off shock of FMD in 2001 when the restocking of farms was responsible for spreading disease. Since then increased testing has discovered that the problem was greater and more geographically spread than previously realised.

An error of the policy disaster school is that it fails to consider the particular and unique characteristics of *M. bovis* that make it so difficult to eradicate. Other livestock diseases have been susceptible to government intervention but it is the materiality of this mycobacterium that has proved to be the most difficult of all to deal with in the long-term.

A rule of experts?

In Chapter 2 we discussed the clash of veterinary and medical knowledges about bTB and we argued that the former struggled for legitimacy into the twentieth century. In the key arena of policy-making in the MAF, veterinarians seem to have been subordinate and this is one plausible explanation for why the disease does not seem to have been a priority in that ministry right through until the end of the 1930s. It was not until 1937/8 that a National Veterinary Service was established, for instance, but by then veterinarians had suffered a set-back when it became obvious that their claim that they could diagnose dangerously tuberculous cows from their udders was spurious. Subsequently they were reduced to administering the TT. Dr Duncan Rabagliati, CVO of West Yorkshire, complained that 'many of the anomalies of our legislation especially with regard to milk and even meat, are due to the fact that the [veterinary] profession was not sufficiently consulted in drawing it up'.[17]

Despite this marginalization of veterinary expertise, the MAF frequently claimed to be basing their livestock disease policies on the best available science. We saw in Chapter 10, for instance, how they invested

---

[17] Rabagliati 1930, 233-34.

money, time and a great deal of hope in the 1930s in the tuberculin research of Basil Buxton at Cambridge. Such claims to be science-based and evidence-based have since become a stock in trade for ministers in their pronouncements about bTB, FMD, BSE and other diseases. But, as Millstone and Van Zwanenberg sensibly comment, 'there can never be a purely scientific justification for *any* policy and ... assertions to the contrary seriously misrepresent real decision-making processes'.[18] We made a similar point at the end of Chapter 10 but there it was not so much a recognition of uncertainty as a constitutive feature of science-based knowledge. There is a difference.

One approach frequently adopted in the British context has been the appointment of committees of experts to make 'non-political' inputs into policy making. One strand of such individuals is drawn from what Jasanoff calls the 'elite tier of civic virtue', people who through a long and distinguished contribution to public life can be said to stand 'above self-interest and even party politics'.[19] A second group is made up of serving or retired academics or other technical experts with the specialist skills relevant to the issue in hand, the assumption being that they will make expert judgements that are neutral and apolitical. A third cohort comes from the various groups with a vested interest in the policy area, usually chosen with at least a nod to balance, although that is very difficult to achieve. Fourth, there is a shadowy group of civil servants from the stakeholder ministries who in effect are delegates protecting their departmental interests. Chapters 9 and 10 made it clear that finding a formula for selecting and running expert advisory committees has proven to be difficult in our policy area.

The problem with many government expert committees over the last 100 years has been that they have often seemed to be slanted towards one vested interest or another. Sometimes this has represented 'political cover' for a minister but on other occasions the results of specialized enquiries have been a political embarrassment, to be ignored or carefully cherry picked for whatever is politically expedient.[20] The current TB Advisory Group (2006-) is mainly veterinarians and the Bovine TB Eradication Group (2008-) is largely farmers and vets. They

---

[18] Millstone and Van Zwanenberg 2001, 100.
[19] Jasanoff 1997.
[20] Grant 2009, 570.

have not stirred up much controversy but academic expert committees such as Zuckerman, Dunnet, Krebs and the ISG have occasionally proved troublesome for government. This is because academics tend to be independently minded and to resent any attempt to massage their findings, but it is also because their lengthy attention to detail is not appreciated in a world that expects (often unrealistically) rapid and definitive results.

Anthony Giddens has commented that one of the features of the present phase of modernity is our increasing inability to know fully the scale and complexity of the risks that face us and therefore there is greater scope for scientific controversies and associated social problems.[21] Certainly we can say that the increased use of technoscience in the dairy industry in the later nineteenth and twentieth centuries added complexity, not just the more scientific approach of dairy factories using more standardised cultures and the advanced technology of the cooler and separator, but also the scientific testing of milk for disease (adulteration and preservatives, colouring) and the scientific notion of cleansing the cowshed which swept through dairy farming in the 1920s. Nevertheless, while it may be true that the science of bTB in recent decades has uncovered new problems, we have never been 'certain' about bTB and so indeterminacy is not just a feature of late modernity.

David Miller argues cogently that the relationship between science and policy, in the BSE drama at least, was one of the policy-makers shaping the science rather than the other way around. This is not just influencing how the science is presented and picking and choosing the 'right' science for the policy, but sometimes even wilfully misrepresenting scientific findings in order the build a particular case. Consider also that civil servants and their political masters control the funding agenda (Table 12.1) and are therefore able to keep warm the kind of science they respect and trust and leave the rest in the cold outside the policy sauna. Miller sees this not as dishonesty but as a discursive construct.[22]

Millstone and Van Zwanenberg reject any distinction between risk assessments by scientists and risk management by politicians because 'it is not possible to construct a risk assessment from available scientific data without embedding it with some prior, socially derived framing

---

[21] Giddens 1991; Miller 1999; Nelkin 1992.
[22] Miller 1999.

assumptions ... all science-based risk assessments are inevitably framed by some set of prior socially-based considerations'. This is also the line taken by Timothy Mitchell in his influential *Rule of Experts*.[23]

If expertise has been unable to make a breakthrough in either knowing or taming bTB maybe we are dealing with a problem that not only brings with it socially and politically embedded issues that are difficult to control for, but also one that is so complex and vast in scale that maybe we should include it in the rare category of 'wicked'.

Bovine TB: a wicked problem?

Pellizzoni has suggested that 'indeterminacy no longer is a problem, but rather becomes a resource.'[24] To illustrate the point he cites the example of ecosystems, which in the original formulation of Eugene Odum were in a state of balance but which are now thought of as dynamic. The same is true of the non-equilibrium economics of the neoliberal world order. In other words, indeterminacy and uncertainty are increasingly accepted, with new fields opening out such as complexity theory to cope with the analytical consequences.

According to Fish, any uncertainty that can be expressed in probabilistic terms is 'risk'. For instance the outcome of drinking raw milk was unknown but the majority of medical practitioners agreed that there was a risk of contracting TB because of its proven bacillary load.[25] This is different from 'strong uncertainty', where a number of outcomes are possible but no statistical calculation can be made. The raw milk problem became uncertain in this sense in the first third of the twentieth century because the MAF preferred not to know the full extent of the problem because of the cost of any nationwide intervention that might follow in the cattle herd. The uncertainty here could have been reduced by collecting accurate data, and so it was essentially epistemic. But there is also 'indeterminacy', where there is an inability to know and where 'outcomes defy prediction because causal chains and networks are open'. This is 'ontological or irreducible uncertainty' perhaps because of the

---

[23] Mitchell 2002.
[24] Pellizzoni 2014, 81.
[25] Fish et al. 2011.

degree of complexity. It may be temporary until research is undertaken, although again that research may uncover even greater complexity.

Governance issues that have multiple framings by different stakeholders and high levels of strong uncertainty are sometimes called 'wicked problems'. Often they are highly complex, such as modern debates about climate change, and with low levels of consensus about which interventions, if any, are appropriate. Even the definition of the problem is difficult in the first place because it may intersect with others. In the absence of resolving the interests represented by cross-cutting frames it becomes difficult for those affected to adjust their behaviour to changing circumstances.[26] Ultimately these problems remain wicked until the policy stagnations are somehow unblocked through the development of new capabilities by some or all of the actors. However, even then the solution of one set of problems may lead to new ones.

Table 15.1 Sources of past indeterminacy and uncertainty in bovine TB in the UK

Representational   • Narratives, constructions, frames and discourses used in particular by MAF and NFU were that bTB was an insoluble problem that could not be solved by large-scale intervention.
Conventional   • Framing and performances of ministries divergent.
Epistemic   • The authority of expertise: clash of medical and veterinary expertise.   • Mode of testing: greater variation than protocol.   • Uncertain locus of responsibility: farmers (e.g. biosecurity of farms, risk-based trading, culling companies) or public purse (compensation for slaughter)?
Ontological   • Koch's views on *M. bovis* contested.   • Pasteurization very controversial.   • Pathogenesis of TB in bovine body unclear, e.g. latency.   • Epidemiology: cattle-to-cattle or wildlife-to-cattle the main source of infection?   • Sensitivity and specificity of skin and blood testing inadequate.   • Protective science: vaccination for cattle not yet available.

Readers of this history of the contested, indecisive and ultimately unsuccessful efforts to rid the British Isles of bTB may judge the disease to be a good example of a wicked problem. It displays some of the characteristics (Table 15.1), including the difficulty of recognising when the problem has been solved. It was declared to have been eradicated in 1960 but within 15-20 years was making a come-back because of the removal of testing resources. This suggests that bTB will in future

---

[26] Termeer et al. 2013.

require continuous management and may never be fully conquered, no matter which solutions are proposed and adopted.

As Whyte and Thompson comment, 'wicked problems are characterized by deep ambiguity in the ontological assumptions and metaphysical categories used in their articulation'.[27] As a result of this, they observe that every wicked problem is unique and it is not possible to turn to precedents for solutions. Again this fits the situation of bTB which over a period of more than 150 years has proven to be the most intractable of all livestock diseases in the UK.

One of the most interesting reviews of wicked problems is by Ney and Verweij, where they pose a number of 'clumsy solutions'. They argue that pluralism is essential because in complex situations no one way of organizing and thinking can succeed. The current dialogue of the deaf between the badger cullers and the anti-cullers suggests that some new form of deliberative institution is probably the only way forward. My feeling is that the recognition of lay expertise will be decisive, to which we can add that it is essential that the particular materiality of *M. bovis* must somehow also be represented.

Situated knowledges and lay expertise

One suggestion that has been made recently about rural policy-making generally is that satisfactory outcomes depend upon expanding inputs to include lay knowledges. This was the spirit of Brian Wynne's work with the farmers of Cumbria whose understanding of their environment proved to be more robust concerning fall-out from the Chernobyl nuclear melt-down than the 'experts' sent in to comment on the cycling of radioactive materials.[28] In our case here we can admire the work of Damian Maye and colleagues on farmers' 'narratives of nature' with regard to bTB, the point being that surely it is right to listen to those in the front line of livestock disease. It is important not to fantasise that somehow veterinary expertise can be forced on them top-down without any discussion, explanation, persuasion and, above all, collaborative goal seeking.[29] As one way into this, Philip Robinson's ethnographic work

---

[27] Whyte and Thompson 2012, 442.
[28] Wynne 1996.
[29] Maye et al. 2014.

is epistemologically exemplary in seeking farmer buy-in specifically to research about bTB that is ultimately in their best interests.[30]

An important point about lay expertise is its close link to place. According to Fish and colleagues, taking it seriously 'may expose higher level weakness in containment practices, such as those embedded in necessarily more synthetic scientific models' and 'it is precisely because local knowledge is so "situated" that it is authoritative at the point of outbreak'.[31] There may be a price to pay here, however, because of potentially 'fundamental mismatches between local and global understandings of an appropriate intervention' and because vested interests are also local and contingent. So, distinguishing self interest from knowledgeable calibration is itself uncertain.

I acknowledge Hinchliffe's point that the inclusivity of deliberative democracy does not necessarily reduce uncertainty.[32] He suggests that it is the lack of a decision that is undemocratic, more than the lack of plurality in decision-making. This is the same as saying that an artificial balancing of interests (including those of microbes) that may lead to the avoidance of hard decisions by government. True, but I am nevertheless convinced that the collaboration of livestock farmers is an essential step towards a solution to the present bTB crisis in the South West of England and South Wales. The question then becomes one of how best to bring this about. There is now a vast literature on what has been called citizen science, distributed deliberation, participatory action, epistemic communities, cooperative research and many other labels that imply a recognition that expertise is not just the preserve of a science establishment but is widely distributed.[33] There is not the space here to review this departure but we can say that engaging with this lay knowledge is now generally agreed to be helpful in policy innovation. A key question is the practical means of elicitation and delivery: there are dozens of methods that have been tried by the public deliberation industry. Another is whether participation should be consultative or co-productive. An exceptionally interesting example of the latter is the apprentice flood modellers who were recruited by Whatmore and Lane

---

[30] Robinson 2014.

[31] Fish et al. 2011, 2032.

[32] Hinchliffe 2001.

[33] Castree 2014; Hinchliffe et al. 2014.

in Pickering, with whose active help a new and effective mode of flood protection was devised.[34]

Inevitably, difficult issues remain. Although well organized by the NFU, livestock farmers are differentiated, for instance by region and risk category. The attitudes of those in a low risk area such as County Durham are different from those in the front line in, say, Gloucestershire. Even in Devon, a county with a great deal of bTB, I know from talking to low intensity farmers there with no cattle disease that their perceptions vary from those of their near neighbours with many reactors. So, who should represent farmers' views?

Another point is that lay expertise may not necessarily be disinterested. This has been shown in the participatory research that has been so popular and to a degree successful in development work in the Global South. The Panglossian bubble surrounding this was burst by Cooke and Kothari in their book, *Participation: the New Tyranny.*[35] They and their contributors found an over-romanticized view of lay knowledge amongst participation activists, and, as Cameron and Gibson, remind us, these so-called 'authentic' local understandings are in fact multiply produced and cannot be guaranteed to be positively transformative.[36]

A vital task for farmer engagement is for policy-makers to understand that livestock practices are time/space contingent. We urgently need to know about the variations that are a product of local agro-ecologies and/ or of specific materialities that, as we have argued in this book, produce the patchwork of possibility spaces in which *M. bovis* thrives. By way of example, Philip Robinson has definitively shown that Northern Ireland is a special case.[37] Eliminating bTB there faces the particular challenge of the 'conacre' grazing regime. Talking to farmers is the only way of producing veterinary understandings of their systems and associated risks, and a dialogue is perhaps the best means of farmers coming to know how bTB sits in their agro-ecosystem. Robinson's work is first-

---

[34] Lane et al. 2011.

[35] Cooke and Kothari 2001.

[36] Cameron and Gibson 2005.

[37] Robinson 2014.

hand confirmation of the recommendation by Leach and Scoones for 'ethnographically-grounded approaches' to zoonotic disease.[38]

Conclusion

The most consistent element to our story has been the microbiological awkwardness of the mycobacterium, *M. bovis*, always just beyond the reach of a full understanding and effective intervention. Seemingly defeated by one intervention after another, its relentless adaptability to new opportunities has always led to recrudescence, like a birthday cake candle that will not blow out. Coupled to this was the political reality that dealing with bTB was so complex, and yet of no obviously immediate and significant economic benefit to anyone amongst the producer and distributive communities, that driving it forward was problematic. It was unlikely to make any politician into a hero and yet it had the potential to wreck careers through the seemingly bottomless pit of resources it could absorb.

Fundamentally it is the long-run, imperfect understanding of the epidemiology and pathogenesis of bTB, coupled with problems of measuring its presence and its impact, that provide the context for the historical slippages that we have discussed in this book. The continuing bTB problem is not due to a 'reluctant state', a failure of governance in a 'policy disaster', a deficit of formal sector expertise, nor is it an example of the 'tragedy of the commons' bringing forward selfish individual motives or special interests. It is none of these. Instead it is an ontological conundrum. Table 15.2 considers the policy options.

I do believe, however, that better cattle control measures coupled with technical improvements in vaccines will significantly reduce the scale of the bTB problem for the UK cattle industry. The danger is that the disease might once again fade from the political priority list. The resilient mycobacterium is always waiting for new opportunities and in 50 years may find a way to spread once more, maybe this time to a new generation of raw milk drinkers.

The post-1971 emphasis upon badgers may well in the long run be seen as a distraction from the principal need, for better cattle control. Yes, badgers harbour bTB and in certain circumstances are responsible

---

[38] Leech and Scoones 2013.

Table 15.2 Research issues and policy options for bTB in UK cattle

Veterinary science:
- Better understanding of latency of disease in bovine bodies required.

Testing:
- Single most cost-effective measure would be improved skin test.
- Combination of skin and blood tests expensive but worth rolling out to high-risk zones.
- Retraining of vets and strong enforcement of testing protocols.

Vaccines:
- Expensive because cattle likely to need annual inoculations.
- Cattle vaccines will need EU approval for international trading, likely to take ten years.
- Injected badger vaccines mixed results. Feed-based not yet available.

Wildlife reservoir:
- Epidemiological role probably exaggerated outside certain limited ecological niches.
- Limited culling probably counter-productive in UK conditions.

Cattle measures the best short-term option:
- Risk-based trading will be important if IT system can be made to work.
- Pre- and post-movement testing is effective.
- Annual testing vital in medium and high-risk areas.

Environment:
- Survival of *M. bovis* in environment underestimated?
- Movement of *M. bovis* in water needs further research.

Biosecurity:
- Need to invest in anti-badger measures questionable in the minds of many farmers.

Abattoir:
- Greater attention to identification of lesions needed.

Farming issues:
- Changes in farming practice so far under-researched: maize, large herds, intensification of grazing.
- Better management of infected slurry and manure.
- Closed housing with poor ventilation likely to be more important than current wisdom allows.

Compensation:
- Need for both carrot and stick.

Risk zoning:
- Identification of county and sub-county risk zones with their own policies.
- Lay knowledge to enable policy alignment with local circumstances.

for up to half of the disease in cattle, in certain areas. But stopping the analysis there is short-sighted. It is far better to see the disease in its ecological system, in which cattle will probably have given the disease to badgers in the first place and the infection has then been exchanged back and forward between species (including humans at one point) for decades, possibly centuries. Culling badgers seems to work best at medium densities, such as in the RoI, where the lesser pressure of numbers means a reduced likelihood of perturbation. It does not seem to work at high densities, as in the problematic areas of the South West of England and South Wales, unless the cull is at a vast scale likely to challenge the skills and resources of anything less than full state mobilization. It seems very unlikely that politicians would ever commit themselves to this since the cost effectiveness would be marginal in terms of reduced disease and the possibility of widespread opposition from the public. I could be proved wrong on this if a charismatic political leader can persuade the public that decimating the badger population of a whole region is worthwhile.

The unseen but resilient *M. bovis* represents a key challenge to the governance of veterinary health. The possibility spaces that remain open to it - such as the poor sensitivity of the TT, our incomplete knowledge of its epidemiology and pathogenesis, and the risks associated with cattle movement and trading - must be narrowed before we can claim that progress towards eradication is at last being made.

REFERENCES

Abernethy, D.A. et al. (2003) Survey of *Mycobacterium bovis* infection in road-traffic-accident badgers in Northern Ireland, in Proceedings of the 9th International Symposium for Veterinary Epidemiology and Economics, Vina de Mer, Chile, 18-21 November 2003

Abernethy, D.A. et al. (2013) Bovine tuberculosis trends in the United Kingdom and Republic of Ireland, 1995 to 2010, *Veterinary Record* 172, 12, 312-26

Addison, C. (1924) *Politics from within, 1911-1918* London: H. Jenkins

Addison, C. (1934) *Four and a half years: a personal diary from June 1914 to January 1919. Volume I: 1914-1916* London: Hutchinson

Adeane, C.R.W. and Gaskell, J.F. (1928) A segregation method for eliminating tuberculosis from cattle, *Journal of Hygiene* 27, 248-56

Aikman, C.M. (1895) Pasteurized milk, *Journal of the British Dairy Farmers' Association* 10, 45-50

Allen, A.R. et al. (2013) The phylogeny and population structure of Mycobacterium bovis in the British Isles, *Infection, Genetics and Evolution* 20, 8-15

Allen, A.R., Skuce, R.A., and McDowell, S.W.J. (2011) *Bovine TB: a review of badger-to-cattle transmission* Belfast: DARDNI

Allen, C.G. (1925) The Public Health (Meat) Regulations, 1924, *Veterinary Journal* 81, 455-58

Allen, J. (2012) A more than relational geography? *Dialogues in Human Geography* 2, 190-93

Amos, W. et al. (2013) Genetic Predisposition to Pass the Standard SICCT Test for Bovine Tuberculosis in British Cattle, *PLoS ONE* 8, 3, e58245

Anderson, B. and McFarlane, C. (2011) Assemblage and geography, *Area* 43, 124-7

Anderson, B. et al. (2012a) On assemblages and geography, *Dialogues in Human Geography* 2, 171-89

Anderson, B. et al. (2012b) Materialism and the politics of assemblage, *Dialogues in Human Geography* 2, 212-15

Anderson, R.M. and Trewhella, W. (1985) Population dynamics of the badger (*Meles meles*) and the epidemiology of bovine tuberculosis (*Mycobacterium bovis*), *Philosophical Transactions of the Royal Society B* 310, 327-81

Animal and Plant Health Agency (2015a) *Bovine tuberculosis: infection status in cattle in GB. Annual surveillance report for the period January to December 2014* Addlestone: APHA

Animal and Plant Health Agency (2015b) *Bovine tuberculosis: infection status in cattle in England. Annual surveillance report for the period January to December 2014* Addlestone: APHA

Animal Health and Veterinary Laboratories Agency (2014a) *Bovine tuberculosis: infection status in cattle in England. Annual surveillance report for the period January to December 2013* Weybridge: AHVLA

Animal Health and Veterinary Laboratories Agency (2014b) *Bovine tuberculosis: infection status in cattle in GB. Annual surveillance report for the period January to December 2013* Weybridge: AHVLA

Anon. (1889a) *Tuberculous meat: proceedings at trial under petitions at the instance of the Glasgow local authority against Hugh Couper and Charles Moore, before Sheriff Berry* Glasgow: Hodge

Anon. (1889b) Sale of diseased meat in Glasgow, *Lancet* i, 1314

Anon. (1889c) Tuberculosis in meat, *Lancet* ii, 965

Anon. (1895a) The cost of suppressing bovine tuberculosis, *Veterinary Record* 8, 213-5

Anon. (1895b) Sixth International Veterinary Congress, *Journal of Comparative Pathology and Therapeutics* 8, 259-65

Anon. (1899) Tuberculosis in meat, *The Times* 16 March, 12d

Anon. (1900) The Copenhagen control-system of milk supply, *British Food Journal* 2, 316

Anon. (1903) The milk supply of large towns: action and inaction of rural and county authorities, *British Medical Journal* i, 678-80, 739-42, 801-02, 876-8, 933-9, 973-7, 1033-6; ii, 1488-92

Anon. (1907) The protection of towns from tuberculosis in milk, *Justice of the Peace* 71, 279

Anon. (1927) Milk traffic by rail: introduction of 3,000-gallon tank wagons, *Modern Transport* 18, 456, 7 and 18

Anon. (1928) The history of the Royal Institute of Public Health: Report of the committee appointed by the Royal Institute of Public Health to consider the best means to ensure a clean milk supply to the consumer, *Journal of State Medicine* 36, 355-60, 421-8, 477-88

Anon. (1931a) Routine veterinary inspection of dairy cows, *Veterinary Record* 11, 1277

Anon. (1931b) Pure milk, *Lancet* i, 387-8

Anon. (1932a) The People's League of Health: the report on a pure milk supply, *Lancet* ii, 151-2

Anon. (1932b) The problem of safe milk, *Lancet* i, 628-9

Anon. (1934) Milk policy: new government scheme, *Lancet* i, 491

Anon. (1937a) The problem of pasteurization: Lords discuss the Poole Bill, *Home Farmer* 4, 3, 16-17

Anon. (1937b) Milk policy, *Economist* 4902, 282-3

Anon. (1939) Nutritive value of raw and pasteurized milk, *British Medical Journal* ii, 9 December, 1144-5

Anon. (1943a) Doctors agree about pasteurization, *British Medical Journal* i, 258-9

Anon. (1943b) A safe milk supply: B.M.A. deputation to the Minister of Food, *British Medical Journal* i, 265

Anon. (1944-45) Discussion on the veterinary and medical control of the milk supply, *Proceedings of the Royal Society of Medicine* 38, 253-60

Anon. (1945a) Milk still unsafe, *British Medical Journal* ii, 160-61

Anon. (1945b) Veterinary and medical control of milk supply, *British Medical Journal* i, 340-41

Anon. (1945c) Milk policy, *Lancet* i, 502-03

Anon. (1945-46) Discussion on the methods to be employed in eradicating tuberculosis of bovine origin from the human and animal populations, *Proceedings of the Royal Society of Medicine* 39, 213-22

Anon. (1947a) Tuberculin and the control of bovine tuberculosis, *Lancet* i, 35-6

Anon. (1947b) A comparison between the double intradermal comparative test and the single intradermal comparative test: a record of work carried out by the veterinary staff of the Ministry of Agriculture and Fisheries, *Veterinary Record* 59, 95-7

Ares, E. (2014b) Badger culling: alternatives *House of Commons Library Note* SN/SC/6447

Ares, E. and Hawkins, O. (2014) Badger culling: TB control policy, *House of Commons Library Note* SN/SC/5873

Arloing, S. (1889) Tuberculosis, *Journal of Comparative Pathology and Therapeutics* 2, 199-218

Armstrong, H.E. (1900) The sale of the flesh of tuberculous cattle for human food, *Veterinary Record* 13, 40-42

Armstrong, J. (2011) *Veterinary expertise*, unpublished PhD thesis, University of Newcastle

Ashby, A.W. (1939) Agriculture and the state, pp 51-86 in Anon. (Ed.) *Agriculture in the twentieth century: essays on research, practice and organization to be presented to Sir Daniel Hall* Oxford: Clarendon Press

Ashby, H. and Wright, G.A. (1889) *Diseases of children, medical and surgical* London: Longmans, Green and Co.

Ashford, D.A., Voelker, L. and Steele, J.H. (2006) Bovine tuberculosis: environmental public health preparedness considerations for the future, pp 305-315 in Thoen, C.O., Steele, J.H. and Gilsdorf, J.H. (Eds) *Mycobacterium bovis infection in animals and humans* Ames, Iowa: Blackwell

Atkins, P.J. (1977) The intra-urban milk supply of London, circa 1790-1914, *Transactions of the Institute of British Geographers* new series 2, 383-99

Atkins, P.J. (1991) Sophistication detected: or, the adulteration of the milk supply, 1850-1914, *Social History* 16, 317-39

Atkins, P.J. (1992) White poison: the health consequences of milk consumption, *Social History of Medicine* 5, 207-27

Atkins, P.J. (2000a) The pasteurization of England: the science, culture and health implications of milk processing, 1900-1950, pp 37-51 in Smith, D. and Phillips, J. (Eds) *Food, science, policy and regulation in the 20th century* London: Routledge

Atkins, P.J. (2000b) Milk consumption and tuberculosis in Britain, 1850-1950, pp 83-95 in A. Fenton (Ed.) *Order and disorder: the health implications of eating and drinking in the nineteenth and twentieth centuries* East Linton: Tuckwell Press

Atkins, P.J. (2004) The Glasgow case: meat hygiene and the foundations of state food policy in the 1890s, *Agricultural History Review* 52, 161-82

Atkins, P.J. (2010a) *Liquid materialities: a history of milk, science and the law* Farnham: Ashgate

Atkins, P.J. (2010b) Lobbying and resistance with regard to policy on bovine tuberculosis: an inside/outside model of Britain, 1900-1939, pp 189-212 in Worboys, M. and Condrau, F. (Eds) *Tuberculosis then and now* Montreal: McGill-Queen's University Press

Atkins, P.J. (2013) Vinegar and sugar: the early history of factory-made jams, pickles and sauces pp 41-54 in Britain, Oddy, D.J. (Ed.)

The Food Industries of Europe in the Nineteenth and Twentieth Centuries
Farnham: Ashgate

Atkins, P.J. and Robinson, P.A. (2013a) Bovine tuberculosis and badgers in Britain: relevance of the past, *Epidemiology and Infection* 141, 1437-44

Atkins, P.J. and Robinson, P.A. (2013b) Coalition culls and zoonotic ontologies, *Environment & Planning A* 45, 1372-86

Ayers, S.H. (1914) The present status of the pasteurization of milk, *American Journal of Public Health* 4, 1, 15-19

Ayers, S.H. (1916) The present status of the pasteurization of milk, *U.S. Department of Agriculture Bulletin* No. 342

Baker, S. (1973) *Milk to market: forty years of milk marketing* London: Heinemann

Balfour, E.B. (1948) *The living soil: evidence of the importance to human health of soil vitality, with special reference to post-war planning* London: Faber & Faber

Bang, B. (1908) Measures against animal tuberculosis in Denmark, pp 850-868 in vol. 4 of *Transactions of the Sixth International Congress on Tuberculosis, Washington, September 28 to October 5 1908* Philadelphia: Fell

Barlow, N.D. et al. (1997) A simulation model for the spread of bovine tuberculosis within New Zealand cattle herds, *Preventative Veterinary Medicine* 32, 57-75

Barnes, R.C. (2001) The rise of corporatist regulation in the English and Canadian Dairy Industries, *Social Science History* 25, 381-406

Basset, J. (1952) *Immunologie et prophylaxie de la tuberculose* Paris: Vigot Frères Éditeurs

Bayliss, R. and Daniels, C. (1988) The Physical Deterioration Report of 1904 and education in home economics, *History of Education Society Bulletin* 41, 25-35

Bechtel, W. and Richardson, R.C. (1998) Vitalism, pp 639-643 in

Craig, E. (Ed.) *Routledge Encyclopedia of Philosophy*, vol. 9 London: Routledge

Beck, U. (1992) *Risk society* London: Sage

Behrend, H. (1893) *Cattle tuberculosis and tuberculous meat* London: F. Calder-Turner

Bellamy, C. (1988) *Administering central-local relations, 1871-1919: the Local Government Board in its fiscal and cultural context* Manchester: Manchester University Press

Benham, P.F.J. (1985) The behaviour of badgers and cattle and some factors that affect the chance of contact between the species, *Applied Animal Behaviour Science* 14, 390-391

Benham, P.F.J. and Broom, D.M. (1989) Interactions between cattle and badgers at pasture with reference to bovine tuberculosis transmission, *British Veterinary Journal* 145, 226-41

Benham, P.F.J. and Broom, D.M. (1991) Responses of dairy cows to badger urine and Faeces on pasture with reference to bovine Tuberculosis transmission, *British Veterinary Journal* 147, 517-32

Bennett, J. (2010) *Vibrant matter: a political ecology of things* Durham, NC: Duke University Press

Bennett, R. (2014) Economic studies of bTB in GB, Sixth International *M. Bovis* Conference, 16-19 June 2014, Cardiff

Bennett, R.M. and Cooke, R.J. (2006) Costs to farmers of a tuberculosis breakdown, *Veterinary Record* 158, 429-32

Berdah, D. (2012) Entre scientifisation et travail de frontières: les transformations des savoirs vétérinaires en France, XVIIIᵉ-XIXᵉ siècles, *Revue d'Histoire Moderne et Contemporaine* 59, 4, 51-96

Bermingham, M.L. et al. (2011) Evidence for genetic variance in resistance to tuberculosis in Great Britain and Irish Holstein-Friesian populations, *BMC Proceedings* 5, Supplement 4, S15

Bermingham, M.L. et al. (2009) Genetics of tuberculosis in Irish Holstein-Friesian dairy herds, *Journal of Dairy Science* 92, 3447-56

Berry, J. (1908) Tuberculous disease of bones and joints in childhood, pp 166-73 in Kelynack, T.N. (Ed.) *Tuberculosis in infancy and childhood* New York: Wood

Bevir, M. and Rhodes, R.A.W. (2003) *Interpreting British governance* London: Routledge

Bibby, J. & Sons (1911) *Bibby's book on milk, section 4. Bovine tuberculosis: cause, cure, and eradication* Liverpool: Bibby

Bibby, J.P. (1944) *The case against the pasteurisation of milk: a statistical examination of the claim that pasteurisation saves lives* London: Staples and Staples

Bickerstaff, K. and Simmons, P. (2004) The right tool for the job? Modelling, spatial relationships, and styles of scientific practice in the UK foot and mouth crisis, *Environment and Planning D: Society and Space* 22, 393-412

Bielby, J. et al. (2014) Badger responses to small-scale culling may compromise targeted control of bovine tuberculosis, *Proceedings of the National Academy of Sciences* 111, 9193-8

Bishop, H.D. (1908) Tuberculosis in Guernsey cattle, *Public Health* 22, 24

Bishop, P.J. and Neumann, G. (1970) The history of the Ziehl-Neelsen stain, *Tubercle* 51, 196-206

Blancou, J. (2003) *History of the surveillance and control of transmissible animal diseases* Paris: Office Internationale des Épizooties

Böhm, M., Hutchings, M.R. and White, P.C.L. (2009) Contact networks in a wildlife-livestock host community: identifying high-risk individuals in the transmission of bovine TB among badgers and cattle, *PLoS ONE* 4, 4, e5016

Boltanski, L. and Thévenot, L. (2006) *On justification: economies of worth* Princeton: Princeton University Press

Bourne, F.J. et al. (2007) Response to 'Tuberculosis in cattle and badgers: a report by the Chief Scientific Adviser' http://archive.defra.gov.uk/foodfarm/farmanimal/diseases/atoz/tb/isg/documents/isg-responsetosirdking.pdf

Bovine TB Risk-Based Trading Group (2013) *Bovine TB risk-based trading: empowering farmers to manage TB trading risks* https://www.gov.uk/government/uploads/system/uploads/attachment_data/file/193647/rbtg-final-report.pdf [accessed 2 March 2015]

Bramwell, A. (1989) *Ecology in the 20th century: a history* New Haven: Yale University Press

Bramwell, B. (1893) *Atlas of clinical medicine*, volume 2 Edinburgh: University of Edinburgh Press

Brittlebank, J.W. (1908) The problem of bovine tuberculosis, *Veterinary Record* 20, 873-80

Brittlebank, J.W. (1925) The control of tuberculosis and the milk supply, *Veterinary Journal* 81, 171-8

Brittlebank, J.W. (1929) Tuberculous bovines and tuberculous milk, *Journal of State Medicine* 37, 517-23

Bromund, T. (2001) Whitehall, the National Farmers' Union, and Plan G, 1956-57, *Contemporary British History* 15, 76-97

Brooking, T.W.H. (1977) *Agrarian businessmen organise: a comparative study of the origins and early phase of development of the National Farmers Union of England and Wales and the New Zealand Farmers' Union, ca 1880-1929*, unpublished PhD thesis, University of Otago

Brooks-Pollock, E. and Keeling, M. (2009) Herd size and bovine tuberculosis persistence in cattle farms in Great Britain, *Preventive Veterinary Medicine* 92, 360-365

Brown, L. and Sampson, H.L. (1926) *Intestinal tuberculosis: its importance, diagnosis and treatment* Philadelphia: Lea & Febiger

Brown, W. (1901) Examination of carcasses in cases of cattle tuberculosis, *Lancet* ii, 205-8

Brunton, L.A. et al (2015) A novel approach to mapping and calculating the rate of spread of endemic bovine tuberculosis in England and Wales, *Spatial and Spatio-temporal Epidemiology* 13, 41-50

Brunton, L.A. (2014) What is driving the spread of endemic bovine TB in Great Britain? Sixth International M. Bovis Conference, 16-19 June 2014, Cardiff

Bryder, L. (1988) *Below the magic mountain: a social history of tuberculosis in twentieth century Britain* Oxford: Clarendon Press

Bryder, L. (1996) 'Not always one and the same thing': the registration of tuberculosis deaths in Britain, 1900-1950, *Social History of Medicine* 9, 253-65

Buckley, W. (1922) Limits of pasteurisation: better milk means more business, *Milk Industry* 2, 8, 79-81

Buckley, W. (1924) Milk and tuberculosis, *Journal of State Medicine* 32, 25-33

Bulloch, W. (1911) *The problem of pulmonary tuberculosis considered from the standpoint of infection, being the Horace Dobell lecture delivered before the Royal College of Physicians of London, November 10th, 1910* London: School Press

Butler, A., Lobley, M. and Winter, M. (2010) *Economic Impact Assessment of Bovine Tuberculosis in the South West of England.* Centre for Rural Policy Research, University of Exeter

Butler, S. (1872) *Erewhon* London: Trübner

Buxton, J.B. (1927) Some notes on the double intradermal tuberculin test in cattle and the potency of tuberculin, *Journal of the Royal Sanitary Institute* 47, 511-19

Buxton, J.B. and Glover, R.E. (1939) *Tuberculin tests in cattle: observations on the intradermal tuberculin test in cattle by special reference to the use of synthetic medium tuberculin* London: HMSO

Buxton, J.B. and Griffith, A.S. (1931) The use of BCG in the vaccination of calves against tuberculosis, *Lancet* i, 393-401

Buxton, J.B. and MacNalty, A.S. (1928) The intradermal tuberculin test in cattle: collected results of experience, *Medical Research Council, Special Report Series* 122

Calmette, A. (1936) *L'infection bacillaire et la tuburculose chez l'homme et chez les animaux* Paris: Masson

Cameron, J. and Gibson, K. (2005) Participatory action research in a poststructural vein, *Geoforum* 36, 315-31

Carmichael, R. (1810) *Essay on the nature of scrofula, with evidence of its origin from disorders of the digestive organs* London: Callow

Carpenter, A. (1879) Remarks on the first principles of sanitary work, *British Medical Journal* ii, 643-8

Carr, J.W. (1898) What is tabes mesenterica in infants? *Lancet* ii, 1662-3

Carrington, D. (2014) UK government conducting secret badger sett-gassing trials, *Guardian* 15 May

Carrique-Mas, J.J., Medley, G.F. and Green, L.E. (2005) Risk of bovine tuberculosis breakdowns in post-foot and mouth disease restocked cattle herds in Great Britain, pp 27-41 in Mellor, D.J., Russell, A.M. and Wood, J.L.N. (Eds) *Preventive medicine: proceedings of a meeting held at Nairn, Inverness, Scotland on March 30-April 1, 2005 Society for Veterinary Epidemiology*

Carrique-Mas, J.J., Medley, G.F. and Green, L.E. (2008) Risks for bovine tuberculosis in British cattle farms restocked after the foot and mouth disease epidemic of 2001, *Preventive Veterinary Medicine* 84, 85-93

Carter, S.P. et al. (2007) Culling-induced social perturbation in Eurasian badgers *Meles meles* and the management of TB in cattle: an analysis of a critical problem in applied ecology, *Proceedings of the Royal Society* B 274, 2769-77

Cassidy, A. (2012) Vermin, victims and disease: UK framings of badgers in and beyond the bovine TB controversy, *Sociologia Ruralis* 52, 192-214

Cassidy, J.P. (2006) The pathogenesis and pathology of bovine tuberculosis with insights from studies of tuberculosis in humans and laboratory animal models, *Veterinary Microbiology* 112, 151-61

Cassidy, J.P. et al. (1998) Early lesion formation in cattle experimentally infected with Mycobacterium bovis, *Journal of Comparative Pathology* 119, 27-44

Castree, N. (2014) *Making sense of nature* Abingdon: Routledge

Chambers, M.A. et al. (2014) Vaccination against tuberculosis in badgers and cattle: an overview of the challenges, developments and current research priorities in Great Britain, *Veterinary Record* 175, 90-96

Chapman, H.R. et al. (1957) Further studies of the effect of processing on some vitamins of the B complex in milk, *Journal of Dairy Research* 24, 191-7

Cheeseman, C.L., Jones, G.., Gallagher, J. and Mallinson, P.J. (1981) The population structure, density and prevalence of TB (*M. bovis*) in badgers (*Meles meles*) from four areas in south-west England, *Journal of Applied Ecology* 18, 795-804

Cheeseman, C.L. et al. (1985) Population ecology and prevalence of tuberculosis in Badgers in an area of Staffordshire, *Mammal Review* 15, 3, 125-135

Cheeseman, C.L., Wilesmith, J.W., Stuart, F.A. (1989) Tuberculosis: the disease and its epidemiology in the badger, a review, *Epidemiology and Infection* 103, 113-125

Christiansen, K.H. et al. (1992) *A case-control study of herds which fail the tuberculin test six months after being derestricted for tuberculosis* Dublin: Tuberculosis Investigation Unit, University College Dublin

Christley, R.M. et al. (2011) Responses of farmers to introduction in England and Wales of pre-movement testing for bovine tuberculosis, *Preventive Veterinary Medicine* 100, 126-33

City of Manchester (1933) *Proceedings of the Council, 1897-1898* Manchester: NP

Claeys, W.L. et al. (2013) Raw or heated cow milk consumption: review of risks and benefits, *Food Control* 31, 251-62

Claridge, J. et al. (2012) Fasciola hepatica is associated with the failure to detect bovine tuberculosis in dairy cattle, *Nature Communications* 3, 853

Clarke, B.R. (1952) *Causes and prevention of tuberculosis* Edinburgh: Livingstone

Clegg, T., Duignan, A. and More, S.J. (2015) The relative effectiveness of testers during field surveillance for bovine tuberculosis in unrestricted low-risk herds in Ireland, *Preventive Veterinary Medicine* 119, 85-9

Clegg, T.A. et al. (2011a) Longer-term risk of *Mycobacterium bovis* in Irish cattle following an inconclusive diagnosis to the Single Intradermal Comparative Tuberculin test, *Preventative Veterinary Medicine* 100, 147-54

Clegg, T.A. et al. (2011b) Shorter term risk of Mycobacterium bovine is Irish cattle following an inconclusive diagnosis to the Single Intradermal Comparative Tuberculin test, *Preventative Veterinary Medicine* 102, 255-64

Clegg, T.A. et al. (2008) Potential infection-control benefit for Ireland from premovement testing of cattle for tuberculosis, *Preventive Veterinary Medicine* 84, 94-111

Clements, E.D., Neal, E.G. and Yalden, D.W. (1988) The National badger sett survey, *Mammal Review* 18, 1-9

Clifton-Hadley, R. and Cheeseman, C.L. (1997) Performance of an ELISA in determining the Mycobacterium bovis status of badger (*Meles meles*) setts, *Epidémiologie et Santé Animale* 31-32, 0.1.04.1-3

Coad, M., Clifford, D. et al. (2010) Repeat tuberculin skin testing leads to desensitisation in naturally infected tuberculous cattle which is associated with elevated interleukin-10 and decreased interleukin-1 beta responses, *Veterinary Research* 41, 2, 14

Cobbett, L. (1917) *The causes of tuberculosis* Cambridge: Cambridge University Press

Cohen, R.L. (1936) *The history of milk prices: an analysis of the factors affecting the prices of milk and milk products* Oxford: Oxford University, Institute for Research in Agricultural Economics

Cohn, M.D. (1993) The philanthropic life of the merchant and humanitarian Nathan Straus, MA thesis, Lehigh University

Coker, R. et al. (2011) Towards a conceptual framework to support one-health research for policy on emerging zoonoses, *Lancet Infectious Diseases* 11, 326-31

Collinge, G.H. (1920) Abattoirs and methods of slaughter, pp 185-237 in Collinge, G.H., Dunlop Young, T. and McDougall, A.P., *The retail meat trade: a practical treatise by specialists in the meat trade. Volume 1* London: Gresham

Collins, C.H. and Grange, J.M. (1983) The bovine tubercle bacillus, *Journal of Applied Bacteriology* 55, 13-29

Collins, C.H. and Grange, J.M. (1987) Zoonotic implications of *Mycobacterium bovis* infection, *Irish Veterinary Journal* 41, 363-6

Collins, E.J.T. (2000) The Great Depression, 1875-1896, pp 138-207 in idem. (Ed.) *The agrarian history of England and Wales, VII: 1850-1914* Cambridge: Cambridge University Press

Committee of Investigation for England on Complaints Made by the Control Milk Distributive Committee and the Parliamentary Committee of the Cooperative Congress as to the Operation of the Milk Marketing Scheme, 1933 [1936] *Report* London: HMSO

Conford, P. (2005) Organic society: agriculture and radical politics in the career of Gerard Wallop, ninth Earl of Portsmouth (1898-1984), *Agricultural History Review* 53, 78-96

Conlan, A.J.K. et al. (2012) Estimating hidden burden of bovine tuberculosis in Great Britain, *PLoS Computational Biology* 8, e1002730

Convery, I. et al. (2008) *Animal disease and human trauma: emotional geographies of disaster* London: Palgrave Macmillan

Cooke, B. and Kothari, U. (2001) *Participation: the new tyranny?* London: Zed

Coole, D. and Frost, S. (2010) *New materialisms: ontology, agency, and politics* Durham, NC: Duke University Press

Cooper, A.F. (1989) *British agricultural policy, 1912-36: a study in Conservative politics* Manchester: Manchester University Press

Corner, L.A. (1994) Post mortem diagnosis of *Mycobacterium bovis* infection in cattle, *Veterinary Microbiology* 40, 53-63

Corner, L.A. et al. (1990) Efficiency of inspection procedures for the detection of tuberculous lesions in cattle, *Australian Veterinary Journal* 67, 389-92

Corner, L.A.L., Murphy, D. and Gormley, E. (2011) *Mycobacterium bovis* infection in the Eurasian badger (*Meles meles*): the disease, pathogenesis, epidemiology and control, *Journal of Comparative Pathology* 144, 1-24

Corry Mann, H.C. (1926) Diets for boys during school age, *Medical Research Council Special Report Series* 105 London: HMSO

Cosivi, O. et al. (1998) Zoonotic tuberculosis due to mycobacterium tuberculosis in developing countries, *Emerging Infectious Diseases* 4, 59-70

Costello, E. et al. (1998) A study of cattle-to-cattle transmission of Mycobacterium bovis infection, *Veterinary Journal* 155, 245-50

Costello, E. et al. (1997) Performance of the single intradermal comparative tuberculin test in identifying cattle with tuberculous lesions in Irish herds, *Veterinary Record* 141, 222-24

Courtenay, O. et al. (2006) Is *Mycobacterium bovis* in the environment important for the persistence of bovine tuberculosis? *Biology Letters* 2, 460-62

Courtenay, O. et al. (2007) Performance of an environmental test to detect Mycobacterium bovis infection in badger social groups *Veterinary Record* 161, 817-18

Coutts, J.A. (1908) Abdominal tuberculosis, pp 102-14 in Kelynack, T.N. (Ed.) *Tuberculosis in infancy and childhood* New York: Wood

Cox, G, Lowe, P. and Winter, M. (1986) The state and the farmer:

perspectives on agricultural policy, pp 1-19 in Cox, G., Lowe, P. and Winter, M. (Eds) *Agriculture: people and policies* London: Allen & Unwin

Cox, G., Lowe, P. and Winter, M. (1990) The political management of the dairy sector in England and Wales, in Marsden, T.K., Lowe, P and Whatmore, S. (Eds) *Labour and locality: uneven development and the rural labour process* London: Fulton

Cox, G., Lowe, P. and Winter, M. (1991) Origins and early development of the National Farmers' Union, *Agricultural History Review* 39, 30-47

Creighton, C. (1880) An infective variety of tuberculosis in man, identical with bovine tuberculosis (perlsucht), *Lancet* i, 943-6

Creighton, C. (1881a) Grounds for believing that the tubercular disease of animals which supply milk and meat for human use, is communicated by such food to man, *Transactions of the Seventh Session of the International Medical Congress held in London August 2nd-9th, 1881* 4, 481-6

Creighton, C. (1881b) *Bovine tuberculosis in man: an account of the pathology of suspected cases* London: H.K. Lewis

Cresswell, P., Harris, S. and Jefferies, D. (1990) *The history, distribution, status and habitat requirements of the badger in Britain* Peterborough: Nature Conservancy Council

Cronjé, G. (1984) Tuberculosis and mortality in England and Wales, 1851-1910, pp 79-101 in Woods, R. and Woodward, J. (Eds) *Urban disease and mortality in nineteenth century England* London: Batsford

Cronshaw, H.B. (1947) *Dairy information* London: Dairy Industries Ltd

Crozier, G.K.D. and Schulte-Hostedde, A.I. (2014) The ethical dimensions of wildlife disease management in an evolutionary context, *Evolutionary Applications* 7, 788-98

Cumming, W.M. (1935) The type of the causal organism in 1,502 recent English and 320 recent Irish cases of pulmonary tuberculosis, *Tubercle* 17, 67-78

Cumming, W.M. et al. (1933) Pulmonary tuberculosis with the bovine type of the bacillus in the sputum, *Journal of Pathology and Bacteriology* 36, 153-68

Cutbill, L.H. and Lynn, A. (1944) Pulmonary tuberculosis of bovine origin, *British Medical Journal* i, 283-5

Dale, H.E. (1939) Agriculture and the civil service, pp 1-20 in Anon. (Ed.) *Agriculture in the twentieth century: essays on research, practice and organization to be presented to Sir Daniel Hall* Oxford: Clarendon Press

Dale, H.E. (1956) *Daniel Hall: pioneer in scientific agriculture* London: Murray

Daniels, A.L. and Loughlin, R. (1920) A deficiency in heat-treated milks, *Journal of Biological Chemistry* 44, 381-97

Daniels, A. L. and Stearns, G. (1924) The effect of heat treatment of milk feedings on the mineral metabolism of infants, *Journal of Biological Chemistry* 61, 225-40

Dant, T. (2004) The driver-car, *Theory, Culture & Society* 21, 4/5, 61-79

Davies, B. (1923) The triumph of pasteurization, *Modern Farming* 6, 9, 12

Davies, B. (1934) Practical and scientific problems of the milk supply and their laboratory control, *Journal of the Royal Sanitary Institute* 54, 486-501

Davies, D.S. (1899) Bacteriology in public health work, *Public Health* 11, 602-11

Davies, L.M. (1938) Milk as it affects the producer, *Journal of the Royal Institute of Public Health & Hygiene* 1, 334-40

Davis, J. (1950) *A dictionary of dairying* London: Hill

Dawson of Penn, Viscount (1942) Report of the committee on tuberculosis in wartime, *MRC Special Report Series* 246

Dawson of Penn, Viscount et al. (1930) Pasteurization of milk, *Lancet* ii, 1315

Dean, G.S. et al. (2005) Minimum infective dose of *Mycobacterium bovis* in cattle, *Infection and Immunity* 73, 6467-71

Dean, M. (1999) *Governmentality: power and rule in modern society* London: Sage

De Certeau, M. (1984) *The practice of everyday life* Berkeley, CA: University of California Press

Defra (2005) *Controlling the spread of bovine tuberculosis in cattle in high incidence areas in England: badger culling* [London:] Defra

Defra (2011) *The Government's policy on Bovine TB and badger control in England* [London:] Defra

Defra (2014a) *Defra response. Pilot Badger Culls in Somerset and Gloucestershire: Report by the Independent Expert Panel* London: Defra

Defra (2014b) *The strategy for achieving Officially Bovine Tuberculosis Free status for England* London: Defra

Defra (2014c) *Animal Health and Welfare Board for England, Annual report: 2013/2014* London: Defra

Defra (2014d) *Draft strategy for achieving 'officially bovine tuberculosis-free' status for England: summary of responses* London: Defra

Defra (2014e) *Defra bovine TB citizen dialogue: cross-cutting summary* [London:] Defra

De Jong, D.A. (1889) The use of the flesh of tuberculous animals, *Journal of Comparative Pathology and Therapeutics* 12, 315-25

Delahay, R.J. et al. (2006) Habitat correlates of group size, bodyweight and reproductive performance in a high-density Eurasian badger (*Meles meles*) population, *Journal of Zoology* 270, 437-47

Delahay, R.J., Cheeseman, C.L., Clifton-Hadley, R.S. (2001) Wildlife disease reservoirs: the epidemiology of Mycobacterium bovis infection in the European badger (*Meles meles*) and other British mammals, *Tuberculosis* 81, 43-9

Delahay, R.J. et al. (2000) The spatio-temporal distribution of *Mycobacterium bovis* (bovine tuberculosis) infection in a high-density badger population, *Journal of Animal Ecology* 69, 428-41

Delahay, R.J. et al. (2003) TB and the badger: culling as a method to control a wildlife disease reservoir, pp 165-71 in Tattersall, F.

H. and Manley, W.J. (Eds) Conservation and conflict: mammals and farming in Britain, *Linnean Society Occasional Publication Series* Settle: Smith

DeLanda, M. (2006) *A new philosophy of society: assemblage theory and social complexity* London: Continuum

De la Rua-Domenech, R. et al. (2006) Ante mortem diagnosis of tuberculosis in cattle: a review of the tuberculin tests, γ-interferon assay and other ancillary diagnostic techniques, *Research in Veterinary Science* 81, 190-210

Delépine, S. (1893) On the value of experimental tuberculosis in diagnosis, *British Medical Journal* ii, 665-6

Delépine, S. (1896) Desirability of legislation in connection with tuberculosis of living domesticated animals and, more specially, cattle, *Journal of State Medicine* 4, 81-6

Delépine, S. (1898) The bacteriological diagnosis of certain infectious diseases in connexion with public health work, *Lancet* i, 346-8

Delépine, S. (1899) Prevention of tuberculosis in cattle: some economic aspects of the question London: Adlard

Delépine, S. (1900) A practical note on the application of the tuberculin test in cattle, *British Medical Journal* ii, 1201-02

Delépine, S. (1901) The communicability of human tuberculosis to cattle, *British Medical Journal* ii, 1224-6

Delépine, S. (1902) How can the tuberculin test be utilised for the stamping out of bovine tuberculosis? pp 235-80 in vol. 2 *Transactions of the British Congress on Tuberculosis for the Prevention of Consumption, London, July 22nd to July 26th, 1901* London: Clowes

Delépine, S. (1909) Report to the Local Government Board on investigations in the Public Health Laboratory of the University of Manchester upon the prevalence and sources of tubercle bacilli in cow's milk, Appendix B, no. 5, Medical Officer of Health to the Local Government Board *Annual Report for 1908-9,* BPP 1909 (Cd. 4935) xxviii.777-880

Delépine, S. (1920) Infection and predisposition in tuberculosis: some of the views held during the last hundred years, *Journal of State Medicine* 28, 107-21

Denny, G.O. and Wilesmith, J.W. (1999) Bovine tuberculosis in Northern Ireland: a case-control study of herd risk factors, *Veterinary Record* 144, 305-10

Department of Health for Scotland (1933) Tuberculous infection in milk, *MRC Special Report Series* 189 London: HMSO

De Vine, B. (1924) The reliability of the Tuberculin Test: its advantages and disadvantages, *Milk Industry* 5, 5, 59-62

De Vine, B. (1927) The Public Health (Meat) Regulations, 1924, *Journal of the Royal Sanitary Institute* 47, 654-62

Dewar, J.R.U. (1895) Tuberculosis, *Veterinarian* 68, 675-88

Diprose, R. (2002) *Corporeal generosity: on giving with Nietzsche, Merleau-Ponty, and Levinas* Albany, NY: SUNY Press

Dixey, R.N. (1937) *Tuberculin tested milk: a study of re-organization for its production* Oxford: Oxford University, Institute for Research in Agricultural Economics

DNV Consulting (2006) Review of TB testing procedures: report for Defra and the Welsh Assembly Government London: Det Norske Veritas

Dodd, F.L. (1904) *The problem of the milk supply* London: Baillière, Tindall & Cox

Dodd, F.L. (1905) Municipal milk supply and public health, *Fabian Tract* No. 122 London: Fabian Society

Doig, A.T. et al. (1938) Laboratory and clinical investigations on Tuberculin Purified Protein Derivative (P.P.D.) and Old Tuberculin (O.T.), *British Medical Journal* i, 992-9

Domingo, M., Vidal, E. and Marco, A. (2014) Pathology of bovine tuberculosis, *Research in Veterinary Science* 97, S20-29

Donaldson, A. et al. (2006) Foot and mouth – five years on: the legacy of the foot and mouth 2001 crisis for farming and the British countryside, *University of Newcastle, Centre for Rural Economy Discussion Paper* 6

Donkin, H.B. (1899) Tuberculosis in childhood, *British Medical Journal* ii, 1046

Donnelly, C.A. (2012) Estimated proportion of confirmed herd breakdowns attributed to infectious badgers, http://bit.ly/XwmDvN

Donnelly, C.A. and Nouvellet, P. (2013) The contribution of badgers to confirmed tuberculosis in cattle in high-incidence areas in England, *PLoS Currents Outbreaks* 10 October

Donnelly, C.A. et al. (2007) Impacts of widespread badger culling on cattle tuberculosis: concluding analyses from a large-scale field trial, *International Journal of Infectious Diseases* 11, 300-08

Donnelly, C.A. et al. (2006) Positive and negative effects of widespread badger culling on tuberculosis in cattle, *Nature* 439, 843-6

Donnelly, C.A. et al. (2003) Impact of localized badger culling on TB incidence in British cattle, *Nature* 426, 834-7

Dormandy, T. (1999) *The white death: a history of tuberculosis* London: Hambledon Press

Drewe, J.A. et al. (2013) Patterns of direct and indirect contact between cattle and badgers naturally infected with tuberculosis, *Epidemiology and Infection* 141, 1467-75

Drewe, J.A., Pfeiffer, D.U. and Kaneene, J.B. (2014) Epidemiology of *Mycobacterium bovis*, pp 63-77 in Thoen, C.O., Steele, J.H. and Kaneene, J.B. (Eds) *Zoonotic tuberculosis: Mycobacterium bovis and other pathogenic mycobacteria* Ames, IA: Wiley-Blackwell

Drewe, J.A. and Smith, N.H. (2014) Molecular eipdemiology of Mycobacterium bovis, pp. 79-88 in Thoen, C.O., Steele, J.H. and Kaneene, J.B. (Eds) *Zoonotic tuberculosis: Mycobacterium bovis and other pathogenic mycobacteria* Wiley

Driscoll, E.E. et al. (2011) A preliminary study of genetic factors that influence susceptibility to bovine tuberculosis in the British cattle herd, *Plos One* 6, 4, e18806

Drobniewski, F. et al. (2003) Audit of scope and culture techniques applied to samples for the diagnosis of *Mycobacterium bovis* by hospital laboratories in England and Wales, *Epidemiology and Infection* 130, 235-237

Dubos, R. and J. (1953) *The white plague: tuberculosis, man and society* London: Gollancz

Duguid, W. (1890) Tuberculosis in animals, and its relation to consumption in man, *Journal of the Royal Agricultural Society of England* series 3, 1, 305-20

Dunleavy, P. (1995) Policy disasters: explaining the UK's record, *Public Policy and Administration* 10, 2, 52-70

Dunlop Young, T. (1929) Meat inspection, pp 241-84 in Collinge, G.H., Dunlop Young, T. and McDougall, A.P., *The retail meat trade: a practical treatise by specialists in the meat trade. Volume 1* London: Gresham

Dunnet, G.M., Jones, D.M. and McInerney, J.P. (1986) *Badgers and bovine tuberculosis - review of policy* London: HMSO

Eaton Jones, T. (1931) Routine veterinary inspection of dairy cattle: mainly from the point of view of tuberculosis, *Medical Officer* 46, 127-28

Ebbatson, R. (1980) *Lawrence and the nature tradition: a theme in English fiction 1859-1914* Brighton: Harvester

Edgar, W.A. (1898/99) Tuberculosis and its suppression, *Veterinary Record* 11, 478

Enock, A.G. (1943) *This milk business: from 1895 to 1943* London: H.K. Lewis

Ensor, R.C.K. (1936) *England 1870-1914* Oxford: Clarendon Press

Enticott, G. (2008a) The spaces of biosecurity: prescribing and negotiating solutions to bovine tuberculosis, *Environment & Planning A* 40, 1568-82

Enticott, G. (2008b) The ecological paradox: social and natural consequences of the geographies of animal health promotion, *Transactions of the Institute of British Geographers* 33, 433-46

Enticott, G. (2011) Techniques of neutralising wildlife crime in rural England and Wales, *Journal of Rural Studies* 27, 200-08

Enticott, G. (2012a) Regulating animal health, gender and quality control: a study of veterinary surgeons in Great Britain, *Journal of Rural Studies* 28, 559-67

Enticott, G. (2012b) The local universality of veterinary expertise and the geography of animal disease, *Transactions of the Institute of British Geographers* 37, 75-88

Enticott, G. (2014) Relational distance, neoliberalism and the regulation of animal health, *Geoforum* 52, 42-50

Enticott, G. et al. (2011) The changing role of veterinary expertise in the food chain, *Philosophical Transactions of the Royal Society B* 366, 1955-65

Enticott, G. and Franklin, A. (2009) Biosecurity, expertise and the institutional void: the case of bovine tuberculosis, *Sociologia Ruralis* 49, 375-93

Enticott, G. and Lee, R. (2015) Buying biosecurity: UK compensation for animal diseases, pp 57-78 in Havinga, T., van Waarden, F. and Casey, D. (Eds) *The changing landscape of food governance: public and private encounters* Cheltenham: Elgar

Enticott, G., Lowe, P. and Wilkinson, K. (2011) Neoliberal reform and the veterinary profession, *Veterinary Record* 169, 327-9

Enticott, G. et al. (2014) Badger vaccination: dimensions of trust and confidence in the governance of animal disease, *Environment and Planning A* 46, 2881-97

Enticott, G. and Vanclay, F. (2011) Scripts, animal health and biosecurity: the moral accountability of farmers' talk about animal health risks, *Health, Risk & Society* 13, 293-309

Environment, Food and Rural Affairs Select Committee (2013a)

Vaccination against bovine TB. Volume I: report, together with formal minutes, oral and written evidence, HC 258 London: Stationery Office

Ernst, W. (1914) *Textbook of milk hygiene* London: Baillière, Tindall & Cox

European Commission, Health & Consumer Protection Directorate-General, Veterinary and International Affairs, Unit G5 -Veterinary Programmes (2012*) Report of the Bovine Tuberculosis Sub-group Meeting held in the United Kingdom 27-28 March 2012* [Brussels]: European Commission

European Commission, Health & Consumer Protection Directorate-General, Veterinary and International Affairs, Unit G5 -Veterinary Programmes (2013) *Working document on eradication of bovine tuberculosis in the EU Accepted by the Bovine Tuberculosis Subgroup of the Task Force on monitoring animal disease eradication* Brussels: European Commission

European Commission, Health & Consumer Protection Directorate-General, Veterinary and International Affairs, Unit G5 -Veterinary Programmes (2014) *Report on Task Force Meeting of the Bovine Tuberculosis Subgroup, 5-6 March 2014, Dublin (Backweston), Ireland* [Brussels]: European Commission

European Food Safety Agency and European Centre for Disease Prevention and Control (2014) The European Union summary report on trends and sources of zoonoses, Zoonotic Agents and Foodborne outbreaks in 2012, *EFSA Journal* 12, 2, 3547

Ewald, F. (1991) Insurance and risks, pp 197-210 in Burchell, G., Gordon, C. and Miller, P. (Eds) *The Foucault Effect: Studies in Governmentality* London: Allen & Unwin

Eyler, J.M. (1979) *Victorian social medicine: the ideas and methods of William Farr* Baltimore: Johns Hopkins University Press

Farm Crisis Network (2009) *Stress and loss: a report on the impact of bovine TB on farming families* West Haddon, Northampton: Farm Crisis Network

Farr, W. (1885) *Vital statistics* London: Royal Sanitary Institute

Feore, S. and Montgomery, W.I. (1999) Habitat effects on the spatial ecology of the European badger (*Meles meles*), *Journal of Zoology* 247, 537-49

Fiddes, E. (1937) *Chapters in the history of Owens College and of the University of Manchester, 1851-1914* Manchester: Manchester University Press

Fish, R. et al. (2011) Uncertainties in the governance of animal disease: an interdisciplinary framework for analysis, *Philosophical Transactions of the Royal Society* B 366, 2023-34

Fishburn, F. (1932) York's experience with tubercular milk, *Journal of the Royal Sanitary Institution* 52, 539-47

Fisher, J.R. (1986) A panzootic of pleuro-pneumonia, 1840-1860, *Historia Medicinae Veterinariae* 11, 26-32

Fisher, J.R. (1993b) Not quite a profession: the aspirations of veterinary surgeons in England in the mid nineteenth century, *Historical Research* 66, 284-302 Chapter 2

Fisher, R. (2013) 'A gentleman's handshake': The role of social capital and trust in transforming information into usable knowledge, *Journal of Rural Studies* 31, 13-22

Fisher, R. et al. (2012) The spatial distribution of bovine tuberculosis in England, *Geography* 97, 68-77

Fishwick, V.C. (1947) *Dairy farming, theory and practice* London: Crosby Lockwood

Fleming, G. (1874) The transmissibility of tuberculosis, *British and Foreign Medico-Chirurgical Journal* 54, 461-86

Fleming, G. (1875) *A manual of veterinary sanitary science and police* 2 vols London: Chapman & Hall

Fleming, G. (1880) *Tuberculosis from a sanitary and pathological point of view* London: Baillière, Tindall & Cox

Fleming, G. (1888) Bovine and human tuberculosis, *Lancet* i, 698

Fletcher, T.W. (1961) The Great Depression in English agriculture, *Economic History Review* 13, 417-32

Food Standards Agency (2014) *Manual for official controls* http://www.food.gov.uk/enforcement/monitoring/meat/manual/#. U9zGlvldV8E

Forbes, J. (1907) Tuberculosis from the public health point of view, *Veterinary Record* 20, 414-18

Forrester, R.B. (1927) The fluid milk market in England and Wales, *Ministry of Agriculture and Fisheries, Economic Series* 16 London: HMSO

Forsyth, T. (2011) Politicizing environmental explanations: what can political ecology learn from sociology and philosophy of science? pp 31-46 in Goldman, M.J., Nadasdy, P. and Turner, M.D. (Eds) *Knowing nature* Chicago: University of Chicago Press

Foucault, M. (1991) Governmentality, pp 85-103 Burchell, G., Gordon, C. and Miller, P. (Eds) *The Foucault effect: studies in governmentality* London: Allen & Unwin

Fowler, J.S. (1908) The milk problem and tuberculosis in infancy and childhood, pp 27-34 in Kelynack, T.N. (Ed.) *Tuberculosis in infancy and childhood* New York: Wood

Fowler, D. (2011) Rolf Gardiner: pioneer of British youth culture, 1920-1939, pp 17-46 in Jefferies, M. and Tyldesley, M. (Eds) *Rolf Gardiner: folk, nature and culture in interwar Britain* Farnham: Ashgate

Fox, P.F. and Kelly, A.L. (2006) Indigenous enzymes in milk: historical aspects, *International Dairy Journal* 16, 500-32

Francis, J. (1947) *Bovine tuberculosis, including a contrast with human tuberculosis* London: Staples Press

Francis, J. (1958) *Tuberculosis in animals and man* London: Cassell

Francis, J. (1972a) Pathogenesis of tuberculosis in cattle, pp 47-51 in *Proceedings of the First International Seminar on Bovine Tuberculosis for the Americas, Santiago, Chile, 21-25 September 1970* Washington, DC: Pan American Health Organization

Francis, J. (1972b) The economic importance of bovine tuberculosis, pp 101-02 in *Proceedings of the First International Seminar on Bovine Tuberculosis for the Americas, Santiago, Chile, 21-25 September 1970* Washington, DC: Pan American Health Organization

Frankena, K., White, P.W., O'Keeffe, J., Costello, E., Martin, S.W., van Grevenhof, I. and More, S.J. (2007) Quantification of the relative efficiency of factory surveillance in the disclosure of tuberculosis lesions in attested Irish cattle, *Veterinary Record* 161, 679-84

Franklin, M. (1994) Food policy formation in the UK/EC, pp 3-8 in Henson, S. and Gregory, S. (Eds) The politics of food: proceedings of an inter-disciplinary seminar held at the University of Reading, 7 July 1993, *University of Reading, Department of Agricultural Economics and Management, Occasional Paper* No. 2

Frederiksen, J.D. (1919) *The story of milk* New York: Macmillan

Freidson, E. (2001) *Professionalism, the third logic* Chicago: University of Chicago Press

French, M. and Phillips, J. (2000) *Cheated not poisoned? Food regulation in the United Kingdom, 1875-1938* Manchester: Manchester University Press

Fyfe, C. (1937) Milk policy: farmers' attitude explained, *The Times* 20 September, 13f

Gaiger, S.H. and Davies, G.O. (1931) Bovine tuberculosis: biological tests of milk, *Veterinary Record* 11, 1072-4

Gairdner, W.T. and Coats, J. (1888) *Lectures to practitioners* London: Longmans, Green and Co.

Gallagher, J. and Clifton-Hadley, R.S. (2000) Tuberculosis in badgers: a review of the disease and its significance for other animals, *Research in Veterinary Science* 69, 203-17

Gannon, B.W., Hayes, C.M. and Roe, J.M. (2007) Survival rate of airborne Mycobacterium bovis, *Research in Veterinary Science* 82, 169-72

Garnett, B.T. (2002) Behavioural aspects of bovine tuberculosis

(Mycobacterium bovis) transmission and infection in badgers (Meles meles), unpublished PhD thesis, University of Sussex

Garnett, B.T., Delahay, R.J. and Roper, T.J. (2002) Use of cattle farm resources by badgers (*Meles meles*) and risk of bovine tuberculosis (*Mycobacterium bovis*) transmission to cattle, *Proceedings of the Royal Society B, Biological Sciences* 269, 1487-91

Gerber, N. and Wieske, P. (1903) Pasteurisation des flacons dans la grande industrie (pasteurisation avec agitation), *Revue Générale du Lait* 2, 8, 167-77

Gervois, M. (1937) *Le bacille de type bovin dans la tuberculose humaine: revue de la documentation actuelle* Lille: Danel

Ghodbane, R. et al. (2014) Long-term survival of tuberculosis complex mycobacteria in soil, *Microbiology* doi: 10.1099/mic.0.073379-0

Giddens, A. (1991) *Modernity and self-identity* Cambridge: Polity

Giddings, P.J. (1974) *Marketing boards and ministers: a study of agricultural marketing boards as political and administrative instruments* Farnborough: Saxon House

Gilbert, B.B. (1965) Health and politics: the British Physical Deterioration Report of 1904, *Bulletin of the History of Medicine* 39, 143-53

Gilbert , M. et al. (2005) Cattle movements and bovine tuberculosis in Great Britain, *Nature* 435, 491-6

Gofton, A. (1925) The problem of the tuberculous cow, *Journal of the Royal Sanitary Institute* 46, 382-7

Gofton, A. (1931) Bovine tuberculosis and the tuberculous infection of milk, *Journal of the Royal Sanitary Institute* 52, 217-22

Golby, P. et al. (2013) Genome-level analyses of Mycobacterium bovis lineages reveal the role of SNPs and antisense transcription in differential gene expression, *BMC Genomics* 14, 710

Good, M. (2014) Integration of science, policy and IT advances in the Irish bovine TB eradication programme: updates and progress

2005-2013, VI International M. bovis Conference, Cardiff, 16-19 June 2014

Good, M. and Duignan, A. (2011) Perspectives on the history of bovine TB and the role of tuberculin in bovine TB eradication, *Veterinary Medicine International* Article ID 410470

Goodchild, A.V. and Clifton-Hadley, R.S. (2001) Cattle-to-cattle transmission of Mycobacterium bovis, *Tuberculosis* 81, 23-41

Goodchild, T. and Clifton-Hadley, R. (2006) The fall and rise of bovine tuberculosis in Great Britain, pp 100-116 in Thoen, C.O., Steele, J.H. and Gilsdorf, M.H.J. (eds) *Mycobacterium Bovis Infection in Animals and Humans*. Chichester: Wiley-Blackwell

Goodchild, A.V. et al. (2003) Association between molecular type and epidemiological features of Mycobacterium bovis in cattle, pp 45-59 in Proceedings, Society for Veterinary Epidemiology and Preventive Medicine, University of Warwick 31 March - 2 April

Goodchild, A.V. et al. (2012) Geographical association between the genotype of bovine tuberculosis in found dead badgers and in cattle herds, *Veterinary Record* 170, 10, 257

Gopal, R. et al. (2006) Introduction of bovine tuberculosis to north-east England by bought in cattle, *Veterinary Record* 159, 265-271

Gordon, S.V. and Behr, M.A. (2015) Comparative mycobacteriology of the Mycobacterium tuberculosis complex, in Chambers, M., Mukundan, H., Larsen, M. and Waters, R. (eds) *Many hosts of mycobacteria: tuberculosis, leprosy, and other mycobacterial diseases of man and animals* Wallingford: CAB International

Gormley, E. et al. (2014) Bacteriological diagnosis and molecular strain typing of *Mycobacterium bovis* and *Mycobacterium caprae*, *Research in Veterinary Science* 97, S30-43

Grange, J.M. (2014) Mycobacterium tuberculosis – the organism, pp 39-53 in Davies, P.D.O., Gordon, S.B. and Davies, G. (Eds) *Clinical tuberculosis* Boca Raton: CRC Press

Grange, J.M. and Bishop, P.J. (1982) 'Über tuberkulose': a tribute to

Robert Koch's discovery of the tubercle bacillus, 1882, *Tubercle* 63, 3-17

Grange, J.M. and Collins, C.H. (1997) Tuberculosis and the cow, *Journal of the Royal Society of Health* 117, 119-22

Grange, J.M. and Yates, M.D. (1994) Zoonotic aspects of *Mycobacterium bovis* infection, *Veterinary Microbiology* 40, 137-51

Grant, W. (1997) BSE and the politics of food, pp 342-54 in Dunleavy, P., Gamble, A., Holliday, I. and Peele, G. (Eds) *Developments in British politics 5* Basingstoke: Macmillan

Grant, W. (2009) Intractable policy failure: the case of bovine TB and badgers, *British Journal of Politics and International Relations* 11, 557-73

Green, D.M. and Kao, R.R. (2007) Data quality of the Cattle Tracing System in Great Britain, *Veterinary Record* 161, 439-43

Green, D.M. et al. (2008) Estimates for local and movement-based transmission of bovine tuberculosis in British cattle, *Proceedings of the Royal Society of London B* 275, 1001-05

Green, H.H. (1946) Weybridge PPD tuberculins, *Veterinary Journal* 102, 267-78

Green, J.W. (1908) Milk pasteurization: probable bearings on proposed legislation, *British Food Journal* 10, 19-20

Green, L. and Medley, G. (2008) Cattle to Cattle Transmission of Bovine Tuberculosis: Risk Factors and Dynamics, *Cattle Practice* 16, 116-21

Green, L.E. et al. (2012) Patterns of delayed detection and persistence of bovine tuberculosis in confirmed and unconfirmed herd breakdowns in cattle and cattle herds in Great Britain, *Preventive Veterinary Medicine* 106, 266-74

Green, L.E. and Cornell, S.J. (2005) Investigations of cattle herd breakdowns with bovine tuberculosis in four counties of England and Wales using VETNET data, *Preventive Veterinary Medicine* 70, 293-311

Greenhough, B. (2014) More-than-human geographies, pp 94-119 in Lee, R. et al. (Eds) *The Sage handbook of human geography* Los Angeles: Sage

Greenhow, E.H. (1858) On the different prevalence of certain diseases in different districts in England and Wales, pp 1-164 in General Board of Health, *Papers relating to the sanitary state of the people of England* London: HMSO

Greger, M. (2007) The human/animal interface: emergence and resurgence of zoonotic infectious diseases, *Critical Reviews in Microbiology* 33, 243-99

Gregson, N. (2011) Book review forum: Vibrant Matter: a Political Ecology of Things, *Dialogues in Human Geography* 1, 402-04

Griffin, J.M. (1993) The role of bought-in cattle in herd breakdowns due to tuberculosis in part of County Cavan during 1989, *Irish Veterinary Journal* 46, 143-8

Griffin, J.M. and Dolan, L.A. (1995) The role of cattle-to-cattle transmission of *Mycobacterium bovis* in the epidemiology of tuberculosis in cattle in the Republic of Ireland: a review, *Irish Veterinary Journal* 48, 228-34

Griffin, J.M., Hahesy, T. and Lynch, K. (1992) The role of farm management practices and environmental factors in chronic TB, *Irish Veterinary Journal* 45, 120-22

Griffin, J.M. et al. (1993) The association of cattle husbandry characteristics, environmental factors and farmer characteristics with the occurrence of chronic bovine tuberculosis in dairy herds in the Republic of Ireland, *Preventive Veterinary Medicine* 17, 145-60

Griffin, J.M. et al. (1996) A case-control study on the association of selected risk factors with the occurrence of bovine tuberculosis in the Republic of Ireland, *Preventive Veterinary Medicine* 27, 75-87

Griffin, J.M. et al. (2005a) Tuberculosis in cattle: the results of the four-area project, *Irish Veterinary Journal* 58, 629-36

Griffin, J.M. et al. (2005b) The impact of badger removal on the control of tuberculosis in cattle herds in Ireland, *Preventive Veterinary Medicine* 67, 237-66

Griffith, A.S. (1911) *Royal Commission on the Relation between Human and Animal Tuberculosis, Final Report, Part II. Appendix,* vols 1-3

Griffith, A.S. (1914) Further investigations of the type of tubercle bacilli occurring in the sputum of phthisical persons, *British Medical Journal* i, 1171-5

Griffith, A.S. (1916a) An investigation of human bone and joint tuberculosis, *Journal of Pathology and Bacteriology* 21, 54-77

Griffith, A.S. (1916b) Investigation of strains of tubercle bacilli derived from sputum, *Lancet* i, 721

Griffith, A.S. (1930) The types of tubercle bacilli occurring in the sputum of phthisical persons, *Journal of Pathology and Bacteriology* 33, 1145-69

Griffith, A.S. (1937) Bovine tuberculosis in man, *Tubercle* 18, 529-43

Griffith, A.S. and Menton, J. (1936) Human tuberculosis of bovine origin in Staffordshire, *British Medical Journal* 1, 524-6

Griffith, A.S. and Munro, W.T. (1944) Human pulmonary tuberculosis of bovine origin in Great Britain, *Journal of Hygiene* 43, 229-40

Griffith, A.S. and Smith, J. (1940) Types of tubercle bacilli in pulmonary tuberculosis in north east Scotland, *Lancet* 2, 291-4

Griffiths, R. (1980) *Fellow travellers of the right: British enthusiasts for Nazi Germany 1933-9* London: Constable

Griffiths, H.I. and Thomas, D.H. (Eds)(1997) The conservation and management of the European badger (*Meles meles*) Strasbourg: Council of Europe

Gurlt, E.F. (1831) *Lehrbuch der pathologischen anatomie* Berlin : Theil

Hacking, I. (1991) How should we do the history of statistics? pp 181-95 in Burchell, G., Gordon, C. and Miller, P. (Eds) *The Foucault effect: studies in governmentality* Chicago: University of Chicago Press

Hall, C.W. and Trout, G.M. (1968) *Milk pasteurization* Westport, CT: AVI Publishing

Hall, S. (2010) Official bovine tuberculosis-free status in Scotland, *Veterinary Record* 166, 245-6

Hamill, J.M. (1933) Milk, *Lancet* ii, 1495-8

Hamill, J.M. (1934) Milk, in Anon. (Ed.) *The preventative aspects of medicine* London: Lancet Ltd

Hamlin, C. (1985) Providence and putrefaction: Victorian sanitarians and the natural theology of health and disease, *Victorian Studies* 28, 381-411

Hammond, R.J. (1954) Food and agriculture in Britain 1939-45: aspects of wartime control Stanford: Stanford University Press

Hammond, R.J. (1956) *Food. Volume 2: studies in administration and control* London: HMSO

Hardie, R.M. and Watson, J.M. (1992) *Mycobacterium bovis* in England and Wales: past, present and future, *Epidemiology and Infection* 109, 23-33

Hardstaff, J.L. et al. (2012) Impact of external sources of infection on the dynamics of bovine tuberculosis in modelled badger populations, *BMC Veterinary Research* 8, 92

Hardstaff, J.L. et al. (2014) Evaluating the tuberculosis hazard posed to cattle from wildlife across Europe, *Research in Veterinary Science* 97, S86-93

Hardy, A. (1988) Diagnosis, death and diet: the case of London, 1750-1909, *Journal of Interdisciplinary History* 18, 387-401

Hardy, A. (1993) *The epidemic streets: infectious disease and the rise of preventative medicine, 1856-1900* Oxford: Clarendon Press

Hardy, A. (1994) 'Death is the cure of all diseases': using the General Register Office cause of death statistics for 1837-1920, *Social History of Medicine* 7, 472-92

Hardy, A. (2002) Pioneers in the Victorian provinces: veterinarians, public health and the urban animal economy, *Urban History* 29, 372-87

Hardy, A. (2003a) Animals, disease and man: making connections, *Perspectives in Biology and Medicine* 46, 200-15

Hardy, A. (2003b) Professional advantage and public health: British veterinarians and state veterinary services, *Twentieth Century British History* 14, 1-23

Hardy, A. (2003c) Reframing disease: changing perceptions of tuberculosis in England and Wales, 1938-70, *Historical Research* 76, 535-56

Hardy, A. (2010) John Bull's beef: meat hygiene and veterinary public health in England in the twentieth century, *Review of Agricultural and Environmental Studies* 91, 369-92

Hardy, A. (2015) *Salmonella infections, networks of knowledge, and public health in Britain, 1880-1975* Oxford: Oxford University Press

Harman, G. (2008) DeLanda's ontology: assemblage and realism, *Continental Philosophy Review* 41, 367-83

Harris, N.B. (2006) Molecular techniques: applications in epidemiologic studies, pp 54-62 in in Thoen, C.O., Steele, J.H. and Gilsdorf, J.H. (Eds) *Mycobacterium bovis infection in animals and humans* Ames, Iowa: Blackwell

Hartman, A.M. and Dryden, L.P. (1965) The vitamins in milk and milk products, pp 261-338 in Webb, B.H. and Johnson, A.H. (Eds) *Fundamentals of dairy chemistry* Westport, Connecticut: Avi Publishing

Harvey, W.C. and Hill, H. (1936, 1967) *Milk production and control* 1st and 4th eds London: H.K. Lewis

Headrick, M.L. et al. (1997) Profile of raw milk consumers in California, *Public Health Reports* 112, 418-22

Heclo, H. and Wildavsky, A. (1981) *The private government of public money: community and policy inside British politics* London: Macmillan

Henry, M. and Roche, M. (2013) Valuing lively materialities: bio-economic assembling in the making of new meat futures, *New Zealand Geographer* 69, 197-207

Hewinson, R.G. et al. (2006) Recent advances in our knowledge of Mycobacterium bovis: a feeling for the organism, *Veterinary Microbiology* 112, 127-39

Higgs, E. (1996a) A cuckoo in the nest? The origins of civil registration and state medical statistics in England and Wales, *Continuity and Change* 11, 115-34

Higgs, E. (1996b) The statistical Big Bang of 1911: ideology, technological innovation and the production of medical statistics, *Social History of Medicine* 9, 409-26

Higgs, E. (2004a) *The information state in England: the central collection of information on citizens since 1500* Basingstoke: Palgrave Macmillan

Higgs, E. (2004b) *Life, death and statistics: civil registration, censuses and the work of the General Register Office, 1836-1952* Hatfield: Local Population Studies

Hill, H. (1943) *Pasteurization* London: H.K. Lewis

Hills, A.F. (1892) *Vital food* London: Vegetarian Society

Hinchliffe, S. (2001) Indeterminacy in-decisions – science, policy and politics in the BSE (Bovine Spongiform Encephalopathy) crisis, *Transactions of the Institute of British Geographers* NS 26, 182-204

Hinchliffe, S. (2008) Reconstituting nature conservation: Towards a careful political ecology, *Geoforum* 39, 88-97

Hinchliffe, S. (2011) Book review forum: Vibrant Matter: a Political Ecology of Things, *Dialogues in Human Geography* 1, 396-9

Hinchliffe, S., Levidow, L. and Oreszczyn, S. (2014) Engaging cooperative research, *Environment and Planning A* 46, 2080-94

Hird, M.J. (2009) *The origins of sociable life: evolution after science studies* Basingstoke: Palgrave Macmillan

Holburn, A. (1905) Some suggestions with a view to the improvement of meat inspection in country districts, *London Congress, Section F, July 1905, the Royal Institute of Public Health*

Holsinger, V.H., Rajkowski, K.T. and Stabel, J.R. (1997) Milk pasteurization and safety: a brief history and update, *Revue Scientifique et Technique International Office of Epizootics* 16, 441-51

Hooker, C. (2001) Sanitary failure and risk: pasteurization, immunization and the logics of prevention, pp 129-52 in Bashford, A. and Hooker, C. (Eds) *Contagion: historical and cultural studies* London: Routledge

Hope, E.W. (1901) Sterilisation and pasteurisation v. tubercle-free herds, *Lancet* ii, 197-198

Hopkins, F.G. (1912) Feeding experiments illustrating the importance of accessory factors in normal dietaries, *Journal of Physiology* 44, 425-60

Hopkins, F.G. (1913) A note concerning the influence of diets upon growth, *Biochemical Journal* 7, 97-9

Hopkins, F.G. (1919) Vitamines: unknown but essential accessory factors of the diet, pp 27-49 in Halliburton, W.D. (Ed.) *Physiology and national needs* London: Constable

Hopkins, F.G. (1920) Note on the vitamine content of milk, *Biochemical Journal* 14, 721-4

Hubsher, R. (1999) *Les maîtres des bêtes: les vétérinaires dans la société française (XVIIIe-XXe siècle)* Paris: Odile Jacob

Humblet, M.F., Boschiroli, M.L. and Saegerman, C. (2009) Classification of worldwide bovine tuberculosis risk factors in cattle: a stratified approach, *Veterinary Research* 40, 5, 1-24

Humblet, M.F. et al. (2010) New assessment of bovine tuberculosis risk factors in Belgium based on nationwide molecular epidemiology, *Journal of Clinical Microbiology* 48, 2802-8

Hunter, P. (2004) *Veterinary medicine: a guide to historical sources* Aldershot: Ashgate

[Hunting, W.] (1894) Tuberculosis: its prevention, *Veterinary Record* 6, 438-9

[Hunting, W.] (1899a) Legislative control of bovine tuberculosis, *Veterinary Record* 11, 472-5

Hutchens, H.J. (1914) Some points on the relationship of bovine to human tuberculosis, *Journal of the Royal Sanitary Institute* 35, 94-102

Hutchings, M.R. and Harris, S. (1997) Effects of farm management practices on cattle grazing behaviour and the potential for transmission of bovine tuberculosis from badgers to cattle, *Veterinary Journal* 153, 149-62

Hutchings, M.R. and Harris, S. (1999) Quantifying the risks of TB infection to cattle posed by badger excreta, *Epidemiology and Infection* 122, 167-73

Hutyra, F. and Marek, J. (1912) *Special pathology and therapeutics of the diseases of domestic animals* Chicago: Eger

Huzard, J.-B. (père)(1795) Essai sur la maladie qui affecte les vaches laitières des faubourgs et des environs de Paris, *Feuille du Cultivateur* 12, 65-71

Huzard, J.-B. (fils)(1834) Rapport à M. le préfet de police, sur la pommelière ou phthisie pulmonaire des vaches laitières de Paris et des environs, *Annales d'hygiène publique et de médecine légale* série 1, 447-56

Independent Scientific Group (2004) *An epidemiological investigation into bovine tuberculosis: towards a science-based control strategy* London: ISG

Independent Scientific Group (2007) *Bovine TB: the scientific evidence. Final Report of the Independent Scientific Group on Cattle TB* London: ISG

Ingold, T. (2012) Toward an ecology of materials, *Annual Review of Anthropology* 41, 427-42

Jackson, A.J. (1956) *Official history of the National Federation of Meat Associations (Incorporated)* Plymouth: Clarke, Domble & Brendon

Jasanoff, S. (1997) Civilization and madness: the great BSE scare of 1996, *Public Understanding of Science* 6, 221-32

Jeffcock, W.P. (1937) *Agricultural politics 1915-1935, being a history of the Central Chamber of Agriculture during that period* Ipswich: Harrison

Jefferies, M. (2011) Rolf Gardiner and German naturism, pp 47-64 in Jefferies, M. and Tyldesley, M. (Eds) *Rolf Gardiner: folk, nature and culture in interwar Britain* Farnham: Ashgate

Jenkins, A. (1970) *Drinka Pinta: the story of milk and the industry that serves it* London: Heinemann

Jenkins, H.E., Woodroffe, R. and Donnelly, C.A. (2008) The effects of annual widespread badger culls on cattle tuberculosis following the cessation of culling, *International Journal of Infectious Diseases* 12, 457-65

Jenkins, H.E., Woodroffe, R. and Donnelly, C.A. (2010) The duration of the effects of repeated widespread badger culling on cattle tuberculosis following the cessation of culling, *PLoS ONE* 5, 2, e9090

Jenkins, H.E. et al. (2007) Effects of culling on spatial associations of Mycobacterium bovis infections in badgers and cattle, *Journal of Applied Ecology* 44, 897-908

Jensen, C.O. (1909) *Essentials of milk hygiene* Philadelphia: Lippincott

Jessop, B. (1990) *State theory: putting the capitalist state in its place* Cambridge: Polity Press

Jin, R. et al. (2013) An association between rainfall and bovine TB in Wicklow, Ireland, *Veterinary Record* 173, 452

Johnston, W.T. et al. (2005) Herd-level risk factors associated with tuberculosis outbreaks among cattle herds in England before the 2001 foot-and-mouth disease epidemic, *Biology Letters* 1, 53-6

Jones, G.R. (1939) Co-ordination between local authorities and the Ministry of Agriculture in the administration of the Agriculture Act, 1937 (Part IV), *Journal of the Royal Sanitary Institute* August, 61-5

Jones, K.E. et al. (2008) Global trends in emerging infectious diseases, *Nature* 451, 990-94

Jones, S.D. (2004) Mapping a zoonotic disease: Anglo-American efforts to control bovine tuberculosis before World War I, *Osiris* 19, 133-48

Jordan, A.G. and Richardson, J.J. (1982) The British policy style or the logic of negotiation? pp 80-110 in Richardson, J.J. (Ed.) *Policy styles in Western Europe* London: Allen & Unwin

Jordan, G., Maloney, W.A. and McLaughlin, A.M. (1994) Characterizing agricultural policy-making, *Public Administration* 72, 505-26

Jordan, L. (1933) The eradication of bovine tuberculosis, Me*dical Research Council, Special Reports Series* no. 184

Judge, J. et al. (2014) Density and abundance of badger social groups in England and Wales in 2011-2013, *Scientific Reports* 4, 3809

Kaneene, J.B. et al. (2014) One Health approach for preventing and controlling tuberculosis in animals and humans, pp 9-20 in Thoen, C.O., Steele, J.H. and Kaneene, J.B. (Eds) *Zoonotic tuberculosis: Mycobacterium bovis and other pathogenic mycobacteria* Ames, IA: Wiley-Blackwell

Kaplan, M.M., Abdussalem and Bijlenga, G. (1962) Diseases transmitted through milk, pp 11-74 in World Health Organization (Eds) Milk hygiene: hygiene in milk production, processing and distribution, *World Health Organisation Monograph Series* no. 48 Geneva: WHO

Karolemeas, K. et al. (2010) Predicting prolonged bovine tuberculosis breakdowns in Great Britain as an aid to control, *Preventive Veterinary Medicine* 97, 183-90

Karolemeas, K. et al. (2011) Recurrence of bovine tuberculosis breakdowns in Great Britain Risk factors prediction, *Preventive Veterinary Medicine* 102, 22-9

Kay, H.D.,et al. (1953) Milk pasteurization: planning, plant, operation, and control Rome: FAO

Kayne, G.G., Pagel, W. and O'Shaughnessy, L. (1939) *Pulmonary tuberculosis* London: Oxford University Press

Kelly, G.E. and More, S.J. (2011) Spatial clustering of TB-infected cattle herds prior to and following proactive badger removal, *Epidemiology and Infection* 139, 1220-29

Kelly, W.R. and Collins, J.D. (1978) The health significance of some infectious agents present in animal effluents, *Veterinary Science Communications* 2, 95-103

Kent, W.R.G. (1950) *John Burns, Labour's lost leader: a biography* London: Williams & Norgate

Kenwood, H. (1926) The trade pasterization of milk and the public health, *Journal of the Royal Sanitary Institute* 47, 355-60, 366

Kerr, H. (1924) *The constitution of genuine pure milk and notes on some other dairy products* Newcastle: City of Newcastle-upon-Tyne, Health Committee

Kilbourne, C.H. (1916) *The pasteurization of milk from the practical viewpoint* New York: Wiley

King, J. (1901) Tuberculosis and the meat supply, Paper read to the British Congress on Tuberculosis, Section IV: Tuberculosis in Animals, *Lancet* ii, 245-7

Kleeberg, H.H. (1984) Human tuberculosis of bovine origin in relation to public health, *Revue Scientifique et Technique International des Epizooties* 3, 11-32

Knorr Cetina, K. (2001) Objectual practice, pp 175-88 in Schatzki, T.R., Knorr Cetina, K. and von Savigny, E. (Eds) *The practice turn in contemporary theory* New York: Routledge

Koch, R. (1890) A further communication on a remedy for tuberculosis, *Journal of Comparative Pathology and Therapeutics* 3, 301-08

Koch, R. (1901) The combating of tuberculosis in the light of experience that has been gained in the successful combating of other infectious diseases, *Journal of Comparative Pathology and Therapeutics* 14, 203-15

Komorowski, E.S. and Early, R. (1992) Liquid milk and cream, pp 1-23 in Early, R. (Ed.) *The technology of dairy products* Glasgow: Blackie

Kon, S.K. (1972) Milk and milk products in human nutrition Rome: FAO

Koolmees, P.A. (1999) The development of veterinary public health in Western Europe, 1850-1940, *Sartoniana* 12, 153-79

Koolmees, P. (2000) Veterinary inspection and food hygiene in the twentieth century, pp 53-68 in Smith, D.F. and Phillips, J. (Eds) *Food, science, policy and regulation in the twentieth century: international and comparative perspectives* London: Routledge

Koolmees, P.A., Fisher, J.R. and Perren, R. (1999) The traditional responsibility of veterinarians in meat production and meat inspection, pp 7-26 in Smulders, F. (Ed.) *Veterinary aspects of meat production, processing and inspection* Utrecht: ECCEAMST

Krebs, J.R. and the Independent Scientific Review Group (1997) *Bovine tuberculosis in cattle and badgers* London: MAFF

Kruuk, H. and Parish, T. (1982) Factors affecting population density, group size and territory size of the European badger, *Meles meles, Journal of Zoology* 196, 31-9

Lampert, L.M. (1965) *Modern dairy products* New York: Chemical Publishing Co.

Lane, R.W. (1933) Sterilized milk, pp 237-246 in Raison, C. (Ed.) *The milk trade: a comprehensive guide to the development of the dairy industry* London: Virtue & Co.

Lane, S. et al. (2011) Doing flood risk science differently: an experiment in radical scientific method, *Transactions of the Institute of British Geographers* NS 36, 15-36

Lane-Claypon, J. E. (1916) *Milk and its hygenic relations* London: Longmans, Green and Co

Langford, E.W. (1922) *Methods of milk production and distribution in the United States and Canada* London: National Farmers' Union

Langmuir, A.D. (1961) Epidemiology of airborne infection, *Bacteriology Review* 25, 173-81

Latour, B. (1988) *The pasteurization of France* Cambridge MA: Harvard University Press

Latour, B. (1993) Ethnography of a 'high-tech' case: about Aramis, pp 372-98 in Lemonier, P. (Ed.) *Technological choices: transformation in material cultures since the neolithic* London: Routledge

Latour, B. (2005) *Reassembling the social: an introduction to Actor-Network Theory* New York: Oxford University Press

Latour, B. and Woolgar, S. (1986) *Laboratory life: the construction of scientific facts* Princeton NJ: Princeton University Press

Law, J. (1994) *Organizing modernity: social order and social theory* Oxford: Blackwell

Law, J. and Lien, M.E. (2013) Slippery: field notes in empirical ontology, *Social Studies of Science* 43, 363-78

Law, J. and Moser, I. (2012) Contexts and Culling, *Science Technology and Human Values* 37, 332-54

League of Nations (1937) *Nutrition: Final report of the Mixed Committee of the League of Nations on the relation of nutrition to health, agriculture and economic policy* Geneva: League of Nations

LeCain, T. (2014) The ontology of absence, pp 62-78 in Olsen, B. and Pétursdóttir, T. (Eds) *Ruin memories: materialities, aesthetics and the archaeology of the recent past* Abingdon: Routledge

Leach, M. and Scoones, I. (2013) The social and political lives of zoonotic disease models: narratives, science and policy, *Social Science & Medicine* 88, 10-17

Legg, S. (2005) Foucault's population geographies: classifications, biopolitics and governmental spaces, *Population, Space and Place* 11, 137-56

Legge, T.M. (1896) *Public health in European Capitals* London: Swan Sonnenschein

Legge, T.M. and Sessions, H. (1898) *Cattle tuberculosis: a practical guide to the farmer, butcher, and meat inspector* London: Baillière, Tindall & Cox

Leighton, G. (1927) *The principles and practice of meat inspection* Edinburgh: Hodge

Leighton, G. and Douglas, L.M. (1910) *The meat industry and meat inspection* 5 vols London: Educational Book Co.

Leighton, G. and McKinlay, P.L. (1930) *Milk consumption and the growth of school children: report on an investigation in Lanarkshire schools* Edinburgh: Department of Health for Scotland

Lenzini, L., Rottoli, P. and Rottoli, L. (1977) The spectrum of human tuberculosis, *Clinical and Experimental Immunology* 27, 230-37

Le Roex, N. et al. (2013) Bovine TB in livestock and wildlife: what's in the genes? *Physiological Genomics* 45, 631-7

Le Roy Ladurie, E. (1967) *Histoire du climat depuis l'an mil* Paris: Flammarion

Lesslie, I.W. et al. (1975) Comparison of the specificity of human and bovine tuberculin PPD for testing cattle. 1. Republic of Ireland; 2. South-eastern England; 3. National trial in Great Britain, *Veterinary Record* 96, 332-41

Lethem, W.A. (1946) Bovine tuberculosis, *The Medical Officer* 75, 82

Linton, D.S. (2005) *Emil von Behring: infectious disease, immunology, serum therapy* Philadelphia: American Philosophical Society

Little, A. (2012) Political action, error and failure: the epistemological limits of complexity, *Political Studies* 60, 3-19

Lloyd, J.S. (1902) The veterinary work done under the Milk Clauses in Manchester, and the difficulties met with, pp 293-301 in *Transactions of the British Congress on Tuberculosis for the Prevention of Consumption, London, July 22nd to July 26th, 1901. Volume 2: report of the state section* London: Clowes

Lloyd, J.S. (1927) Tuberculous infection in milk as affected by recent legislation, *Journal of the Royal Society for the Promotion of Health* 48, 319-27

Loat, L. (1938a) *Compulsory pasteurization of milk would be disastrous* London: National Anti-Vaccination League

Loat, L. (1938b) The vivisectionists and the milk supply, *Anti-Vivisection Journal* April; reprinted as pamphlet London: London & Provincial Anti-Vivisection Society

Lodge, M. and Matus, K. (2014) Science, badgers, politics: advocacy coalitions and policy change in bovine tuberculosis policy in Britain, *Policy Studies Journal* 42, 367-90

Lomax, E. (1977) Heredity or acquired disease? early nineteenth century debates on the cause of infantile scrofula and tuberculosis, *Journal of the History of Medicine and Allied Sciences* 32, 4, 356

London Butchers' Trade Society (1899) *Inspections of meat and milk* [London: LBTS]

London County Council, Central Public Health Committee (1933) *Milk supply coming into London: infection with tubercle bacilli* London: LCC

López, M.P. (2014) Speculative experiments: what if Simondon and Harman individuate together? *Speculations* 5, 225-47

Louckx, K. and Vanderstraeten, R. (2014) State-istics and statistics: exclusion categories in the population census (Belgium, 1846-1930), *Sociological Review* 62, 530-46

Lowe, R. (2011) *The official history of the British civil service: reforming the civil service, volume I: The Fulton years, 1966-81* London: Routledge

Luckin, B. (1980) Death and survival in the city, approaches to the history of disease, *Urban History Yearbook* 7, 53-62

Luhmann, N. (1979) *Trust and power* Chichester: Wiley

Lydtin, A., Fleming, G. and Hertsen, M. van [1883] *The influence of heredity and contagion on the propagation of tuberculosis: and the prevention of injurious effects from consumption of the flesh of tuberculous animals* London: Baillière, Tindall & Cox

Lyle Cummins, J. (1925) A warning note on the control of tuberculosis and the milk supply, *Veterinary Journal* 81, 190-91

Lymington, Viscount (1938) *Famine in England* London: Witherby

Lymington, Viscount (1941) The policy of husbandry, pp 12-31 in

Massingham, H.J. (Ed.) *England and the farmer: a symposium* London: Faber

McAllan, J. (1925) Common difficulties in meat inspection, *Journal of the Royal Sanitary Institute* 46, 391-94

McCallan, L., McNair, J. and Skuce, R. (2014) A review of the potential role of cattle slurry in the spread of bovine tuberculosis [Belfast]: Bacteriology Branch, Veterinary Sciences Division, Agri-food and Biosciences Institute

McCarthy, D.J. (1908) Tuberculous affections of the nervous system in infancy and childhood, pp 43-54 in Kelynack, T.N. (Ed.) *Tuberculosis in infancy and childhood* New York: Wood

McCollum, E.V. (1957) *A history of nutrition: the sequence of ideas in nutrition investigations* Boston: Houghton Mifflin

McCorry, T. et al. (2005) Shedding of Mycobacterium bovis in the nasal mucus of cattle infected experimentally with TB by the intranasal and intratracheal routes, *Veterinary Record* 157, 613-18

MacDonald, D.W., Riordan, P. and Mathews, F. (2006) Biological hurdles to the control of TB in cattle: a test of two hypotheses concerning wildlife to explain the failure of control, *Biological Conservation* 131, 268-86

McDonald, R.A. et al. (2008) Perturbing implications of wildlife ecology for disease control, *Trends in Ecology and Evolution* 23, 53-6

Macewen, H.A. (1910) *The public milk supply* London: Blackie

[McFadyean, J.] (1888a) Tuberculosis in Scotland, *Journal of Comparative Pathology and Therapeutics* 1, 98

[McFadyean, J.] (1888b) Congress for study of tuberculosis in man and animals, *Journal of Comparative Pathology and Therapeutics* 1, 262-75

[McFadyean, J.] (1888c) New decree regarding tuberculosis in France, *Journal of Comparative Pathology and Therapeutics* 1, 288

[McFadyean, J.] (1888d) The connection between human and animal tuberculosis, *Journal of Comparative Pathology and Therapeutics* 1, 352-5

[McFadyean, J.] (1889a) The tuberculous meat cases at Glasgow, *Journal of Comparative Pathology and Therapeutics* 2, 138-9

[McFadyean, J.] (1889b) Important trial regarding tuberculous carcases at Glasgow, *Journal of Comparative Pathology and Therapeutics* 2, 180-95

[McFadyean, J.] (1890a) Inspection of meat at Liverpool, *Journal of Comparative Pathology and Therapeutics* 3, 159-61

McFadyean, J. (1890b) Experiments with expressed muscle juice from tuberculous carcasses, pp 13-19 in *Annual Report, Veterinary Department* London

[McFadyean, J.] (1891a) The inspection of tuberculous meat, *Journal of Comparative Pathology and Therapeutics* 4, 349-51

[McFadyean, J.] (1891b) Sanitary control of milk supply in Edinburgh, *Journal of Comparative Pathology and Therapeutics* 4, 271-2

[McFadyean, J.] (1895a) How are we to deal with bovine tuberculosis?, *Journal of Comparative Pathology and Therapeutics* 8, 239-42

[McFadyean, J.] (1895b) The prevention of tuberculosis in cattle, *Journal of Comparative Pathology and Therapeutics* 6, 353

[McFadyean, J.] (1895c) Ought tuberculosis to be included in the Contagious Diseases (Animals) Act? *Journal of Comparative Pathology and Therapeutics* 8, 145-8

[McFadyean, J.] (1895d) The danger of tuberculous meat, *Journal of Comparative Pathology and Therapeutics* 8, 237-9

[McFadyean, J.] (1896) The butcher as meat inspector, *Journal of Comparative Pathology and Therapeutics* 9, 222-3

[McFadyean, J.] (1897) Medical Officers as Veterinary Inspectors, *Journal of Comparative Pathology and Therapeutics* 10, 166-8

[McFadyean, J.] (1898) The relationship between human and bovine tuberculosis, *Journal of Comparative Pathology and Therapeutics* 11, 344-50

[McFadyean, J.] (1900a) The requirements of an efficient meat inspection, *Journal of Comparative Pathology and Therapeutics* 13, 244-5

[McFadyean, J.] (1900b) The frequency of tuberculosis among British cattle, *Journal of Comparative Pathology and Therapeutics* 13, 68-71

McFadyean, J. (1901) The Tuberculin Test, *Journal of Comparative Pathology and Therapeutics* 14, 68-73

McFadyean, J. (1910) What is the common method of infection in tuberculosis? *Journal of Comparative Pathology and Therapeutics* 23, 239-50, 289-303

McFadyean, J. (1921) Special discussion on 'the eradication of tuberculosis from man and animals', *Proceedings of the Royal Society of Medicine* 14 (Gen Rep), 11-25

McFadyean, J. (1927) The prevention of tuberculosis in animals, *Veterinary Record* 7, 859-64

MacFadyen, N. (1938) Pasteurisation of milk, *British Medical Journal* i, 148-9, 259

Macgregor, A.S.M. (1890) *The milk supply of Copenhagen* Edinburgh: Scott Ferguson Burness

MacGregor, W.T. (1935) The unification of control of animal diseases and of the meat and milk supply, *Journal of State Medicine* 43, 156-65

McHugh, F.G. (1943) The milk supply of the future, *Journal of the Royal Sanitary Institute* 63, 111-16

McIlroy, S.G., Neill, S.D. and McCracken, R.M. (1986) Pulmonary lesions and *Mycobacterium bovis* excretion from the respiratory tract of tuberculin reacting cattle, *Veterinary Record* 118, 718-21

Mackintosh, J., Pennington, S. and Williams, R.S. (1915) The supply of non-tuberculous dairy stock, *Journal of Hygiene* 15, 51-63

Mackenzie, L. (1899) The hygienics of milk, *Edinburgh Medical Journal* 5, 372-8 and 563-76

MacLeod, R.M. (1968) Treasury control and social administration, *Occasional Papers on Social Administration* 23 London: Bell

MacNutt, J.S. (1917) *The modern milk problem in sanitation, economics and agriculture* New York: Macmillan

Maddock, E.C.G. (1933) Studies on the survival time of the bovine tubercle bacillus in soil, soil and dung, in dung and on grass, with experiments on the preliminary treatment of infected organic matter and the cultivation of the organism, *Journal of Hygiene* 33, 103-17

Maddock, E.C.G. (1934) Further studies on the survival time of the bovine tubercle bacillus in soil, soil and dung, in dung and on grass, with experiments on feeding guinea-pigs and calves on grass artificially infected with bovine tubercle bacilli *Journal of Hygiene* 34, 372-9

Maddock, E.C.G. (1936) Experiments on the infectivity for healthy calves of bovine tubercle bacilli discharged in dung upon pasture. Part I: from tubercular calves fed with emulsions of tubercle bacilli, 1933-4. Part II: from tubercular cows passing tubercle bacilli in their dung, 1935-6, *Journal of Hygiene* 36, 594-601

Maitland, M.L.C. (1937) Rapid detection of B. tuberculosis in milk, *Lancet* i, 1297-9

Malcolm, J. (1901) Veterinary dairy inspection, *Journal of Comparative Pathology and Therapeutics* 14, 29-37

Maloney, W.A., Jordan, G. and McLaughlin, A.M. (1994) Interest groups and public policy: the insider/outsider model revisited, *Journal of Public Policy* 14, 17-38

Martin, B. (1991) *Scientific knowledge in controversy: the social dynamics of the fluoridation debate* Albany: State University of New York Press

Martin, J. (2000) *The development of modern agriculture: British farming since 1931* Basingstoke: Macmillan

Matless, D. (1995) 'The art of right living': landscape and citizenship,

1918-39, pp 93-122 in Pile, S. and Thrift, N.J. (Eds) *Mapping the subject: geographies of cultural transformation* London: Routledge

Matless, D. (1998) *Landscape and Englishness* London: Reaktion

Matthews, A.H.H. (1915) *Fifty years of agricultural politics, being the history of the Central Chamber of Agriculture 1865-1915* London: King

Matthews, S. (2005) Cattle clubs, insurance and plague in the mid-nineteenth century, *Agricultural History Review* 53, 192-211

Matthews, S. (2010) Underwriting disaster: risk and the management of agricultural crisis in mid-nineteenth century Cheshire, *Agricultural History Review* 58, 217-35

Mattick, A.T.R. (1944) Bacteriological aspects of milk processing and distribution, *Proceedings of the Nutrition Society* 2, 141-9

Mattick, E.C.V. and Golding, J. (1931) Relative value of raw and heated milk in nutrition, *Lancet* i, 662-7

Mattick, E.C.V. and Golding, J. (1936) Relative value of raw and heated milk in nutrition, *Lancet* i, 1132-34; ii, 702-06

Maye, D. et al. (2014) Animal disease and narratives of nature: farmers' reactions to the neoliberal governance of bovine tuberculosis, *Journal of Rural Studies* 36, 401-10

Mba Medie, F. et al. (2011) *Mycobacterium tuberculosis* complex mycobacteria as amoeba-resistant organisms, *PLoS ONE* 6, e20499

Medical Research Council (1925) Tuberculin tests in cattle with special reference to the intradermal test, *Medical Research Council, Special Report Series* 94 London: HMSO

Medical Research Council (1932) Vitamins: a survey of our present knowledge, *Medical Research Council, Special Report Series* 167 London: HMSO

Medical Research Council (1952) National tuberculosis survey 1949-1950: background and methods of survey, *Lancet* i, 775-85

Mendelson, A. (2011) In bacteria land: the battle over raw milk, *Gastronomica* 11, 1, 35-43

Menton, J. (1930) Bovine tuberculosis in relation to the public milk supply, *Medical Officer* 43, 153-5

Menzies, F.D. et al. (2011) A comparison of badger activity in two areas of high and low bovine tuberculosis incidence of Northern Ireland, *Veterinary Microbiology* 151, 112-19

Menzies, F.D. and Neill, S.D. (2000) Cattle-to-cattle transmission of bovine tuberculosis, *Veterinary Journal* 160, 92-106

Meyer-Renschhausen, E. and Wirz, A. (1999) Dietetics, health reform and social order: vegetarianism as a moral physiology. The example of Maximilian Bircher-Benner (1867-1939), *Medical History* 43, 323-41

Meyn, A. (1952) Die Bekämpfung der Rindertuberkulose in der Bundesrepublik, *Monatshefte der Tierheilkunde* 4, 510-26

Michel, A.L., Müller, B. and van Helden, P.D. (2010) *Mycobacterium bovis* at the animal-human interface: a problem, or not? *Veterinary Microbiology* 140, 371-81

Milk Nutrition Committee (1937) *Milk experiments reported to the Milk Nutrition Committee. Part I. The effect of commercial pasteurisation on the nutritive value of milk, as determined by laboratory experiment* Reading: National Institute for Research in Dairying

Milk Nutrition Committee (1938a) *Milk and Nutrition: new experiments reported to the Milk Nutrition Committee. Part II. The effects of dietary supplements of pasteurised and raw milk on the growth and health of school children (interim report)* Reading: National Institute for Research in Dairying

Milk Nutrition Committee (1938b) *Milk and Nutrition: new experiments reported to the Milk Nutrition Committee. Part III. The effect of commercial pasteurisation on the nutritive value of milk as determined by experiments on calves* Reading: National Institute for Research in Dairying

Milk Nutrition Committee (1939) *Milk and Nutrition. New experiments reported to the Milk Nutrition Committee. Part IV. The Effects of dietary supplements of pasteurised and raw milk on the growth and health of school children (final report); summary of all researches carried out by the Committee and practical conclusions* Reading: National Institute for Research in Dairying

Mill, A.C. et al. (2012) Farm-scale risk factors for bovine tuberculosis incidence in cattle herds during the Randomized Badger Culling Trial, *Epidemiology and Infection* 140, 219-30

Miller, D. (1999) Risk, science and policy: definitional struggles, information management, the media and BSE, *Social Science and Medicine* 49, 1239-55

Millstone, E. and Van Zwanenberg, P. (2001) Politics of expert advice: lessons from the early history of the BSE saga, *Science and Public Policy* 28, 99-112

Ministry of Agriculture and Fisheries (1933) Report of the Reorganization Commission on Milk [Chairman: E. Grigg], *Ministry of Agriculture and Fisheries, Economic Series* 38

Ministry of Agriculture and Fisheries (1953) *Tuberculosis (Attested Herds) Scheme: ear marking of cattle* Tolworth: MAF

Ministry of Agriculture, Fisheries and Food (1965) *Animal health: a centenary, 1865-1965* London: HMSO

Ministry of Health (1931) A memorandum on bovine tuberculosis in man, with special reference to infection by milk, *Reports on Public Health and Medical Subjects* 63

Mitchell, A. et al. (2008) An analysis of the effect of the introduction of pre-movement testing for bovine TB in England and Wales, pp 172-90 in Society for Veterinary Epidemiology and Preventive Medicine (Eds) *Proceedings of a meeting held at Liverpool, UK, on the 26th-28th March 2008*

Mitchell, A. et al. (2005) Characteristics of cattle movements in Britain – an analysis of records from the Cattle Tracing System, *Animal Science* 80, 265-73

Mitchell, A.P. (1914) Report on tuberculous milk in Edinburgh, *British Medical Journal* ii, 71-2

Mitchell, A.P. et al. (2006) An analysis of single intradermal comparative cervical test (SICCT) coverage in GB cattle population, pp 70-86 in Mellor, D.J., Russell, A.M. (Eds) *Proceedings of the Conference of the Society for Veterinary Epidemiology and Preventive Medicine, Exeter*

Mitchell, B.R. (1988) *British historical statistics* Cambridge: Cambridge University Press

Mitchell, T. (2002) *Rule of experts* Oakland, CA: University of California Press

Mol, A. (2002) *The body multiple* Durham, NC: Duke University Press

Monaghan, M.L. et al. (1994) The tuberculin test, *Veterinary Microbiology* 40, 111-24

Mond, Sir R.L. (1914) *Mid-Cheshire Farmers' Association. Sterilization of milk: its danger to infants. Lecture at Knutsford reprinted from the Knutsford Division Guardian* Knutsford: Mackie & Co.

Monrad, J.H. (1901) *Pasteurization and milk preservation, with a chapter on selling milk* Winnetka, IL: Author

Montgomerie, R.F. (1937) The incidence of tuberculosis in cattle breeding districts, *Journal of the Royal on the Sanitary Institute* 57, 514-20

Mooney, G. (2009) Diagnostic spaces: workhouse, hospital and home in mid-Victorian London, *Social Science History* 33, 357-90

Moore, S.G. (1921) *This concerns you* London: St Catherine's Press

Moore, J.A.H. and Roper, T.J. (2003) Temperature and humidity in badger *Meles meles* setts, *Mammal Review* 33, 308-13

Moore, V.A. (1913) *Bovine tuberculosis and its control* Ithaca: Carpenter

Moore-Colyer, R.J. (2001) Back to basics: Rolf Gardiner, H. J. Massingham and A Kinship in Husbandry, *Rural History* 12, 85-108

Moore-Colyer, R.J. (2004) Towards 'mother earth': Jorian Jenks, organicism, the right and the British Union of Fascists, *Journal of Contemporary History* 39, 353-71

Moore-Colyer, R.J. (2011) Rolf Gardiner, farming and the English landscape, pp 95-119 in Jefferies, M. and Tyldesley, M. (Eds) *Rolf Gardiner: folk, nature and culture in interwar Britain* Farnham: Ashgate

Moore-Colyer, R.J. and Conford, P. (2004) A 'Secret Society'? The internal and external relations of the Kinship in Husbandry, 1941-1952, *Rural History* 15, 189-206

Morris, R.S., Pfeiffer, D.U. and Jackson, R. (1994) The epidemiology of *Mycobacterium bovis* infections, *Veterinary Microbiology* 40, 153-77

Mullen, E.M. et al. (2013) Foraging Eurasian badgers *Meles meles* and the presence of cattle in pastures. Do badgers avoid cattle? *Applied Animal Behaviour Science* 144, 130-37

Munro, R. (2014) *Pilot badger culls in Somerset and Gloucestershire: report by the Independent Expert Panel* London: Defra

Munro, W.T. (1945) Diet and tuberculosis, *Proceedings of the Nutrition Society* 3, 155-6

Munroe, F.A. et al. (1999) Risk factors for the between-herd spread of Mycobacterium bovis in Canadian cattle and cervids between 1985 and 1994, *Preventive Veterinary Medicine* 41, 119-33

Murhead, R.H. and Burns, K.J. (1974) Tuberculosis in wild badgers in Gloucestershire: epidemiology, *Veterinary Record* 95, 522-55

Murphy, D. et al. (2011) Tuberculosis in cattle herds are sentinels for Mycobacterium bovis infection in European badgers (*Meles meles*): the Irish Greenfield Study, *Veterinary Microbiology* 151, 120-25

Myers, J.A. (1940) *Man's greatest victory over tuberculosis* Springfield, IL: Thomas

Myers, J.A. (1977) *Captain of all those men of death: tuberculosis historical highlights* St Louis, MO: W.H. Green

Myers, J.A. and Steele, J.H. (1969) *Bovine tuberculosis: control in man and animals* St Louis, Missouri: W.H. Green

National Audit Office (2003) *Livestock identification and tracing in England:*

report by the Conptroller and Auditor General London: Stationery Office

National Farmers' Union (2012) NFU Conference 2012, February 21-22, The ICC, Birmingham, http://www.nfuonline.com/News/NFU-Conference-2012/NFU-Conference-2012,-February-21-22,-The-ICC,-Birmingham/ [accessed 12 June 2012]

National Milk Conference Committee (1926) *Report of the proceedings of the National Milk Conference. Subject: milk in relation to public health* London: National Clean Milk Society

National Veterinary Association (1891) *Proceedings of the ninth general meeting of the National Veterinary Association held at the Guildhall, Doncaster on Tuesday and Wednesday, July 21st and 22nd, 1891* Birmingham: G. Jones & Son

Naylor, R., Maye, D., Ilbery, B., Enticott, G. and Kirwan, J. (2014) Researching controversial and sensitive issues: using visual vignettes to explore farmers' attitudes towards the control of bovine tuberculosis in England, *Area* 46, 285-93

Neill, S.D., Bryson, D.G. and Pollock, J.M. (2001) Pathogenesis of tuberculosis in cattle, *Tuberculosis* 81, 79-86

Neill, S.D. et al. (1988) Excretion of Mycobacterium bovis by experimentally infected cattle, *Veterinary Record* 123, 340-43

Neill S. D. et al. (1989) Transmission of tuberculosis from experimentally infected cattle to in-contact calves, *Veterinary Record* 124, 269-71

Neill, S.D. et al. (1994) Pathogenesis of *Mycobacterium bovis* infection in cattle, *Veterinary Microbiology* 40, 41-52

Neill, S.D., Skuce, R.A. and Pollock, J.M. (2005) Tuberculosis – new light from an old window, *Journal of Applied Microbiology* 98, 1261-9

Nelkin, D. (Ed.)(1992) *Controversy: politics of technical decisions* Newbury Park: Sage

Newman, G. (1926) Report on public health, *British Medical Journal* ii, 566

Newsholme, A. (1910) *The prevention of tuberculosis* London: Methuen

Newsholme, A. (1935) *Fifty years in public health* London: Allen & Unwin

Newton, J. (1924) The unreliability of the Tuberculin Test, *Milk Industry* 5, 5, 59-61

Newton, J. (1932) Pasteurized or raw milk?, *The Cooperative News* 26 November, 11

Ney, S. and Verweij, M. (2015) Messy institutions for wicked problems: how to generate clumsy solutions, *Environment and Planning C* forthcoming

Nimmo, R. (2010) *Milk, modernity and the making of the human* London: Routledge

Niven, J. (1902) The administration of the Manchester Milk Clauses, pp 282-93 in *Transactions of the British Congress on Tuberculosis for the Prevention of Consumption, London, July 22nd to July 26th, 1901. Volume 2: report of the state section* London: Clowes

Niven, J. (1908) Eradication of tuberculosis, *Veterinary Record* 20, 762-9

Niven, J. (1923) *Observations on the history of public health effort in Manchester* Manchester: Heywood

Nocard, E. (1895) *The animal tuberculoses and their relation to human tuberculosis* London: Baillière, Tindall & Cox

Norris, F.J. (1928) Milk: safeguards required to ensure its freedom from bovine infection, *Journal of State Medicine* 36, 714-25

North, C. (1922) Safeguarding milk, pp 159-79 in National Milk Conference Committee (Eds) *Report of the proceedings of the National Milk Conference* London: National Clean Milk Society

North, R. (1943) Poisoned milk - the facts, *The Sunday Pictorial* 23 May, 5

Nugent, G. (2011) Maintenance, spillover and spillback transmission of bovine tuberculosis in multi-host wildlife complexes: a New Zealand case study, *Veterinary Microbiology* 151, 34-42

O'Connor, C.M., Haydon, D.T. and Kao, R.R. (2012) An ecological and comparative perspective on the control of bovine tuberculosis in Great Britain and the Republic of Ireland, *Preventive Veterinary Medicine* 104, 185-97

Oddy, D.J. (2003) *From plain fare to fusion food: the British diet from the 1890s to the 1990s* Woodbridge: Boydell & Brewer

Office International des Épizooties (2009) Bovine tuberculosis, Chapter 2.4.7 in *Manual of diagnostic tests and vaccines for terrestrial animals* Paris: OIE

O'Hare, A. et al. (2014) Estimating epidemiological parameters for bovine tuberculosis in British cattle using a Bayesian partial-likelihood approach, *Proceedings of the Royal Society B* 281, 20140248

Olea-Popelka F. et al. (2006) A case study of bovine tuberculosis in an area of County Donegal, *Irish Veterinary Journal* 59, 683-90

Olea-Popelka, F.J. et al. (2008) Risk factors for disclosure of additional tuberculous cattle in attested clear herds that had one animal with a confirmed lesion of tuberculosis at slaughter during 2003 in Ireland, *Preventive Veterinary Medicine* 85, 81-91

Olea-Popelka, F.J. et al. (2005) Spatial relationship between *Mycobacterium bovis* strains in cattle and badgers in four areas in Ireland, *Preventive Veterinary Medicine* 71, 57-70

Olmstead, A.L. and Rhode, P.W. (2004a) An impossible undertaking: the eradication of bovine tuberculosis in the United States, *Journal of Economic History* 64: 734-72

Olmstead, A.L. and Rhode, P.W. (2004b) The "Tuberculous Cattle Trust": Disease Contagion in an Era of Regulatory Uncertainty, *Journal of Economic History* 64, 929-63

Olmstead, A.L. and Rhode, P.W. (2007) Not on my farm! Resistance to bovine tuberculosis eradication in the United States, *Journal of Economic History* 67, 768-809

Olmstead, A.L. and Rhode, P.W. (2012) The eradication of bovine tuberculosis in the United States in a comparative perspective, pp 7-30 in Zilberman, D., Otte, J., Roland-Holst, D. and Pfeiffer, D. (Eds) *Health and animal agriculture in developing countries* New York: Springer

Ó'Máirtín, D. et al. (1998) The effect of a badger removal programme on the incidence of tuberculosis in an Irish cattle population, *Preventive Veterinary Medicine* 34, 47-56

O'Reilly, L.M. and Daborn, C.J. (1995) The epidemiology of *Mycobacterium bovis* infections in animals and man: a review, *Tubercle and Lung Disease* 76, Supplement 1, 1-46

Ormerod, P. (2014) Non-respiratory tuberculosis, pp 167-87 in Davies, P.D.O., Gordon, S.B. and Davies, G. (Eds) *Clinical tuberculosis* Boca Raton: CRC Press

Orr, J.B. (1936) *Food, health and income* London: Macmillan

Palmer, M.V. and Waters, W.R. (2011) Bovine tuberculosis and the establishment of an eradication programme in the United States: role of veterinarians, *Veterinary Medicine International* Article ID 816345

Palmer, M.V. et al. (2012) Mycobacterium bovis: a model pathogen at the interface of livestock,wildlife, and humans, *Veterinary Medicine International* Article ID 236205

Parker, H.N. (1917) *City milk supply* New York: McGraw Hill

Paterson, A.B. (1948) The production of bovine tuberculoprotein, *Journal of Comparative Pathology* 58, 302-13

Pattison, I. (1981) *John McFadyean: a great British veterinarian* London: J.A. Allen

Pattison, I. (1984) *The British veterinary profession, 1791-1948* London: J.A. Allen

Pellizzoni, L. (2014) Metaphors and problematizations: notes for a research programme on new materialism, *Tecnoscienza* 5, 2, 73-91

Pennington, C. (1982) Tuberculosis, pp 86-99 in Checkland, O.

and Lamb, M. (Eds) *Health care as social history: the Glasgow case* Aberdeen: Aberdeen University Press

People's League of Health (1932a) *Report of a special committee appointed by the People's League of Health (Inc.) to make a survey of tuberculosis of bovine origin in Great Britain* London: People's League of Health

People's League of Health [1932b] *The need for a safe milk supply: some medical opinions* London: People's League of Health

People's League of Health (1934) *Milk for school children: report of a Special Committee of the Medical, Science and Veterinary Councils of the People's League of Health (Incorporated)* London: People's League of Health

People's League of Health (1943) *A safe milk supply: memorandum of the People's League of Health on the compulsory pasteurization of milk* London: People's League of Health

Pérez-Lago, L., Navarro, Y. and García-de-Viedma, D. (2014) Current knowledge and pending challenges in zoonosis caused by *Mycobacterium bovis*: a review, *Research in Veterinary Science* 97, S94-100

Perren, R. (1978) *The meat trade in Britain 1840-1914* London: Routledge & Kegan Paul

Perren, R. (1989) The manufacture and marketing of veterinary products from 1850-1914, *Veterinary History* 6, 2, 43-61

Petersen, G. (1938) The principles of prophylaxis of bovine tuberculosis in Denmark, *Bulletin de l'Office International des Epizooties* 15, 662-9

Pfeiffer, D.U. (2013) Epidemiology caught in the causal web of bovine tuberculosis, *Transboundary and Emerging Diseases* 60, Supp. 1, 104-10

Phillips, B. (1846) *Scrofula: its nature, its causes, its prevalence, and the principles of treatment* London: Baillière

Phillips, C.J.C. et al. (2000) TB and cattle husbandry: the role of cattle husbandry in the development of a sustainable policy to control

M.bovis infection in cattle: report of the Independent Husbandry Panel London: MAFF

Phillips, C.J.C. et al. (2002) Genetic and management factors that influence the susceptibility of cattle to *Mycobacterium bovis* infection, *Animal Heath Research Reviews* 3, 3-13

Phillips, C.J.C. et al. (2003) The transmission of *Mycobacterium bovis* infection to cattle, *Research in Veterinary Science* 74, 1-15

Pickering, A. (1995) *The mangle of practice* Chicago: University of Chicago Press

Pickering, A. (2005) Decentring sociology: synthetic dyes and social theory, *Perspectives on Science* 13, 352-405

Picton, L.J. (1938) Pasteurisation of milk, *British Medical Journal i*, 812

Plimmer, R.H.A. and Plimmer, V.G. (1925) *Food, health and vitamins* London: Longmans, Green & Co.

Plimmer, V.G. and Plimmer, R.H.A. (1922) *Vitamins and the choice of food* London: Longmans, Green & Co.

Pollock, J.I. (2006) Two controlled trials of supplementary feeding of British school children in the 1920s, *Journal of the Royal Society of Medicine* 99, 323-7

Pollock, J.M. and Neill, S.D. (2002) Mycobacterium bovis infection and tuberculosis in cattle, *Veterinary Journal* 163, 115-27

Pollock, J.M. et al. (2006) Pathogenesis of bovine tuberculosis: the role of experimental models of infection, *Veterinary Microbiology* 112, 141-50

Ponnuswamy, A. (2014) Respiratory tuberculosis, pp 129-50 in Davies, P.D.O., Gordon, S.B. and Davies, G. (Eds) *Clinical tuberculosis* Boca Raton: CRC Press

Ponting, C. (1986) *Whitehall: tragedy and farce* London: Hamilton

Pool, W.A. (1946) Discussion on the methods to be employed in eradicating tuberculosis of bovine origin from the human and animal populations, *Proceedings of the Royal Society of Medicine* 39, 213-22

Pope, L.C. et al. (2007) Genetic evidence that culling increases badger movement: implications for the spread of bovine tuberculosis, *Molecular Ecology* 16, 4919-29

Pritchard, D.G. (1988) A century of bovine tuberculosis 1888-1988: conquest and controversy, *Journal of Comparative Pathology* 99, 357-99

Pullinger, E.J. (1934) The incidence of tubercle bacilli and *Brucella abortus* in milk, *Lancet* i, 967-71

Rabagliati, D.S. (1930) Veterinary science in relation to state and municipal control, *Journal of the Royal Sanitary Institution* 51, 233-41

Rabagliati, D.S. (1932) The veterinary profession and the milk supply, *Veterinary Record* 12, 572, 1403-07

RADAR (2008) *The cattle book 2008* York: Defra

Raison, C. and Ashby, A.W. (1934) *The Milk Marketing Board: its objects and regulations briefly described, together with a producer retailers guide to the Milk marketing scheme* London: Virtue & Co Ltd

Ramírez-Villaescusa, A.M. et al. (2009) Herd and individual animal risks associated with bovine tuberculosis skin test positivity in cattle in herds in south west England, *Preventive Veterinary Medicine* 92 (2009) 188-98

Ramírez-Villaescusa, A.M. et al. (2010) Risk factors for herd breakdown with bovine tuberculosis in 148 cattle herds in the south west of England, *Preventive Veterinary Medicine* 95, 224-30

Ravenel, M.P. (1902) The intercommunicability of human and bovine tuberculosis, *Journal of Comparative Pathology and Therapeutics* 15, 112-43

Redford, A. and Russell, I.S. (1940) *The history of local government in Manchester. Volume III: the last half century* London: Longmans, Green & Co.

Reilly, L.A. and Courtenay, O. (2007) Husbandry practices, badger sett density and habitat composition as risk factors for transient and persistent bovine tuberculosis on UK cattle farms, *Preventive Veterinary Medicine* 80, 129-42

Reilly, L.V. (1950) Human tuberculosis of bovine origin in Northern Ireland, *Journal of Hygiene* 48, 464-71

Reviriego Gordejo, F.J. and Vermeersch, J.P. (2006) Towards eradication of bovine tuberculosis in the European Union, *Veterinary Microbiology* 112, no. 2-4, 101-09

Rheinberger, H-J. (1997) *Toward a history of epistemic things* Stanford, CA: Stanford University Press

Rheinberger, H-J. (2010) *Epistemology of the concrete* Durham, NC: Duke University Press

Rhodes, R.T. (1929) Milk and Dairies Order, 1926, *Journal of the Royal Sanitary Institute* 50, 25-35

Rich, A.R. (1944) *The pathogenesis of tuberculosis* Springfield, IL: Thomas

Richardson, J.J. (Ed.)(1993) *Pressure groups* Oxford: Oxford University Press

Richardson, J.J., Gustafsson, G. and Jordan, G. (1982) The concept of policy style, pp 1-16 in Richardson, J.J. (Ed.) *Policy styles in western Europe* London: Allen & Unwin

Richardson, J.J., Jordan, A.G. and Kimber, R.H. (1978) Lobbying, administrative reform and policy styles: the case of land drainage, *Political Studies* 26, 47-64

Ritchie, J.N. (1945) The progress of eradication of tuberculosis from cattle in Great Britain, *Proceedings of the Nutrition Society* 3, 180-85

Ritchie, J.N. Sir (1959) *Britain's achievement in the eradication of bovine tuberculosis: the George Scott Robertson Memorial Lecture, the Queen's University of Belfast* Belfast: Boyd

Ritchie, M. et al. (2011) *Bovine TB: time for a rethink* [np:] Rethink Bovine TB

Ritz, N. et al. (2008) Influence of BCG vaccine strain on the immune response and protection against tuberculosis, *FEMS Microbiology Reviews* 132, 821-41

Riviere, C. (1917) *Tuberculosis and how to avoid it* London: Methuen

Reviriego Gordejo, F.J. and Vermeersch, J.P. (2006) Towards eradication of bovine tuberculosis in the European Union, *Veterinary Microbiology* 112, 101-09

Roadhouse, C.L. and Henderson, J.L. (1941) *The market-milk industry* New York: McGraw-Hill

Robbe-Austerman, S. and Turcotte, C. (2014) New and current approaches for isolation, identification, and genotyping of Mycobacterium bovis, pp 89-98 in Thoen, C.O., Steele, J.H. and Kaneene, J.B. (Eds) *Zoonotic tuberculosis: Mycobacterium bovis and other pathogenic mycobacteria* Ames, IA: Wiley-Blackwell

Robbins, P. (2012) *Political ecology* Chichester: Wiley-Blackwell

Robbins, P. and Marks, B. (2010) Assemblage geographies, pp 176-95 in Smith, S.J. et al. (Eds) *The SAGE handbook of social geographies* London: SAGE

Roberts, A.E. (1973) Feeding and mortality in the early months of life; changes in medical opinion and popular feeding practice, 1850-1900, unpublished Ph.D. thesis, University of Hull

Roberts, T. (1986) A retrospective assessment of human health protection benefits from removal of tuberculous beef, *Journal of Food Protection* 49, 293-8

Robertson, J. (1909) The prevention of tuberculosis among cattle, Paper read to the Society of Medical Officers of Health April 2nd 1909, *Lancet* i, 1113-4

Robbins, P. (2012) *Political ecology* Chichester: Wiley-Blackwell

Robbins, P. and Marks, B. (2010) Assemblage geographies, pp 176-95 in Smith, S.J., Pain, R., Marston, S.A. and Jones, J.P. (Eds) *The SAGE handbook of social geographies* London: Sage

Robinson, A. (1923) An analysis of the Milk & Dairies (Amendment) Act, 1922, *Medical Officer* 29, 30-31

Robinson, P.A. (2014) A political ecology of bovine tuberculosis eradication in Northern Ireland, unpublished PhD thesis, University of Durham

Robinson, S.E., Everett, M.G. and Christley, R.M. (2007) Recent network evolution increases the potential for large epidemics in the British cattle population, *Journal of the Royal Society Interface* 4, 669-74

Rodriguez-Campos, S. et al. (2014) Overview and phylogeny of *Mycobacterium tuberculosis* complex organisms: Implications for diagnostics and legislation of bovine tuberculosis, *Research in Veterinary Science* 97, S5-19

Roper, T.J. (1925) False statements: a denial and an explanation, *Milk Industry* 5, 11, 42-3

Roper, T.J. (2010) *Badger* London: Collins

Rose, M. (2002) The seductions of resistance: power, politics, and a performative style of systems, *Environment and Planning D: Society and Space* 20, 383-400

Rose N. (1991) Governing by numbers: figuring out democracy, *Accounting, Organizations and Society* 16, 673-92

Rosenau, M.J. (1912) *The milk question* Boston: Houghton Mifflin

Rosenkrantz, B.G. (1985) The trouble with bovine tuberculosis, *Bulletin of the History of Medicine* 59, 155-75

Rowland, P. (1971) *The last liberal governments: unfinished business, 1911-1914* London: Barrie & Jenkins

Ruddock-West, T. (1937) Demonstration of tubercle bacilli in milk by cultural method, *Journal of the Royal Sanitary Institute* 57, 524-7

Russell, J.B. (1889) *On the sanitary requirements of a dairy farm* Glasgow: Macdougall

Salmon, D.E. (1906) Tuberculosis of the food producing animals, *Bulletin, United States Department of Agriculture, Bureau of Animal Industry* 38

Sanderson, I. (2009) Intelligent policy making for a complex world: pragmatism, evidence and learning, *Political Studies* 57, 699-719

Savage, G. (1987) Friend to the worker: social policy at the Ministry of Agriculture between the wars, *Albion* 19, 193-208

Savage, G. (1996) *The social construction of expertise: the English civil service and its influence, 1919-1939* Pittsburgh, PA: University of Pittsburgh Press

Savage, W.G. (1912) *Milk and the public health* London: Macmillan

Savage, W.G. (1926a) The working of the 1924 meat regulations in rural areas, *Journal of State Medicine* 34, 716-22

Savage, W.G. (1926b) Recent legislation and the problem of human tuberculosis of bovine origin, *Journal of State Medicine* 34, 497-507

Savage, W.G. (1927a) Bovine tuberculosis and the Tuberculosis Order, *Veterinary Journal* 83, 227-38

Savage, W.G. (1927b) Bovine tuberculosis and the Tuberculosis Order, 1925, *Lancet* i, 722-5

Savage, W.G. (1928) Milk and tuberculosis, *Journal of the Royal Sanitary Institute* 49, 339-45

Savage, W.G. (1929a) *The prevention of human tuberculosis of bovine origin* London: Macmillan

Savage, W.G. (1929b) Methods for the reduction of human tuberculosis of bovine origin, *British Medical Journal* ii, 492-5

Savage, W.G. (1931a) Pasteurisation in relation to milk distribution, *Lancet* i, 543-6

Savage, W.G. (1931b) Routine veterinary inspection of dairy cattle: mainly from the point of view of tuberculosis, *Medical Officer* 46, 128-2

Savage, W.G. (1932) Laboratory tests and milk control, *Medical Officer* 49, 231-2

Savage, W.G. (1938) Safety factor of designated and other types of liquid milk, *Lancet* i, 42-3

Savage, W.G. (1949) Milkborne infections in Great Britain, *British Journal of Social Medicine* 3, 45-55

Scanlon, M.P. and Quinn, P.J. (2000) The survival of *Mycobacterium bovis* in sterilised cattle slurry and its relevance to the persistence of this pathogen in the environment, *Irish Veterinary Journal* 53, 412-15

Schaafsma, G. (1995) Effects of light exposure, storage and packaging on the nutrient content of milk, *International Dairy Federation Nutrition Newsletter* 4, 2

Scantlebury, M. et al. (2006) Individual trade-offs between nutrition and risk of interspecific transmission of disease by grazing: cows, badger latrines and bovine tuberculosis, *Behaviour* 143, 141-58

Schatzki, T. (2010) Materiality and social life, *Nature and Culture* 5, 2, 123-49

Schatzki, T. (2015) Practice theory as flat ontology, forthcoming in Schäfer, H. (Ed.) *Praxistheorie: ein soziologisches forschungsprogramm* Bielefeld: Transcript

Schiller, I. et al. (2010) Bovine tuberculosis: a review of current and emerging diagnostic techniques in view of their relevance for disease control and eradication, *Transboundary and Emerging Diseases* 57, 205-20

Schiller, I. et al. (2011) Bovine tuberculosis in Europe from the perspective of an officially tuberculosis free country: Trade, surveillance and diagnostics, *Veterinary Microbiology* 151, 153-9

Schneider, G.W. and Winslow, R. (2014) Parts and wholes: the human microbiome, ecological ontology, and the challenges of community, *Perspectives in Biology and Medicine* 57, 208-23

Schonfield, J.K. et al. (1982) Human-to-human spread of infection by *M. bovis, Tubercle* 63, 143-4

Scott, J.C. (1985) *Weapons of the weak: everyday forms of peasant resistance* New Haven: Yale University Press

Scott Henderson, J. (1951) *Report of the Committee on Cruelty to Wild Animals* London: HMSO

Self, P. and Storing, H.J. (1962) *The state and the farmer* London: Allen & Unwin

Self, R. (Ed.)(2000) *The Neville Chamberlain diary letters. Volume 2: the reform letters, 1921-27* Aldershot: Ashgate

Seligman, R. (1932) Pasteurization methods, *Journal of the Royal Sanitary Institute* 53, 19-30

Sessions, H. (1905) *Cattle tuberculosis: a practical guide to the agriculturalist and inspector* London: Baillière, Tindall & Cox

Seyfarth, D. and Seyfarth, H.-J. (1998) The dispute on the pathogenesis of bovine 'perlsucht' (Pearls disease) in the nineteenth century, *Historia Medicinae Veterinariae* 23, 3/4, 86-7

Shaw, W.V. (1919) Report on the pasteurization of milk in England, in *Departmental Committee of Production and Distribution of Milk*, Third Interim Report BPP 1919 (Cmd. 315) xxv.634

Shennan, T. (1914) The morbid anatomy of tuberculosis in man, *Lancet* i, 595-603, 673-8

Shittu, A. et al. (2013) Factors associated with bovine tuberculosis confirmation rates in suspect lesions found in cattle at routine slaughter in Great Britain, 2003-2008, *Preventive Veterinary Medicine* 110, 395-404

Shove, E., Pantzar, M. and Watson, M. (2012) *The dynamics of social practice: everyday life and how it changes* London: SAGE

Sigurdsson, J. (1945) *Studies on the risk of infection with bovine tuberculosis to the rural population: with special reference to pulmonary tuberculosis* Copenhagen: Munksgaard

Simon, J. (1863) Diseases of livestock in their relation to the public supplies of meat and milk, in *Fifth Report of the Medical Officer of the Privy Council*, 1862, BPP 1863 (161) xxv.21-32

Simondon, G. (1964) *L'individu et sa genese physico-biologique* Paris: Presses Universitaires De France

Simondon, G. (2009) The position of the problem of ontogenesis, *Parrhesia* 7, 4-16

Sims Woodhead, G. (1888) Tuberculosis and tabes mesenterica, *Lancet* ii, 51-4

Sims Woodhead, G. (1891) The relations of diseases of animals to those of man, *Journal of the Royal Agricultural Society of England* series 3, 2, 634-40

Singh, H. and Bennett, R.J. (2002) Milk and milk processing, pp 1-38 in Robinson, R.K. (Ed.) *Dairy microbiology handbook* New York: Wiley-Interscience

Sjögren, I. and Sutherland, I. (1975) Studies of tuberculosis in man in relation to infection in cattle, *Tubercle* 56, 113-27

Skuce, R.A., Allen, A.R. and McDowell, S.W.J. (2011) *Bovine tuberculosis (TB): a review of cattle-to-cattle transmission, risk factors and susceptibility* Belfast: DARDNI

Skuce, R.A., Allen, A.R. and McDowell, S.W.J. (2012) Herd-Level risk factors for bovine tuberculosis: a literature review, *Veterinary Medicine International* ID 621210

Skuce, R.A. et al. (2010) *Mycobacterium bovis* genotypes in Northern Ireland: herd-level surveillance (2003 to 2008), *Veterinary Record* 167, 684-9

Skuce, R.A. et al. (2005) Discrimination of isolates of *Mycobacterium bovis* in Northern Ireland on the basis of variable numbers of tandem repeats (VNTRs), *Veterinary Record* 157, 501-504

Smart, N. (1999) *The National Government, 1931-40* Basingstoke: Macmillan

Smith, E.B. (1923) Notes on Section 2, Milk & Dairies (Amendment) Act, 1922, *Medical Officer* 30, 129-30

Smith, F.B. (1988) *The retreat of tuberculosis, 1850-1950* London: Croom Helm

Smith, G.C. et al. (2001) A model of bovine tuberculosis in the badger

Meles meles: the inclusion of cattle and the use of a live test, *Journal of Applied Ecology* 38, 520-35

Smith, G.C. et al. (2006) Modelling disease dynamics and management scenarios, pp 53-77 in Delahay, R.J., Smith, G.C. and Hutchings, M.R. (Eds) *Management of disease in wild mammals* Tokyo: Springer

Smith, G.C. et al. (1995) Modelling bovine tuberculosis in badgers in England: preliminary results, *Mammalia* 59, 639-50

Smith, J. (1950) Milk-borne disease, *Journal of Dairy Research* 17, 91-105

Smith, J. (1959) Milk-borne disease, *Journal of Dairy Research* 26, 88-104

Smith, M.J. (1988) Consumers and agricultural policy: a case of long term exclusion, *University of Essex, Department of Government, Essex Papers in Politics and Government* 48

Smith, M.J. (1989) The Annual Review: the emergence of a corporatist institution? *Political Studies* 37, 81-96

Smith, M.J. (1990) *The politics of agricultural support in Britain: the development of the agricultural policy community* Aldershot: Dartmouth

Smith, M.J. (1993) *Pressure, power and policy: state autonomy and policy networks in Britain and the United States* New York: Harvester Wheatsheaf

Smith, M.J. (1998) Reconceptualizing the British state: theoretical and empirical challenges to central government, *Public Administration* 76, 45-72

Smith, N.H. et al. (2006a) Ecotypes of the *Mycobacterium tuberculosis* complex, *Journal of Theoretical Biology* 239 (2006) 220-25

Smith, N.H. et al. (2006b) Bottlenecks and broomsticks: the molecular evolution of *Mycobacterium bovis*, *Nature Reviews Microbiology* 4, 670-81

Smith, N.H. et al. (2009) Myths and misconceptions: the origin and evolution of Mycobacterium tuberculosis, *Nature Reviews Microbiology* 7, 537-44

Smith, N.H. and Upton, P. (2012) Naming spoligotype patterns for the RD9-deleted lineage of the Mycobacterium tuberculosis complex, *Infection, Genetics and Evolution* 12, 873-6

Smythe, R.H. (1927) The eradication of bovine tuberculosis, *Veterinary Record* 7, 548-9

Society for General Microbiology (2008) *Independent overview of bovine tuberculosis research in the United Kingdom* London: Defra

Society of Dairy Technology (1953) *Pasteurizing plant manual* London: Society of Dairy Technology

Speake, S.W. (2011) Infectious milk: issues of pathogenic certainty within ideational regimes and their biopolitical implications, *Studies in History and Philosophy of Biological and Biomedical Sciences* 42, 530-41

Spencer, A. (2008) The changing governance of UK animal health policy 1997-2008, unpublished PhD thesis, University of Nottingham

Spencer, A. (2011) One body of evidence, three different policies: bovine tuberculosis policy in Britain, *Politics* 31, 91-9

Spinage, C. A. (2003) *Cattle plague: a history* New York: Kluwer

Stamp, J.T. (1943) Tuberculosis of the bovine udder, *Journal of Comparative Pathology and Therapeutics* 53, 220-30

Stamp, J.T. (1944) A review of the pathogenesis and pathology of bovine tuberculosis with special reference to practical problems, *Veterinary Record* 56, 443-6

Stamp, J.T. (1948) Bovine pulmonary tuberculosis, *Journal of Comparative Pathology and Therapeutics* 58, 9-23

Stamp, J.T. and Wilson, A. (1946) Some aspects of the pathogenesis of bovine tuberculosis based on abattoir returns, *Veterinary Record* 58, 11-15

Stanziani, A. (2005) *Histoire de la qualité alimentaire (XIXe-XXe siècle)* Paris: Seuil

Stead, D.R. (2004) Risk and risk management in English agriculture, c. 1750-1850, *Economic History Review* 57, 334-61

Steele, J.H. (2000) History, trends, and extent of pasteurization, *Journal of the American Veterinary Medical Association* 15, 175-8

Stiles, H.J. (1913) The necessity for a more thorough control of the milk supply in combating surgical tuberculosis in childhood, *British Medical Journal* 11, 370-71

Still, G.F. (1899) Observations on the morbid anatomy of tuberculosis in childhood, *British Medical Journal* ii, 455-8

Still, G.F. (1901) Abdominal tuberculosis in children, *Clinical Journal* 19, 113-20

Stirland, R.M. (1984) Auguste Sheridan Delépine, 1855-1921, pp 107-112 in Elwood, W.J. and Tuxford, A.F. (Eds) *Some Manchester doctors* Manchester: Manchester Medical Society

Stocking, S.H. and Holstein, L.W. (1993) Constructing and reconstructing scientific ignorance, *Knowledge: Creation, Diffusion, Utilization* 15, 186-210

Stockman, S. (1925) Tuberculosis and the milk supply, *Veterinary Record* 5, 39-41

Sutherland, H. (1938) Pasteurisation of milk, *British Medical Journal i*, 704, 812, 918, 1028

Swaving, A.J. (1928) Guarantees as to purity, genuineness and composition of the Dutch milk and milk products, pp 157-77 in *World's Dairy Congress – 1928: report of proceedings, Great Britain, June 26th-July 12th* London: World's Dairy Congress Committee

Swithinbank, H. and Newman, G. (1903) *Bacteriology of milk* London: Murray

Szmaragd, C. et al. (2012) Impact of imperfect test sensitivity on determining risk factors: the case of bovine tuberculosis, *PLoS ONE* 7, e43116

Szmaragd, C. et al. (2013) Factors associated with herd restriction and de-restriction with bovine tuberculosis in British cattle herds, *Preventive Veterinary Medicine* 111, 31-41

Szreter, S. (1991) The GRO and the public health movement in Britain, 1837-1914, *Social History of Medicine* 4, 435-64

Tamime, A. (Ed.)(2009) *Milk processing and quality management* Oxford: Blackwell

Taylor, D. (1976) The English dairy industry, 1860-1930, *Economic History Review* 2nd series 29, 585-601

Taylor, D. (1987) Growth and structural change in the English dairy industry, c.1860-1930, *Agricultural History Review*, 35, 47-64

Taylor, E.M.M. (1979) The politics of Walter Elliot, unpublished PhD thesis, University of Edinburgh

Termeer, C.J.A.M. et al. (2013) Governance capabilities for dealing wisely with wicked problems, *Administration & Society* 20, 10, 1-31

Thévenot, L. (2006) Convention school, pp 111-15 in Beckert, J. and Zafirovski, M. (Eds) *International encyclopedia of economic sociology* Abingdon: Routledge

Thoen, C.O. and Barletta, R.G. (2014) Pathogenesis of tuberculosis caused by Mycobacterium bovis, pp 51-62 in Thoen, C.O., Steele, J.H. and Kaneene, J.B. (Eds) *Zoonotic tuberculosis: Mycobacterium bovis and other pathogenic mycobacteria* Ames, IA: Wiley-Blackwell

Thoen, C., LoBue, P., and de Kantor, I. (2006) The importance of *Mycobacterium bovis* as a zoonosis, *Veterinary Microbiology* 112, 339-45

Thoen, C., LoBue, P. and de Kantor, I. (2010) Why has zoonotic tuberculosis not received much attention? *International Journal of Tuberculosis and Lung Disease* 14, 1073-4

Thoen, C., LoBue, P., and Enarson, D.A. (2014) Tuberculosis in animals and humans: an introduction, pp 3-7 in Thoen, C.O., Steele, J.H. and Kaneene, J.B. (Eds) *Zoonotic tuberculosis: Mycobacterium bovis and other pathogenic mycobacteria* Ames, IA: Wiley-Blackwell

Thoen, C.O. et al. (2009) Tuberculosis: a re-emerging disease in animals and humans, *Veterinaria Italiana* 45, 135-81

Thomson, J. and Fordyce, A.D. (1908) On the relative prevalence of abdominal and meningeal tuberculosis in children in different countries as shown by clinical hospital statistics, pp 115-19 in Kelynack, T.N. (Ed.) *Tuberculosis in infancy and childhood* New York: Wood

Thorne Thorne, Sir R. (1899) *The administrative control of tuberculosis* London: Baillière, Tindall & Cox

Thornton, H. (1949, 1962) *Text book of meat inspection, including the inspection of rabbits and poultry* 1st and 4th eds London: Baillière, Tindall & Cox

Thwaites, G. (2014) Tuberculosis of the central nervous system, pp 151-65 in Davies, P.D.O., Gordon, S.B. and Davies, G. (Eds) *Clinical tuberculosis* Boca Raton: CRC Press

Tolhurst, B.A. et al. (2009) Behaviour of badgers (*Meles meles*) in farm buildings: Opportunities for the transmission of *Mycobacterium bovis* to cattle? *Applied Animal Behaviour Science* 117, 103-13

Tolhurst, B.A. et al. (2008) The behavioural responses of badgers (*Meles meles*) to exclusion from farm buildings using an electric fence, *Applied Animal Behaviour Science* 113, 224-35

Transactions of the British Congress on Tuberculosis for the Prevention of Consumption, London, July 22nd to July 26th, 1901 London: Clowes

Transactions of the Sixth International Congress on Tuberculosis, Washington, September 28 to October 5 1908, 6 vols Philadelphia: Fell

Trentmann, F. (1994) Civilization and its discontents: English neo-romanticism and the transformation of anti-modernism in twentieth century western culture, *Journal of Contemporary History* 29, 583-625

Tsairidou, S. et al. (2014) Genomic prediction for tuberculosis resistance in dairy cattle, *Plos One* 9, 5, e96728

Tustin, P.B. (1929) Retail aspects of milk hygiene, *Journal of the Royal Sanitary Institute* 50, 312-15, 322-3

Van Arendonk, J.A.M. and Liinamo, A.E. (2003) Dairy cattle production in Europe, *Theriogenology* 59, 563-9

Vanclay, F. and Enticott, G. (2011) The role and functioning of cultural scripts in farming and agriculture, *Sociologia Ruralis* 51, 256-71

Van Loon, J. (2002) A contagious living fluid objectification and assemblage in the history of virology, *Theory, Culture and Society* 19, 107-24

Van Zwanenbeg, P. and Millstone, E. (2003) BSE: a paradigm of policy failure, *Political Quarterly* 74, 27-37

Van Zwanenberg, P. and Millstone, E. (2005) *BSE: risk, science and governance* Oxford: Oxford University Press

Varnam, A.H. (1994) *Milk and milk products: technology, chemistry, and microbiology* London: Chapman & Hall

Verma, R. (2006) The status of *Mycobacterium bovis* in India, pp 161-72 in Thoen, C.O., Steele, J.H. and Gilsdorf, M.J. (Eds) *Mycobacterium bovis infection in animals and humans* Ames, IA: Blackwell

Vernon, M.C. (2010) Spatial spread of farm animal diseases, unpublished PhD thesis, University of Cambridge

Vernon, M.C. (2011) Demographics of cattle movements in the United Kingdom, *BMC Veterinary Research* 7, 31

Vernon, M.C. and Keeling, M.J. (2009) Representing the UK's cattle herd as static and dynamic networks, *Proceedings of the Royal Society B* 276, 469-76

Vial, F., Johnston, W.T. and Donnelly, C.A. (2011) Local cattle and badger populations affect the risk of confirmed tuberculosis in British cattle herds, *PLoS ONE* 6, 3, e18058

Vial, F. et al. (2013) Bovine tuberculosis risk factors for British herds before and after the 2001 foot-and-mouth epidemic: what have we learned from the TB99 and CCS2005 studies? *Transboundary and Emerging Diseases* DOI: 10.1111/tbed.12184

Vicente, J. et al. (2007) Social organization and movement influence the incidence of bovine tuberculosis in an undisturbed high-density badger *Meles meles* population, *Journal of Animal Ecology* 76, 348-60

Vincent, R. (1911) *On the production of pure milk: an account of the methods employed at the Infants' Hospital farm* London: P.S. King

Virilio, P. (2007) *The original accident* Cambridge: Polity

Volkova, V.V. et al. (2010) Potential for transmission of infections in networks of cattle farms, *Epidemics* 2, 116-22

Vordermeier, M. et al. (2012) The influence of cattle breed on susceptibility to bovine tuberculosis in Ethiopia, *Comparative Immunology Microbiology and Infectious Diseases* 35, 227-32

Vordermeier, H.M. et al. (2014) Vaccination of domestic animals against tuberculosis: Review of progress and contributions to the field of the TBSTEP project, *Research in Veterinary Science* 97, S53-60

Waddington, K. (2001) The science of cows: tuberculosis, research and the state in the United Kingdom, 1890-1914, *History of Science* 39, 355-81

Waddington, K. (2004) To stamp out 'so terrible a malady': bovine tuberculosis and tuberculin testing in Britain, 1890-1939, *Medical History* 48, 29-48

Waddington, K. (2005) *The bovine scourge: meat, tuberculosis and the public's health, 1860s-1914* Woodford: Boydell

Waddington, K. (2011) The dangerous sausage: diet, meat and disease in Victorian and Edwardian Britain, *Cultural and Social History* 8, 51-71

Wagener, K. (1949) Das problem der rindertuberkulose, *Zentralblatt für Bakteriologie* 154, 3-12

Walley, T. (1889) Tuberculosis in milk, *British Medical Journal* ii, 338-9

Walley, T. (1890) *A practical guide to meat inspection* Edinburgh: Pentland

Wang, C.Y. (1916) Isolation of tubercle bacilli from sputum and determination of their type, *Journal of Pathology and Bacteriology* 21, 14

Ward, A.I. et al. (2008) A survey of badger access to farm buildings and facilities in relation to contact with cattle, *Veterinary Record* 163, 107-11

Ward, A.I., Judge, J. and Delahay, R.J. (2010) Farm husbandry and badger behaviour: opportunities to manage badger to cattle transmission of Mycobacterium bovis? *Preventive Veterinary Medicine* 93, 2-10

Warren, M., Lobley, M. and Winter, M. (2013) Farmer attitudes to vaccination and culling of badgers in controlling bovine tuberculosis, *Veterinary Record* 173, 2, 40

Wasserstein, B. (1992) *Herbert Samuel: a political life* Oxford: Oxford University Press

Watts, P.S. and Robertson, J. (1950) The influence of the Attested herds scheme on the local incidence and degree of tuberculosis in slaughtered cows and calves, *Veterinary Record* 62, 127-31

Weber, N. et al. (2013) Badger social networks correlate with tuberculosis infection, *Current Biology* 23, R915-16

Weisbecker, A. (2007) A legal history of raw milk in the United States, *Journal of Environmental Health* 69, 8, 62-3

West, G.P. (Ed)(1988) *Black's veterinary dictionary* London: Black

Westergaard, J.M. (2007) Overview of control and surveillance problems with bovine tuberculosis worldwide, *Bulletin of the International Dairy Federation* 416, 67-74

Westhoff, D.C. (1978) Heating milk for microbial destruction: a historical outline and update, *Journal of Food Protection* 41, 122-30

Whipple, A.C. (2010) 'Into every home, into every body': organicism and anti-statism in the British anti-fluoridation movement, 1952-1960, *Twentieth Century British History* 21, 330-49

Whipple, D.L., Bolin, C.A. and Miller, J.M. (1996) Distribution of lesions in cattle infected with *ycobacterium bovis*, *Journal of Veterinary Diagnosis and Investigation* 8, 351-4

White, P.C.L. and Benhin, J.K.A. (2004) Factors influencing the incidence and scale of bovine tuberculosis in cattle in southwest England, *Preventive Veterinary Medicine* 63, 1-7

White, P.C.L. and Harris, S. (1995) Bovine tuberculosis in badger (*Meles meles*) populations in South West England - the use of a spatial stochastic simulation model to understand the dynamics of the disease, *Philosophical Transactions of the Royal Society of London,* B 349, 391-413

White, P.W. et al. (2013) The importance of 'neighbourhood' in the persistence of bovine tuberculosis in Irish herds, *Preventive Veterinary Medicine* 110, 346-55

Whyte, K.P. and Thompson, P.B. (2012) Ideas for how to take wicked problems seriously, *Journal of Agricultural and Environmental Ethics* 25, 441-5

Wilesmith, J.W. (1983) Epidemiological features of bovine tuberculosis in cattle herds in Great Britain, *Journal of Hygiene* 90, 159-76

Wilkinson, D. et al. (2009) Cost-benefit analysis model of badger (*meles meles*) culling to reduce cattle herd tuberculosis breakdowns in Britain, with particular reference to badger perturbation, *Journal of Wildlife Diseases* 45, 1062-88

Wilkinson, K. (2007) Evidence-based policy and the politics of expertise: a case study of bovine tuberculosis, University of Newcastle, Centre for Rural Economy, *Discussion Paper Series* No. 12

Wilkinson, K. (2011) Organised chaos: an interpretive approach to evidence-based policy making in Defra, *Political Studies* 59, 959-77

Williams, N. (1996) The reporting and classification of causes of death in mid-nineteenth-century England: the example of Sheffield, *Historical Methods* 29, 58-71

Williams, R.S. and Hoy, W.A. (1927) Tubercle bacilli in the faeces of apparently healthy cows, *Journal of Hygiene* 27, 37-9

Williams, R.S. and Hoy, W.A. (1928) The frequency of the appearance of tubercle bacilli in the faeces of three apparently healthy cows, *Journal of Hygiene* 28, 89-91

Williams, R.S. and Hoy, W.A. (1930) The viability of *B. Tuberculosis (bovinus)* on pasture land, in stored faeces and in liquid manure, *Journal of Hygiene* 30, 413-19

Williams, R.S. and Mattick, A.T.R. (1922) The dangers of pasteurized milk, *Modern Farming* 6, 8, 5-6

Wilson, A. (1896/7) Tuberculosis from a farmer's point of view, *Veterinary Record* 9, 292-3

Wilson, G.J., Harris, S. and McLaren, G. (1997) *Changes in the British badger population, 1988 to 1997* London: Peoples Trust for Endangered Species

Wilson, G.S. (1942) *The pasteurization of milk* London: Arnold

Wilson, G.S., Minett, F.C. and Carling, H.F. (1937) The nutritive value of raw and pasteurized milk for calves, *Journal of Hygiene* 37, 243-53

Winnifrith, Sir J. (1962) *The Ministry of Agriculture, Fisheries and Food* London: Allen & Unwin

Wint, G.R.W. et al. (2002) Mapping bovine tuberculosis in Great Britain using environmental data, *Trends in Microbiology* 10, 441-4

Wint, W. et al. (2004) *Exploratory investigation of cattle movement records in britain to enhance animal disease surveillance and control strategies, Final Project Report: SE3034* London: Defra

Wolfe, D.M. et al. (2009) The risk of a positive test for bovine tuberculosis in cattle purchased from herds with and without a recent history of bovine tuberculosis in Ireland, *Preventive Veterinary Medicine* 92, 99-105

Wood, D.R. (1930) The examination of milk for tubercle bacilli: a survey of experience and results, *Analyst* 55, 544-9

Woodroffe, R. et al. (2006) Effects of culling on badger *Meles meles* spatial organization: implications for the control of bovine tuberculosis, *Journal of Applied Ecology* 43, 1-10

Woodroffe, R. et al. (2009) Bovine tuberculosis in cattle and badgers in localized culling areas, *Journal of Wildlife Diseases* 45, 128-43

Woodroffe, R. et al. (2005) Spatial association of *Mycobacterium bovis* infection in cattle and badgers *Meles meles*, *Journal of Applied Ecology* 42, 852-62

Woodroffe, R. et al. (2009) Social group size affects *Mycobacterium bovis* infection in European badgers (*Meles meles*), *Journal of Animal Ecology* 78, 818-27

Woodroffe, R., Macdonald, D.W. and da Silva, J. (1995) Dispersal and philopatry in the European badger, *Meles meles*. *Journal of Zoology* **237**, 227-39

Woods, A. (2004a) Why slaughter? The cultural dimensions of Britain's foot and mouth disease control policy, 1892-2001, *Journal of Agricultural & Environmental Ethics* 17, 341-62

Woods, A. (2004b) *A manufactured plague? The history of foot and mouth disease in Britain* London: Earthscan

Woods, A. (2013) From practical men to scientific experts: British veterinary surgeons and the development of government scientific expertise, c. 1878-1919, *History of Science* 51, 457-80

Woolhouse, M.E. and Gowtage-Sequeria, S. (2005) Host range and emerging and re-emerging pathogens, *Emerging Infectious Diseases* 11, 1842-7

Worboys, M. (1991) Germ theories of disease and British veterinary medicine, 1860-1890, *Medical History* 35, 308-27

Worboys, M. (1992) 'Killing and curing': veterinarians, medicine and germs in Britain, 1860-1900, *Veterinary History* 7, 53-71

Worboys M. (2000) *Spreading germs: disease theories and medical practice in Britain, 1865-1900* Cambridge: Cambridge University Press

World Health Organization (2014a) Tuberculosis, *Fact Sheet* 104 Geneva: WHO

World Health Organization (2014b) *Global tuberculosis report 2014* Geneva: WHO

Wray C. (1975) Survival and spread of pathogenic bacteria of veterinary importance within the environment, *Veterinary Bulletin* 45, 543-50

Wright, D.M. et al. (2013) Detectability of bovine TB using the tuberculin skin test does not vary significantly according to pathogen genotype within Northern Ireland, *Infection, Genetics and Evolution* 19, 15-22

Wright, G.A. (1908) Tuberculosis of the cervical glands in childhood, pp 160-65 in Kelynack, T.N. (Ed.) *Tuberculosis in infancy and childhood* New York: Wood

Wright, N.C. (1929) The incidence of tuberculous infection in the milk supplies of Scottish cities, *British Medical Journal* ii, 452-4

Wright, N.C. (1933) *Some implications of compulsory pasteurization: contribution to a discussion on 'milk production and distribution' read at the meeting of the British Association for the Advancement of Science, Leicester, 1933* Ayr: Hannah Dairy Research Institute

Wright, N.C. (1967) *Mycobacterium tuberculosis* in pasteurized milk, *British Medical Journal* ii, 108

Wu, H. et al. (2015) TALE nickase-mediated SP110 knockin endows cattle with increased resistance to tuberculosis, *Proceedings of the National Academy of Sciences* doi: 10.1073/pnas.1421587112

Wynne, A.J. (1953) Costs of attestation in dairy herds, *University of Leeds, Department of Agriculture, Economics Section, Farmers' Report* No. 115

Wynne, B. (1996) May the sheep safely graze? A reflexive view of the expert-lay knowledge divide, pp 44-83 in Lash, S., Szerszynski, B. and Wynne, B. (Eds) *Risk, environment and society: towards a new ecology* London: Sage

Wynne, F.E. (1928) The present position of the milk supply, *Journal of the Royal Sanitary Institute* 49, 3-9

Yeats, W.B. (1928) *The tower* London: Macmillan

Youmans, G.P. (1979) *Tuberculosis* Philadelphia: W.B. Saunders & Co.

Young, J. S., Gormley, E. and Wellington, E.M.H. (2005) Molecular detection of Mycobacterium bovis and Mycobacterium bovis BCG (Pasteur) in soil, *Applied Environmental Microbiology* 71, 1946-52

Zinsstag, J. et al. (2006) *Mycobacterium bovis* in Africa, pp 199-210 in Thoen, C.O., Steele, J.H. and Gilsdorf, M.J. (Eds) *Mycobacterium bovis infection in animals and humans* Ames, IA: Blackwell

Zuckerman, Lord (1980) *Badgers, cattle and tuberculosis* London: HMSO

Main Parliamentary Papers

Wilson Committee. *Departmental Committee to Inquire into Pleuro-Pneumonia and Tuberculosis in the United Kingdom* [Chairman: J. Wilson], BPP 1888 (C. 5461, C. 5461-I) xxxii.267, 295

RC1. *Royal Commission to Inquire into Effect of Food Derived from Tuberculous Animals on Human Health*, BPP 1895 (C. 7703) xxxv.615; 1896 (C. 7992) xlvi.11

RC2. *Royal Commission to Inquire into Administrative Procedures for Controlling Danger to Man Through Use as Food of Meat and Milk of Tuberculous Animals* [Chairman: H. Maxwell], BPP 1898 (C. 8824, C. 8831) xlix.333, 365

RC3. *Royal Commission on the Relation Between Human and Animal Tuberculosis* [Chairmen: Sir Michael Foster, Sir William Power]. *Interim Report*, BPP 1904 (Cd. 2092) xxxix.129; *Second Interim Report, part I*, BPP 1907 (Cd. 3322) xxxviii.1; *Second Interim Report, part II*, BPP 1907 (Cd. 3584) xxxviii.99; BPP 1907 (Cd. 3660) xxxix.1; BPP 1907 (Cd. 3661) xl.1; BPP 1907 (Cd. 3378) xl.643; BPP 1908 (Cd. 3758) lvii.1; *Third Interim Report*, BPP 1909 (Cd. 4483) xlix.365; *Final Report, Part I*, BPP 1911 (Cd. 5761) xlii.173; *Final Report, Part II*, BPP 1911 (Cd. 5790) xlii. 231; BPP 1911 (Cd. 5791) xliii.1; BPP 1911 (Cd. 5893) xliii.495; BPP 1911 (Cd. 5894) xliv.1; BPP 1911 (Cd. 5975) xliv. 465; BPP 1913 (Cd. 6904) xl.71; BPP 1914-16 (Cd. 7941) xxxvii.255; BPP 1913 (Cd. 6796) xl.105

First Astor Committee. *Departmental Committee on Tuberculosis* [Chairman: Waldorf Astor], Interim Report BPP 1912-13 (Cd. 6164) xlviii.1; Final Report BPP 1912-13 (Cd. 6641) xlviii.29; Appendix BPP 1912-13 (Cd. 6654) xlviii.47

Second Astor Committee. *Departmental Committee on Production and Distribution of Milk* [Chairman: Waldorf Astor], First Interim Report, BPP 1917-18 (Cd. 8608) xvi.1003; Second Interim Report, BPP 1917-18 (Cd. 8886) xvi.1011; Report to the Food Controller, BPP 1918 (Cd. 9095) xii.125; Third Interim Report, BPP 1919 (Cmd. 315) xxv.615; Final Report, BPP 1919 (Cmd. 483) xxv.645

Grigg Commission. Ministry of Agriculture and Fisheries (1933) *Report of the Reorganization Commission on Milk* [Chairman: Sir Edward Grigg], Ministry of Agriculture and Fisheries, Economic Series 38 London: HMSO

Hopkins Committee. *Report of the Economic Advisory Council on Milch Cattle Diseases [Chairman: Sir Frederick Gowland Hopkins]*, BPP 1933-4 (Cmd. 4591) ix.427

Cutforth Commission. *Milk: Report of the Reorganization Commission for Milk* [Chairman: Arthur E. Cutforth] (1936) Ministry of Agriculture and Fisheries, Economic Series 44 London: HMSO

Perry Committee. *Report of the Committee Appointed by the Minister of Food to Investigate the Present Cost of Distributing Milk in Great Britain* [Chairman: Lord Perry](1940) London: Ministry of Food

Memorandum on Milk Policy, BPP 1941-42 (Cmd. 6362) ix.69

Measures to Improve the Quality of the Nation's Milk Supply, BPP 1942-43 (Cmd. 6454) xi.149.

Williams Committee. *Ministry of Food, Report of the Committee on Milk Distribution* [Chairman: W.D.A. Williams], BPP 1947-8 (Cmd. 7414) xiii.543-642

INDEX

www.ingramcontent.com/pod-product-compliance
Lightning Source LLC
Chambersburg PA
CBHW060534220326
41599CB00022B/3511